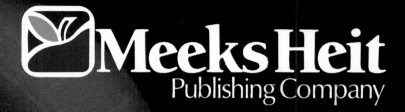

Meeks Heit
Publishing Company

Totally
Awesome®
Health

Course 3

Linda Meeks
The Ohio State University

Philip Heit
The Ohio State University

Meeks Heit Publishing Company
Editorial, Sales, and Customer Service
6833 Clark State Road
Blacklick, OH 43004
(614) 939-1111

Director of Editorial: Julie DeVillers
Managing Editor: Ginger Panico
Project Editor: Heather L. Allen
Director of Illustration: Deborah Rubenstein
Director of Graphics: Elizabeth S. Kim
Graphics Associate: DanniElena Wolfe Hernández
Art Consultant: Jim Brower
Director of Production: Sally Meckling
Designer: Mary Geer
Photographers: Roman Sapecki, Lew Lause
Illustrator: Dave Odell

Unit 10 outlines emergency care procedures that reflect the standard of knowledge and accepted practices in the United States at the time this book was published. It is the teacher's responsibility to stay informed of changes in emergency care procedures in order to teach current accepted practices. The teacher also can recommend that students gain complete, comprehensive training from courses offered by the American Red Cross.

Printed in the United States of America

4 5 6 7 8 9 10   99

Library of Congress Catalog Number: 98-066098

ISBN: 1-886693-86-2

About Meeks Heit Publishing Company

Professor Linda Meeks   **Dr. Philip Heit**

Linda Meeks and Philip Heit are emeritus professors of Health Education in the College of Education at The Ohio State University. Linda and Philip are America's most widely published health education co-authors. They have collaborated for more than 20 years, co-authoring more than 200 health books that are used by millions of students preschool through college. Together, they have helped state departments of education as well as thousands of school districts develop comprehensive school health education curricula. Their books and curricula are used throughout the United States as well as in Canada, Japan, Mexico, England, Puerto Rico, Spain, Egypt, Jordan, Saudi Arabia, Bermuda, and the Virgin Islands. Linda and Philip train professors as well as educators in state departments of education and school districts. Their book, *Comprehensive School Health Education: Totally Awesome® Strategies for Teaching Health,* is the most widely used book for teacher training in colleges, universities, and school districts. Thousands of teachers throughout the world have participated in their Totally Awesome® Teacher Training Workshops. Linda and Philip have been the keynote speakers for many teacher institutes and wellness conferences. They are personally and professionally committed to the health and well-being of youth.

Advisory Board

Medical Reviewers

Donna Bacchi, M.D., M.P.H.
Associate Professor of
  Pediatrics
Director, Division of
  Community Pediatrics
Texas Tech University
  Health Sciences Center
Lubbock, Texas

Albert J. Hart, Jr., M.D.
Mid-Ohio OB-GYN, Inc.
Westerville, Ohio

Reviewers

Kymm Ballard, M.A.
Physical Education, Athletics,
  and Sports Medicine
  Consultant
North Carolina Department
  of Public Instruction
Raleigh, North Carolina

Kay Bridges
Health Educator
Gaston County Public Schools
Gastonia, North Carolina

Reba Bullock, M.Ed.
Coordinator, Sexual
Assault Prevention Project
Maryland State Department
  of Education
Baltimore, Maryland

Anthony S. Catalano, Ph.D.
K–12 Health Coordinator
Melrose Public Schools
Melrose, Massachusetts

Galen Cole, M.P.H., Ph.D.
Division of Health
  Communication
Office of the Director
Centers for Disease Control
  and Prevention
Atlanta, Georgia

Brian Colwell, Ph.D.
Professor
Department of HLKN
Texas A&M University
College Station, Texas

Tommy Fleming, Ph.D.
Director of Health and
  Physical Education
Texas Education Agency
Austin, Texas

Denyce Ford, M.Ed., Ph.D.
Coordinator, Comprehensive
  School Health Education
District of Columbia Public
  Schools
Washington, D.C.

Elizabeth Gallun, M.A.
Supervisor of Drug Programs
Prince George's County
  Public Schools
Upper Marlboro, Maryland

Linda Harrill-Rudisill, M.A.
Chairperson of Health
  Education
Southwest Middle School
Gastonia, North Carolina

Janet Henke
Middle School Team Leader
Baltimore County Public
  Schools
Baltimore, Maryland

Russell Henke
Coordinator of Health
Montgomery County Public
  Schools
Rockville, Maryland

Larry Herrold, M.S.
Supervisor, Office of Health
  and Physical Education
  K–12
Baltimore County Schools
Baltimore, Maryland

Susan Jackson, B.S., M.A.
Health Promotion Specialist
Healthworks, Wake Medical
  Center
Raleigh, North Carolina

Joe Leake, CHES
Curriculum Specialist
Baltimore City Public Schools
Baltimore, Maryland

Debra Ogden, M.A.
Coordinator of Health,
  Physical Education, Driver
  Education, and Safe and
  Drug-Free Programs
Collier County Public
  Schools
Naples, Florida

Diane S. Scalise, R.N., M.S.
Coordinator, Health
  Education Services
The School Board of
  Broward County
Fort Lauderdale, Florida

Michael Schaffer, M.A.
Supervisor of Health
  Education and Wellness
Prince George's County
  Public Schools
Upper Marlboro, Maryland

Merita Thompson, Ed.D.
Professor of Health
  Education
Eastern Kentucky University
Richmond, Kentucky

Linda Wright, M.A.
Project Director
HIV/AIDS Education
  Program
District of Columbia
  Public Schools
Washington, D.C.

Mental and Emotional Health

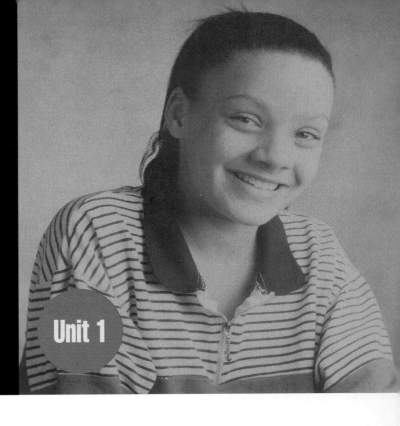

Unit 1

Family and Social Health

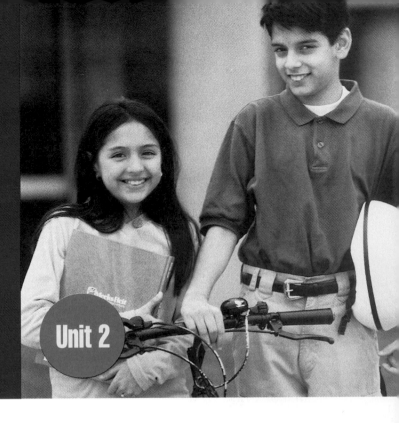

Unit 2

Growth and Development

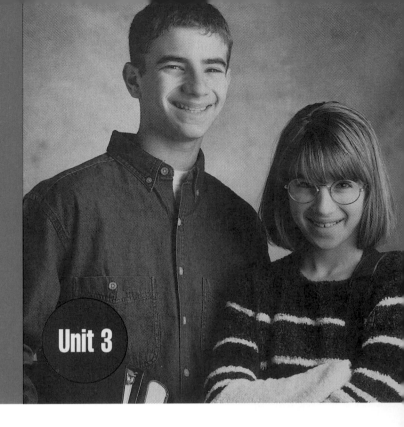

Unit 3

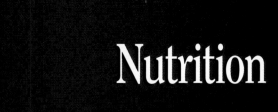

Nutrition

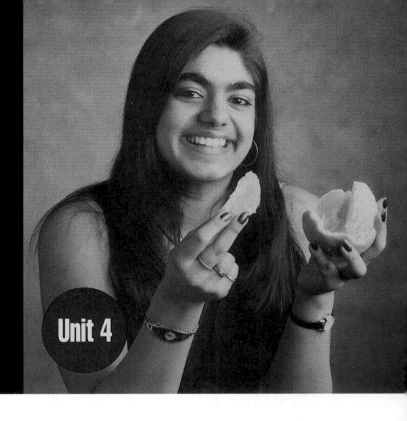

Unit 4

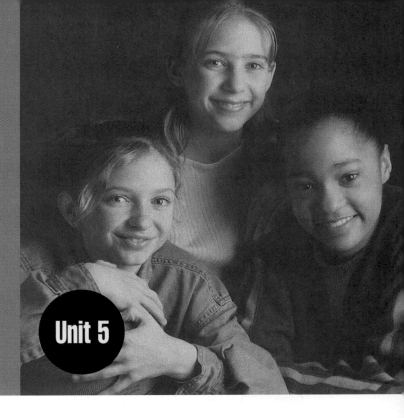

Personal Health and Physical Activity

Unit 5

Alcohol, Tobacco, and Other Drugs

Say No!

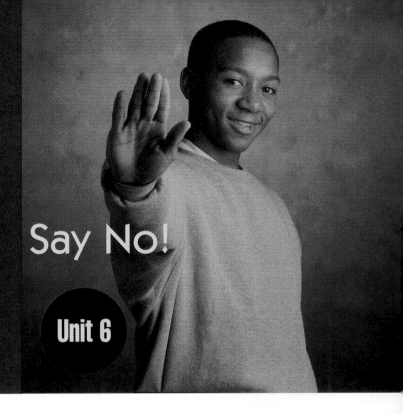

Unit 6

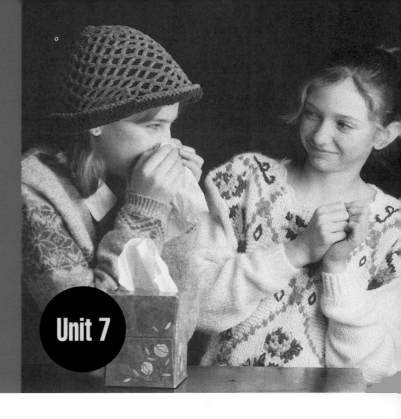

Communicable and Chronic Diseases

Unit 7

Consumer and Community Health

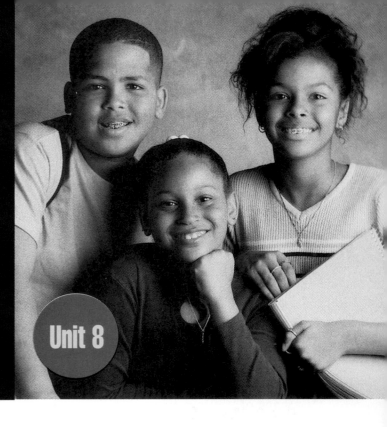

Unit 8

Environmental Health

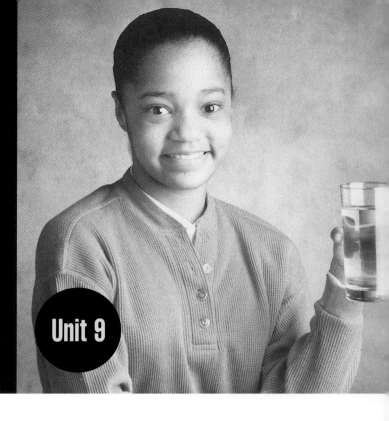

Unit 9

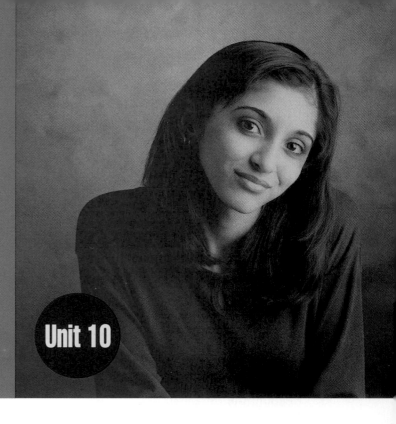

Injury Prevention and Safety

Unit 10

Lesson 49 Staying Safe During Extreme Weather Conditions and Natural Disasters 544

Lesson 50 The Teen's Guide to First Aid 552

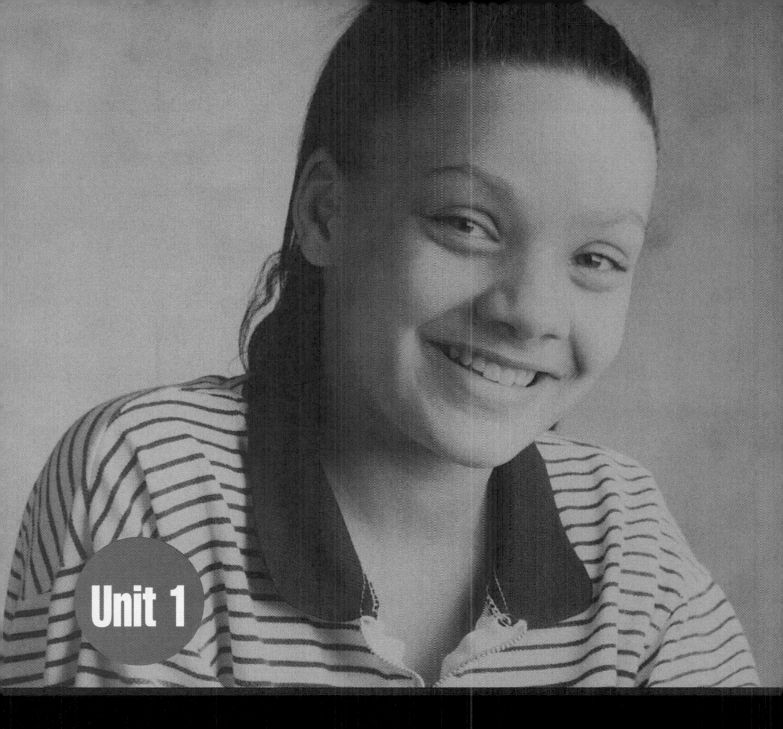

Unit 1

Mental and Emotional Health

The Totally Awesome® Teen

Vocabulary

health

wellness

physical health

mental-emotional health

family-social health

The Wellness Scale

life skills

health knowledge

healthful behaviors

risk behaviors

health awareness

Health Behavior Inventory

self-responsibility for health

self-discipline

health behavior contract

health literate person

Life Skills

- **I will take responsibility for my health.**
- **I will gain health knowledge.**
- **I will practice life skills for health.**

To be totally awesome is to be terrific, extraordinary, and very special. When you feel totally awesome, you take care of yourself. You strive to have optimal health. **Health** is the quality of life that includes physical, mental-emotional, and family-social health. **Wellness** is another term for health. **Physical health** is the condition of the body. **Mental-emotional health** is the condition of the mind and the ways that a person expresses feelings. **Family-social health** is the condition of one's relationships with others.

The Lesson Objectives

- Use *The Wellness Scale* to explain how the actions you choose influence your health.
- Complete a *Health Behavior Inventory* to evaluate whether or not you are practicing life skills for health.
- Design a health behavior contract to take responsibility for your health.
- Explain the skills you need to be a health literate person.

The Wellness Scale

The Wellness Scale is a scale that shows the range of health from optimal health to premature death. Optimal health is achieved by practicing life skills. **Life skills** are healthful actions that are learned and practiced for a lifetime. Some examples of life skills are the following:

1. **I will follow guidelines for motor vehicle safety.**
2. **I will follow a dental health plan.**
3. **I will develop healthful eating habits.**

Life skills help you:
- maintain and improve health;
- prevent disease;
- reduce risk behavior.

The Wellness Scale

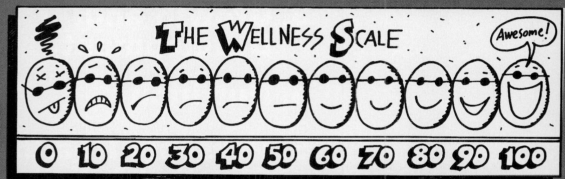

The actions you choose influence your health and well-being.

- I do anything my friend tells me to do.
- I gossip about my friends.
- I get mad at my grandmother when she forgets to do things.
- I pig out on French fries when I am depressed.
- I skipped my last dental appointment.
- I sneak cigarettes.
- I let my friend pierce another hole in my ear.
- I don't wear a safety belt.
- I bought the instant weight-loss cream advertised in a magazine.
- I never use sunscreen.

- I talk to my parents or guardian when I feel depressed.
- I stay away from gangs and people who are in gangs.
- I read to my younger sister to help her learn.
- I eat low-fat foods when I go out to eat.
- I go to basketball practice three times a week.
- I do not drink alcohol.
- I know that heart disease runs in my family.
- I know how to give rescue breathing.
- I volunteer at the annual blood drive.
- I recycle my soda cans.

Health status is the sum total of the positive and negative influences of behaviors, situations, relationships, and decisions, and the use of resistance skills.

Life Skills

This book has ten content areas for health. Life skills are identified for each of the ten content areas.

Ten Content Areas for Health

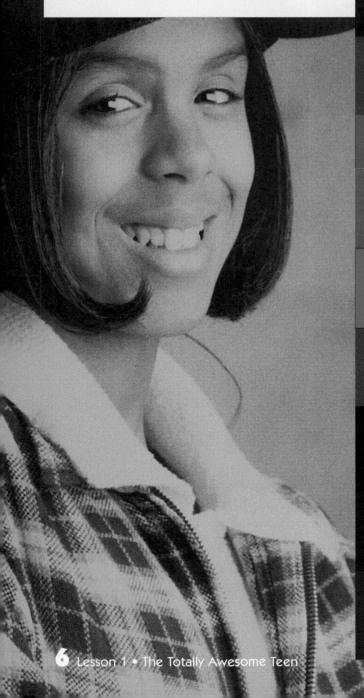

1. **Mental and Emotional Health**

2. **Family and Social Health**

3. **Growth and Development**

4. **Nutrition**

5. **Personal Health and Physical Activity**

6. **Alcohol, Tobacco, and Other Drugs**

7. **Communicable and Chronic Diseases**

8. **Consumer and Community Health**

9. **Environmental Health**

10. **Injury Prevention and Safety**

Healthful Behaviors

Health knowledge is needed to develop each life skill. **Health knowledge** is the information and understanding a person has about health.

Health knowledge helps you tell the difference between healthful behaviors and risk behaviors. **Healthful behaviors** are actions that:

- **promote health;**
- **prevent illness, injury, and premature death;**
- **and improve the quality of the environment.**

Risk Behaviors

Risk behaviors are voluntary actions that:

- **threaten health;**
- **increase the likelihood of illness and premature death;**
- **and harm the quality of the environment.**

Researchers at the Centers for Disease Control and Prevention have studied risk behaviors. They have identified six categories of risk behaviors in teens:

1. Behaviors that result in unintentional and intentional injuries

2. Tobacco use

3. Alcohol and other drug use

4. Sexual behaviors that result in HIV infection, other sexually transmitted diseases, and unintended pregnancies

5. Diet choices that contribute to disease

6. Lack of physical activity

Health Behavior Inventory

Health awareness is the knowledge a person gains about his or her health behavior. It can be gained by studying health and by completing health behavior inventories. A *Health Behavior Inventory* is a personal assessment tool that contains a list of life skills to which a person responds, "YES, I practice this life skill," or "NO, I do not practice this life skill."

The life skills listed are not of equal value. For example, "I do not use tobacco products," influences health more than "I participate in school clubs and community activities that promote health and safety." Although both of these life skills are important, one life skill influences health more than the other.

Directions: On a sheet of paper, number from 1 to 20. Read each life skill carefully. If you practice the life skill, write a (+) next to the same number on your paper. Each (+) indicates a positive action to promote your health. If you do not practice the life skill, write a (-) next to the same number on your paper. A health behavior contract is needed for each (-) response to a life skill.

Mental and Emotional Health

1. I communicate with others in healthful ways.
2. I follow a plan to manage stress.

Family and Social Health

3. I make healthful adjustments to family changes.
4. I have healthful relationships.

Growth and Development

5. I keep my body systems healthy.
6. I practice habits that promote healthful aging.

Nutrition

7. I evaluate food labels.
8. I maintain a desirable weight and body composition.

Personal Health and Physical Activity

9. I follow a dental health plan.
10. I have regular examinations.

Alcohol, Tobacco, and Other Drugs

11. I avoid tobacco use and secondhand smoke.
12. I do not drink alcohol.

Communicable and Chronic Diseases

13. I keep a personal health record.
14. I choose behaviors to reduce my risk of cancer.

Consumer and Community Health

15. I choose healthful entertainment.
16. I am a health advocate by being a volunteer.

Environmental Health

17. I help keep noise at a safe level.
18. I precycle, recycle, and dispose of waste properly.

Injury Prevention and Safety

19. I follow guidelines for motor vehicle safety.
20. I am skilled in first aid procedures.

Health Behavior Contract

Self-responsibility for health is the priority a person assigns to being healthy. **Self-discipline** is the effort or energy with which a person follows through on intentions or promises. A **health behavior contract** is a written plan to develop the habit of following a specific life skill.

Follow a...

Health Behavior Contract

Name: Your Name   **Date:** Today's Date

Life Skill: I will follow a dental health plan.

Effect On My Health: Following a dental health plan will help keep my teeth strong. I will have fewer cavities and less plaque. My teeth will be whiter.

My Plan: I will brush my teeth three times a day. I will use a fluoride toothpaste. I will floss my teeth once a day. I will use the correct toothbrushing and flossing techniques. I will make a check mark on my calendar on the days I follow my dental health plan.

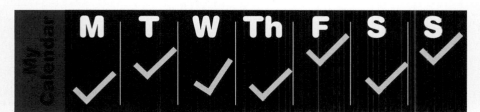

My Calendar: M T W Th F S S — ✓ ✓ ✓ ✓ ✓ ✓ ✓

How My Plan Worked: (Complete after one week.) _____

Four Steps to Follow to Make a Health Behavior Contract

1. Identify the life skill for which a habit needs to be formed.

2. Write a few statements describing how the life skill will affect your health.

3. Make a specific plan to follow and a method of recording your progress.

4. Evaluate the results you experienced.

Health Literacy

A **health literate person** is a person who is skilled in:

1. **effective communication;**
2. **self-directed learning;**
3. **critical thinking;**
4. **and responsible citizenship.**

The symbols below illustrate the four skills needed to be a health literate person. Next to each symbol, there is a description of the skill.

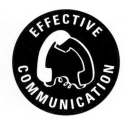

Effective Communication is skill in expressing knowledge, beliefs, and ideas. It includes expressing oneself in different ways—oral, written, artistic, graphic, and technological. It also includes showing empathy and respect for others.

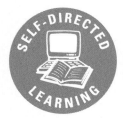

Self-Directed Learning is skill in gathering and using health knowledge. It involves having current information about health.

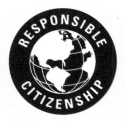

Critical Thinking is skill in evaluating information from reliable sources before making decisions. It includes knowing how to make responsible decisions.

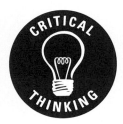

Responsible Citizenship is skill in practicing responsible behavior. It involves choosing behavior that is healthful, is safe, is legal, is respectful of self and others, follows family guidelines, and demonstrates character. It includes behaviors that promote a healthful community, nation, and world.

For information on health literacy, read *The National Health Education Standards: Achieving Health Literacy* by The Joint Committee on Health Education Standards, 1995. Questions can be directed to The American Cancer Society, 1599 Clifton Road NE, Atlanta, Georgia 30329 (1-800-ACS-2345).

What's Awesome/What's Not

Life Skill

I will practice life skills for health.

Materials: Paper, pen or pencil

Directions: The beginning of a What's Awesome/What's Not chart appears below. Copy the chart on a separate sheet of paper. Add four more items to each column.

What's Awesome . . . What's Not

Healthful behavior . . . . Risk behavior

Avoiding alcohol . . . . Drinking alcohol

Getting regular
physical activity . . . . Being a couch potato

Lesson 1

Review

Vocabulary

Write a separate sentence using each of the vocabulary words listed on page 4.

Health Content

Write responses to the following:

1. Draw and label *The Wellness Scale.* **page 5**
2. What are three ways life skills help you? **page 5**
3. What are ten content areas for health? **page 6**
4. What is the difference between healthful behaviors and risk behaviors? **page 7**
5. What are the six categories of risk behaviors in teens identified by the Centers for Disease Control and Prevention? **page 7**
6. How can completing a *Health Behavior Inventory* help you practice life skills? **page 8**
7. What are two ways you can gain health awareness? **page 8**
8. What are the four parts of a health behavior contract? **page 9**
9. What are three ways you can stay motivated when using a health behavior contract? **page 9**
10. What are four skills you need to be a health literate person? **page 10**

Empowered Decision-Making

Vocabulary

empowered

inactive decision-making style

reactive decision-making style

proactive decision-making style

The Responsible Decision-Making Model™

peer pressure

resistance skills

The Model for Using Resistance Skills

- **I will make responsible decisions.**
- **I will use resistance skills when appropriate.**

To be **empowered** means to be inspired because a person feels some sense of control over behavior and decisions. Taking responsibility for decisions is essential to gaining the feeling of empowerment. Teens usually have one of three decision-making styles. In this lesson, you will learn to use a decision-making style that helps you make responsible decisions.

The Lesson Objectives

- Describe the three decision-making styles.
- Use *The Responsible Decision-Making Model™* to make decisions.
- State the seven resistance skills to say NO to negative peer pressure.

Decision-Making Styles

An **inactive decision-making style** is one in which a person fails to make choices, and this failure determines what will happen. Teens with this decision-making style do not know what they want to do. They put off making difficult decisions. Eventually, they have to live with whatever happens. They do not gain the self-confidence they would have if they had made a decision and had been accountable for it.

A **reactive decision-making style** is one in which a person allows others to make decisions. Teens who use this style are easily influenced by what others think, do, or suggest. They lack self-confidence and have a need to be liked by others. They give control of their decisions to others.

A **proactive decision-making style** is one in which a person:

- **examines the decision to be made;**
- **identifies and evaluates actions to take;**
- **selects an action;**
- **and takes responsibility for the consequences of this action.**

Teens who have a proactive decision-making style take responsibility for their decisions and behavior. They use criteria to determine what to do. *The Responsible Decision-Making Model*™ is a series of steps to follow to assure that decisions lead to actions that:

- **promote health;**
- **protect safety;**
- **follow laws;**
- **show respect for self and others;**
- **follow guidelines set by responsible adults such as parents or a guardian;**
- **and demonstrate good character.**

The Responsible Decision-Making Model™

1. **Describe the situation that requires a decision.**
2. **List possible decisions you might make.**
3. **Share the list of possible decisions with a trusted adult.**
4. **Evaluate the consequences of each decision. Ask questions.**

Will this decision result in an action that:

- is healthful;
- is safe;
- is legal;
- shows respect for self and others;
- follows the guidelines of responsible adults such as my parents or guardian;
- demonstrates that I have good character?

5. **Decide which decision is responsible and most appropriate.**
6. **Act on your decision and evaluate the results.**

Resistance Skills

Peer pressure is influence that people of similar age or status place on others to encourage them to make certain decisions or to behave in certain ways. Peer pressure can be negative or positive. Peers might pressure you to stay away from a gang. This is positive peer pressure. Suppose peers pressure you to smoke a cigarette. This is negative peer pressure.

Resistance skills are skills that are used when a person wants to say NO to an action or to leave a situation. Resistance skills can be used when peer pressure is negative. Suppose you want to say NO, but you do not know how to say NO and stick to your decision. *The Model for Using Resistance Skills* is a list of suggested ways to resist negative peer pressure.

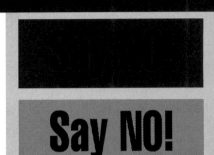

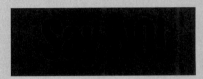

Say NO!

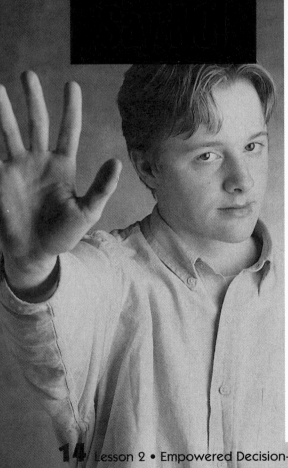

The Model for Using Resistance Skills

1. Say NO in an assertive way.

2. Give reasons for saying NO.

3. Use nonverbal behavior to match verbal behavior.

4. Avoid being in situations in which there will be pressure to make harmful decisions.

5. Avoid being with people who make harmful decisions.

6. Resist pressure to engage in illegal behavior.

7. Influence others to make responsible decisions.

Apply...

The Responsible Decision-Making Model™

You are walking to school with a friend and are going to be late. You approach a field with a "No Trespassing" sign. Gang members often hang out in this field. Going through the field would be a shortcut to school. Your friend says, "Let's cut through the field just once. I'll get detention if I'm late."

Answer the following questions on a separate sheet of paper. Write "Does not apply" if a question does not apply to this situation.

1. Is it healthful to cut across the field? Why or why not?
2. Is it safe to cut across the field? Why or why not?
3. Is it legal to cut across the field? Why or why not?
4. Will you show respect for yourself and others if you cut across the field? Why or why not?
5. Will your parents or guardian approve if you cut across the field? Why or why not?
6. Will you demonstrate good character if you cut across the field? Why or why not?

What is the responsible decision to make in this situation?

Lesson 2

Review

Vocabulary

Write a separate sentence using each of the vocabulary words listed on page 12.

Health Content

Write responses to the following:

1. What does it mean to be empowered? **page 12**
2. What are the three decision-making styles? **page 13**
3. What are the steps in *The Responsible Decision-Making Model™*? **page 13**
4. What is the difference between positive peer pressure and negative peer pressure? **page 14**
5. What are seven resistance skills you can use to resist negative peer pressure? **page 14**

Superb Mental Fitness

Vocabulary

character

addictive behavior

personality

heredity

environment

mental alertness

self-control

self-respect

responsibility

realistic standard

addictive behavior

compulsive

perfectionism

eating disorder

multiple addiction

enabler

formal intervention

relapse

Life Skills

- **I will develop good character.**
- **I will choose behaviors that promote a healthy mind.**

As a totally awesome teen, you will want to strive for superb mental fitness. Mental fitness is achieved by being mentally alert. Developing good character and avoiding addictive behaviors also contribute to mental fitness. **Character** is a person's use of self-control to act on responsible values. **Addictive behavior** is behavior that is repeated, is difficult to stop, and has harmful effects. When mental fitness is threatened, help is needed.

The Lesson Objectives

- Describe how your personality is influenced.
- Explain how you can have mental alertness.
- Discuss the benefits of having good character.
- Give examples of addictive behaviors.
- Identify sources of help for addictive behaviors.

Personality

Personality is a person's unique blend of physical, mental, social, and emotional traits. Your personality is unique to you. Everyone has a personality. You might describe yourself as funny, talkative, or quiet. These are personality traits. Your personality determines how you respond to the challenges of life.

Personality is influenced by heredity and environment. **Heredity** is the sum of the traits that have been transmitted from parents. Traits influenced by heredity include hair color and body type. Your personality traits also are influenced by the environment in which you live. **Environment** is everything living and nonliving that is around a person. It includes people and places, such as your family and your neighborhood. It also includes the experiences you have had. You might be athletic because family members participate in sports with you.

Mental Alertness

Mental alertness is the ability to think clearly, to reason, and to solve problems. Mental alertness allows you to face challenges without being overwhelmed. It allows you to concentrate and remember information. An athlete participates in a training program to have a well-conditioned body. A training program also is needed to have a well-conditioned mind. Your training program for mental alertness might include reading or working crossword puzzles to learn new vocabulary words. It might include choosing healthful entertainment that stimulates your thinking.

Character

Character is a person's use of self-control to act on responsible values. **Self-control** is the degree to which a person regulates his or her own behavior. Having good character provides you with several benefits.

- **You develop self-respect.**
  Self-respect is a high regard for oneself because one behaves in responsible ways. **Responsibility** is the quality of being reliable and dependable. When you have self-respect, you value your relationships with others. You not only respect yourself, but you respect others. You choose behavior to strengthen your relationships. Because your actions are worthy, others treat you with respect. You make responsible decisions. You do not give in to negative peer pressure.

- **You set and meet realistic standards.**
  A **realistic standard** is a requirement a person sets for himself or herself that can reasonably be achieved. All through your life, you will face having to do things you might not feel like doing. Even now, you might want to stay up late to watch television. You might want to pig out on dessert every night. You might want to play on your computer and not clean your room. When you have good character, you do things even if you do not feel like doing them. You discipline yourself. You get things done. You expect yourself to meet the standards you have set. You meet your standards of getting adequate sleep, of keeping a healthful body weight, and of being a responsible family member. If you do not meet your standards, you are gentle on yourself. You might need to re-evaluate your standards to make them realistic.

You might need to ask your parents or guardian to help you. But you do not stop trying to meet the standard. You do not quit.

- **You own your behavior.** You take responsibility for your actions. If you hurt someone, you do not pretend you did not. You say, "I'm sorry" and try to make it up to the person. If you did not do your homework, you do not make up an excuse and lie to your teacher. Everyone makes mistakes. Teens who are mature own up to their mistakes and keep trying to act responsibly. If you act responsibly, you can be proud of yourself.

The Top Ten List of Ways to Improve Your Self-Respect

1. **Set goals and make plans to reach them.**

2. **Develop a skill or talent.**

3. **Make a list of things you do well.**

4. **Work to do your best in school.**

5. **Get involved in school clubs and activities.**

6. **Develop a trusting relationship with at least one adult.**

7. **Choose friends who encourage you to do your best.**

8. **Spend time with friends and adults who provide support.**

9. **Volunteer to help another person.**

10. **Keep a neat appearance.**

Follow a...

Health Behavior Contract

Name: _____ **Date:** _____

Copy the health behavior contract on a separate sheet of paper.

DO NOT WRITE IN THIS BOOK.

Life Skill: I will develop good character.

Effect On My Health: When I have good character, I act in responsible ways. I take care of my health. I do not give in to negative peer pressure. I treat people with respect. I do my best. I can rest easy because I am honest. I do not have unnecessary guilt. Unnecessary guilt is feeling badly even if one has done nothing wrong.

My Plan: I will set realistic standards. I will use the list on page 18 for examples of ways to improve my self-respect and make up some of my own. I will write my standards in a journal. Over the next week, I will identify actions I take that demonstrate I have good character. I will describe these actions in my journal.

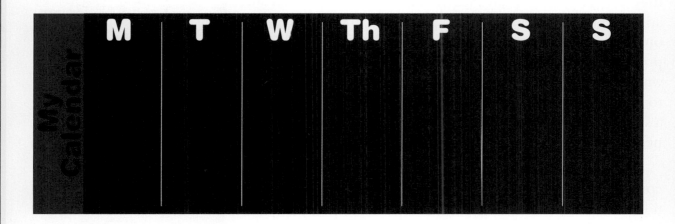

My Calendar	M	T	W	Th	F	S	S

How My Plan Worked: (Complete after one week.) I will review the actions that I took to demonstrate good character. If I make mistakes, I will think of ways I can prevent them from happening again.

Addictive Behaviors

The teen years include many daily challenges. When you are mentally fit, you face these daily challenges though they might be annoying, painful, or difficult.

Some teens are unable to accept responsibility for daily challenges. When problems arise, they want to avoid negative feelings they might experience if they faced these challenges. They want to improve their mood. Addictive behavior is behavior that is repeated, is difficult to stop, and has harmful effects. Practicing addictive behavior is a harmful way to cope with or avoid problems. Addictive behavior differs from a harmful habit. You can change a harmful habit by becoming aware of it and deciding to control and change it. Addictive behavior is compulsive. To be **compulsive** is to have an irresistible urge to repeat a behavior.

Although people of any age can have addictive behavior, let us focus on teens. Often, teens who have addictive behavior are unaware of the reasons they behave the way they do. They might have learned addictive behavior from adults who were trying to avoid problems. They viewed one or more addictive behaviors as ways to cope with problems. They began to use addictive behaviors to cope with their problems. Some teens take a healthful behavior to an extreme and it becomes an addiction. They repeat a specific behavior instead of making the effort that is necessary to solve their problems.

It might be helpful to examine examples of addictions common among teens. Some teens have shopping addiction. When they feel bad, they go on a shopping spree or buy something they cannot afford. They spend money on items they do not need or want. They escape their problems and feel temporary relief from their pain. Soon they feel depressed, lonely, and confused, and again, they feel an intense urge to shop and spend.

I will choose behaviors that promote a healthy mind.

I will choose behaviors that promote a healthy mind.

I will choose behaviors that promote a healthy mind.

Some teens suffer from gambling addiction. They are unable to control the urge to gamble even at the risk of losing money, going into debt, and ruining family relationships. Although buying lottery tickets is illegal for minors, lottery addiction is a problem for some teens. They find ways to purchase lottery tickets. They get a temporary "high" from believing they might win. However, purchasing lottery tickets does not solve their problems. Soon they feel depressed and out of control again. The cycle begins again with the urge to purchase more lottery tickets.

Teens also can become addicted to a healthful behavior by having an obsession with the behavior rather than facing their problems. For example, teens need to study, work hard, and try to do things well. Extra effort contributes to positive self-esteem. However, some teens are obsessed with being perfect as a way of coping. They are never satisfied with their performance. **Perfectionism** (per·FEK·shuh·ni·zum) is an addiction in which a person is obsessed with doing things without fault. A teen with this addiction might do the same tasks over and over. Each time, the teen is not quite satisfied with the outcome. The teen believes, "I will be OK if I am perfect."

Some teens are addicted to exercise. Exercise is a healthful way to maintain fitness and reduce the effects of stress. Teens who are addicted to exercise cannot seem to exercise enough. School activities, family, and social events are neglected. Some teens are addicted to losing weight. It is healthful for teens to manage their weight to feel good about their bodies and appearance. However, teens with low self-esteem might take dieting to extremes as a way of coping. They believe, "I am fat. I will be OK if I lose more weight." These teens develop eating disorders. An **eating disorder** is a food-related dysfunction in which a person changes eating habits in a way that is harmful to the mind and body. Different kinds of eating disorders will be examined in Unit 4.

I will choose behaviors that promote a healthy mind.

I will choose behaviors that promote a healthy mind.

I will choose behaviors that promote a healthy mind.

You might be surprised to learn that some teens are addicted to relationships. These teens often feel neglected and need attention. They cling to a relationship for temporary relief from their feelings of loneliness. They become obsessed with a person and expect this person to be totally devoted to them. When they feel depressed or have self-doubts, they rely on the relationship to change their mood. They give control of their feelings and self-worth to another person. They become confused and mistake relationship addiction for genuine love.

Teens can have other addictions to try to change their mood and cope with problems. Teens might smoke cigarettes, drink alcohol, or use other drugs. You will learn more about these addictions in Unit 6.

Some teens develop multiple addictions. A **multiple addiction** is a condition in which a person has more than one addiction.

Sources of Help

Many sources of help are available for people who have an addiction and for those who care about them. An **enabler** is a person who knowingly or unknowingly supports the harmful behavior of another person. A teen enabler might have a friend or a family member who has an addiction. Teen enablers usually are sincerely trying to help the person who has an addiction. However, enablers often take no positive action. They might want to protect the person by pretending the condition does not exist or by covering up for the person. They might feel embarrassed. The person with the addiction continues with the addiction. Teen enablers need to speak with a counselor or trusted adult. They need to change their enabling behavior. Programs are available to help teen enablers change their behavior.

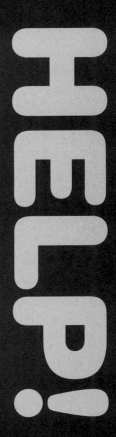

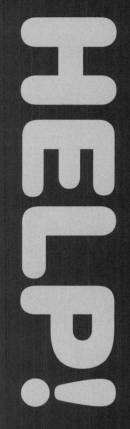

Teens who have addictions also need help. These teens often deny their addictions and refuse to get help. **Formal intervention** is an action by people, such as family members, who want a person to get treatment. During a formal intervention, people share their reactions and feelings. They set limits and explain why treatment is necessary.

There are many different approaches to treatment. One approach is individual therapy or treatment that involves only a trained professional and the person. Other approaches include group therapy and family therapy. In group therapy, a trained professional works with two or more people from different families at one time. In family therapy, a trained professional works with the person and his or her family members. Some teens who have addictions need treatment in a hospital or other recovery facility. They might need treatment for physical health problems that result from their addictive behavior.

Addictions are difficult to overcome. Many people who have an addiction must learn to manage this behavior for the rest of their lives. **Relapse** is the return to addictive behavior after a period of having stopped it. Teens who are recovering from an addiction need to learn the importance of sticking with their plan for recovery. Support programs are available for teens with addictions. These programs emphasize the need for continued support.

Lesson 3

Review

Vocabulary

Write a separate sentence using each of the vocabulary words listed on page 16.

Health Content

Write responses to the following:

1. What are two factors that influence personality? **page 17**
2. What are three activities that promote mental alertness? **page 17**
3. What are ways you can benefit from having good character? **page 18**
4. What are six addictive behaviors common in teens? **pages 20–22**
5. What kinds of therapy are available to teens with addictions? **page 23**

Confident Communication

Vocabulary

communication

feelings

I-message

you-message

active listening

anger

anger cues

hidden anger

anger management skills

self-statements

nonverbal behavior

mixed message

Life Skill • **I will communicate with others in healthful ways.**

Communication is the sharing of feelings, thoughts, and information with another person. Communication involves skill in speaking, listening, and observing. When you have effective communication skills, other people understand your thoughts and feelings. They are then more capable of responding to you. **Feelings** are emotions, such as excitement, sadness, happiness, and anger. You need to recognize and express these feelings to have optimal health and healthful relationships.

The Lesson Objectives

- Construct I-messages to express feelings.
- Outline skills for active listening.
- Describe anger cues and signs of hidden anger.
- Explain how to use anger management skills.
- Discuss how nonverbal behavior and mixed messages affect communication.
- Identify guidelines for using the telephone responsibly.
- State ways you can develop writing skills.

I-Messages and You-Messages

Look at the sidebar to learn ways to express feelings. I-messages can be used to express feelings in healthful ways. An **I-message** is a statement that contains:

1. **a specific behavior or event;**
2. **the effect that the behavior or event has on the individual;**
3. **and the feeling that results.**

When you use an I-message, you assume responsibility for sharing feelings. The other person can respond without feeling defensive.

A **you-message** is a statement that blames or shames another person. A you-message puts down the other person and might cause the person to feel defensive.

Active Listening

Active listening is a type of listening in which a person lets others know that (s)he heard and understood what was said. You can use four ways to show that you have listened carefully.

1. **Ask for more information.**
2. **Repeat what the other person said using your own words.**
3. **Summarize the main idea or ideas expressed.**
4. **Acknowledge the feelings that the person expressed and thank the person for sharing his or her feelings.**

Suppose you and your friend are going to a basketball game. Your friend is late picking you up for the game. Because your friend is late, you will miss part of the game. You are very angry. What might you say?

Suppose you say:

"You are always late and inconsiderate."

This is a you-message. A you-message blames or shames another person. Your friend might feel attacked and become defensive. It will be difficult to resolve the situation.

Suppose you say:

"Because I had to wait for you, I will miss part of the game, and I feel angry."

This is an I-message. An I-message contains a specific behavior (because I had to wait for you), the effect of the behavior (I will miss part of the the game), and a feeling (I feel angry). It allows your friend to respond to your feelings in a positive way. Your friend could respond by saying, "I'm sorry I was late," or by explaining the reason.

Expressing Anger

Communication skills affect your health and your relationships. They help you get along better with others. When you are unable to communicate effectively, your health and relationships suffer.

Suppose you are unable to express feelings of anger. **Anger** is a feeling of being irritated and annoyed. Anger is usually a response to being hurt or frustrated. **Anger cues** are body changes that occur when a person is angry. Anger cues include:

- **rapid breathing;**
- **increase in heart rate;**
- **rise in blood pressure;**
- **increase in sweating;**
- **dryness of the mouth.**

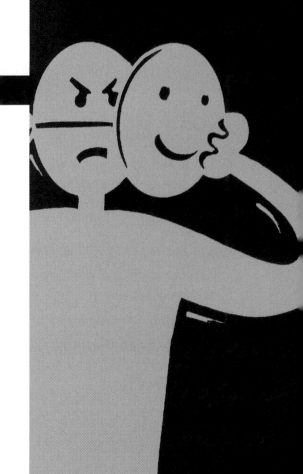

Hidden Anger

Hidden anger is anger that is not expressed or that is expressed in a harmful way. When your anger is not expressed, anger cues continue to cause wear and tear on your body. You might begin to express hidden anger by:

- **being very negative;**
- **making cruel remarks to others;**
- **being defensive;**
- **being depressed.**

If you behave in these ways, you will have difficulty in your relationships. Other people might respond to you in a negative way. These ways of behaving do not reduce your anger. Meanwhile, hidden anger continues to build. It might be expressed in outbursts, temper tantrums, and fights.

Anger Management Skills

Anger management skills are ways of expressing anger without doing something harmful. When you feel angry, you use these skills rather than blowing up or acting out.

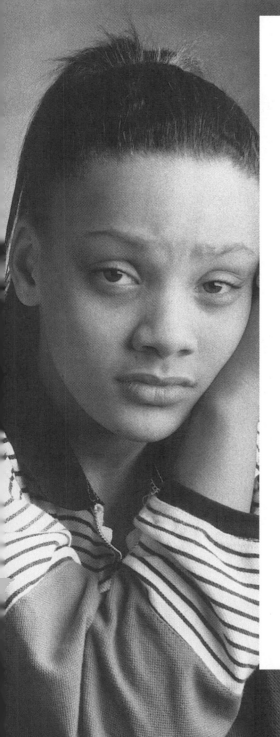

1. **Talk with your parents, guardian, or mentor.**
Adults can help you understand why you are feeling angry. They can help you express anger in healthful ways.

2. **Use self-statements to control your anger.**
Self-statements are words a person says to remind himself or herself to stay in control. They remind you not to blow up. Try saying: "I am not going to let this get to me."

3. **Use I-messages to express angry feelings.** Using I-messages keeps communication open. A person who has made you angry will not feel threatened. The person is more likely to respond to your feelings.

4. **Use active listening techniques.** When you use active listening, you allow another person to express feelings without interrupting them. The other person does not feel ignored. When you express your angry feelings, the person is more likely to listen to you.

5. **Get involved in physical activity.** Physical activity helps to reduce tension. Run, dance, or swim to blow off steam. Scream into a pillow. Squeeze a tennis ball.

6. **Do something creative.** Creative activities can be a positive outlet for expressing anger. Write a poem, draw a picture, or mold some clay.

7. **Write a letter to express your angry feelings.**
Describing your feelings can help you learn the reasons you feel the way you do. Then you will be able to tell another person why you feel a certain way without making harmful remarks. Read the letter at a later date. Decide if it is appropriate to mail the letter. If you decide not to mail the letter, the act of writing it will still have reduced some of your anger.

Nonverbal Behavior

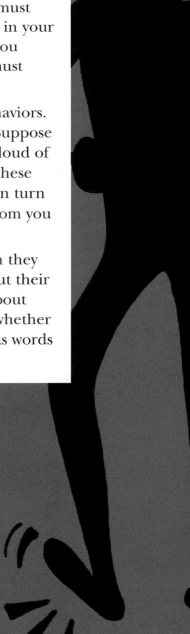

Nonverbal behavior is the use of actions rather than words to express thoughts and feelings. You might shake your head YES or NO to agree or disagree with someone. A smile or a frown might indicate that you like or dislike something. Tapping your foot or chewing on a pencil might show that you are stressed.

These actions send a message to people who observe you. Think about the impression you want to make. Do you want to convey self-confidence? If you do, you must stand and walk with confidence. You cannot slouch in your chair. You cannot slump as you enter a room. Do you want to appear healthy and energized? Then you must smile and have a cheerful bounce to your walk.

Consider the message you send with harmful behaviors. Suppose someone sees you holding a can of beer. Suppose someone sees you smoking a cigarette. There is a cloud of smoke around you. You create an impression with these nonverbal behaviors. These nonverbal behaviors can turn other people off. They might decide to stay away from you even though you have never had a conversation.

Pay attention to the actions of other people when they are speaking. Remember, their actions tell you about their thoughts and feelings. Their actions also tell you about their values. Their nonverbal behavior is a clue to whether or not they value health. Actions are as important as words in the communication process.

Mixed Messages

It is important to avoid sending mixed messages. A **mixed message** is a message that conveys two different meanings. A mixed message can be sent in two ways:

1. Your words and tone of voice convey two different meanings.

2. Your words and actions convey two different meanings.

Suppose you are speaking with a classmate. Your classmate has just won the science fair. How might you send a mixed message?

You might congratulate your classmate, but sound very insincere. As you congratulate your classmate, you frown and avoid eye contact.

I will communicate with others in healthful ways.

I will communicate with others in healthful ways.

I will communicate with others in healthful ways.

Telephone Tips

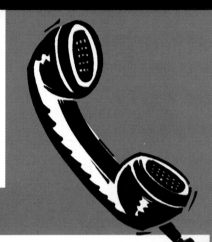

Many teens enjoy talking to their friends on the telephone. Daily events, opposite sex relationships, and social plans are the topics of conversation. Your conversations with friends are important. However, you must remember the telephone serves many purposes. Other family members might conduct business on the telephone. Other people might call your home to leave important messages. Practice the following telephone tips.

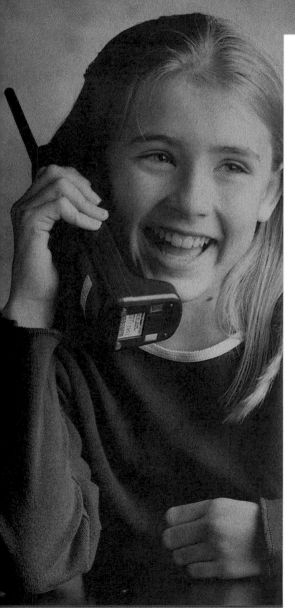

- Ask your parents or guardian for guidelines for using the telephone.

- Be certain your friends know your family's telephone guidelines. Ask them to respect these guidelines. For example, your family might not want friends calling before or after a certain hour.

- Respect the telephone guidelines of your friends' families. Do not call friends early in the morning or late at night unless you have permission.

- Respect other family members' rights to use the phone. Limit the time you spend on the telephone.

- Answer the phone in a polite way. Recognize that your parents or guardian might get work-related calls.

- Keep a notepad and pen by the telephone to write down messages for other family members.

- Keep a list of emergency telephone numbers next to the telephone.

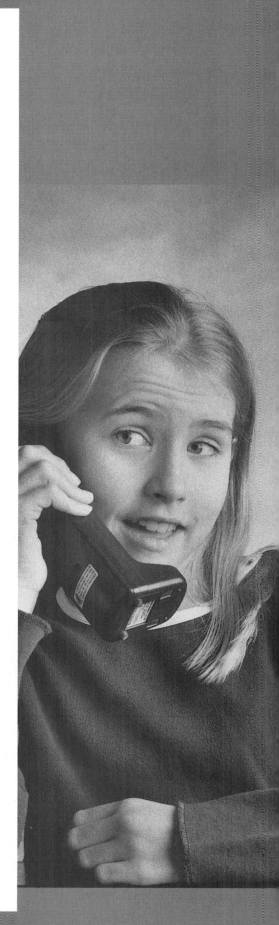

- Answer the telephone in a safe way. Do not give your name, address, or telephone number to a stranger. If a caller says, "Who is this?" respond, "To whom am I speaking?"

- Do not answer surveys or give other information over the telephone without the approval of your parents or guardian.

- Do not give out credit card information over the phone.

- Do not purchase items from television shopping programs or commercials without permission from your parents or guardian.

- Do not make long-distance calls without permission from your parents or guardian.

- Use good manners when calling another person. Say, "This is Melissa Smith. May I please speak with Alicia?"

- Do not make prank calls.

- Do not hang up without speaking if you dial a wrong number. Say, "I am sorry, I dialed the wrong number."

- Be cautious when taping a message to be played if you have an answering machine. Avoid giving out too much information. For example, you would not want to say, "This is the Jones family. We are gone for the weekend, but leave a message." This would alert others that no one is home.

- Use good manners when leaving a message on someone else's answering machine. Keep your message short. Avoid personal messages, because you do not know who will play back the message.

Written Communication

Writing is an important way to express your ideas, thoughts, and feelings. You can take your time and give thought to what you want to say.

You can reread what you have written to be certain you were clear. Writing is a skill that must be developed. Set time aside each week to write. Practice the Six Tips for Written Communication.

Six Tips for Written Communication

1. Use correct grammar and spelling.

2. Try using new vocabulary words to express yourself.

3. Keep a dictionary handy for correct spelling.

4. Keep a thesaurus on hand to look up new words to replace words with which you are familiar.

5. Use a spell check program if you are writing on the computer.

6. Use appropriate greetings and closings when writing to another person.

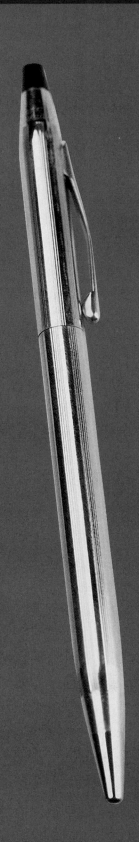

Take Time to Write!

- **Write letters to family members and friends to keep in touch.**

- **Write a pen pal in another city, state, or country.**

- **Include a short note when you send a birthday or greeting card.**

- **Send e-mail to another teen.**

- **Keep a journal.**

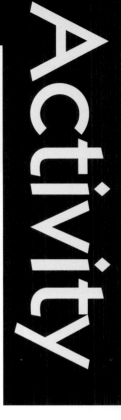

Get the Message

Life Skill

I will communicate with others in healthful ways.

Materials: Paper, pen or pencil

Directions: Complete this activity to demonstrate the effect I-messages and you-messages have on others.

1. Write a brief description of a situation which might make you feel anger. For example, you might write, "My best friend had a party and (s)he did not invite me."

2. After your teacher collects the descriptions and mixes them up, pick one at random.

3. Write a you-message and an I-message to respond to the situation on your slip.

4. Share your messages with your class. Choose a student to role play how (s)he would respond to each message.

5. Discuss with your class which message helped you express your feelings in a healthful way and why.

Lesson 4

Review

Vocabulary

Write a separate sentence using each of the vocabulary words listed on page 24.

Health Content

Write responses to the following:

1. What are three parts of an I-message? **page 25**
2. What is the difference between an I-message and a you-message? **page 25**
3. What are four ways to show active listening? **page 25**
4. What are five anger cues? **page 26**
5. What are four ways hidden anger might be expressed? **page 26**
6. What are seven anger management skills? **page 27**
7. What are three examples of nonverbal behavior? **page 28**
8. What are two ways to send a mixed message? **page 29**
9. What are 17 tips for using the telephone? **pages 30–31**
10. What are six tips for written communication? **page 32**

Successful Stress Management

Vocabulary

stress

stressor

general adaptation syndrome (GAS)

alarm stage

adrenaline

resistance stage

exhaustion stage

eustress

distress

stress management skills

depression

resilient

suicide

suicide prevention skills

Life Skills
- **I will follow a plan to manage stress.**
- **I will be resilient during difficult times.**

   Stress is the response of the body to the demands of daily living. A **stressor** is a source or cause of stress. Stressors can be physical, mental, or social. Having an illness is a physical stressor. Having difficult homework assignments is a mental stressor. Having an argument with a friend is a social stressor. Understanding stress and knowing what to do when it occurs help you remain healthy.

The Lesson Objectives

- Describe the general adaptation syndrome and how it relates to health.
- Outline techniques to help you manage stress.
- Discuss causes and signs of depression in teens.
- State steps you can take when a person shows signs of suicide.

The Stress Response

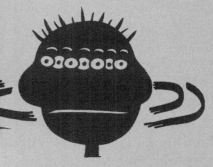

The **general adaptation syndrome (GAS)** is a series of changes that occur in the body when stress occurs. The GAS occurs in three stages.

1. The **alarm stage** is the first stage of the GAS in which adrenaline is secreted into the bloodstream. **Adrenaline** (uh·DREN·uhl·un) is a hormone that prepares the body for quick action.

2. The **resistance stage** is the second stage of the GAS in which the body attempts to return to normal. Adrenaline is no longer secreted. Heart rate and blood pressure decrease. Digestion begins again. The muscles relax and respiration returns to normal.

3. The **exhaustion stage** is the third stage of the GAS in which wear and tear on the body increases the risk of diseases and accidents. This stage of the GAS is usually not experienced if people know how to manage stress.

It is important to understand how you respond to various stressors. **Eustress** (YOO·stres) is a healthful response to a stressor. **Distress** is a harmful response to a stressor. The following example will help you tell the difference between eustress and distress. Suppose your teacher announces you will have a difficult test. Your adrenaline begins to flow. You respond by studying hard and learning the material. The extra energy produced by adrenaline helps you perform well. After the test, you relax and feel confident. Your body functions return to normal (the resistance stage). You have experienced eustress.

You might have a different response when the test is announced. You might experience distress. You might worry so much that it is difficult to study or to sleep. During the test, you feel tired and anxious. After the test, you worry about the grade you will receive. You have experienced distress.

When you experience distress, you are at risk for moving to the exhaustion stage of the GAS. Distress increases the risk of having certain diseases and being involved in accidents.

General Adaptation Syndrome (GAS)

ALARM STAGE
- **Pupils dilate**
- **Hearing sharpens**
- **Saliva decreases**
- **Heart rate increases**
- **Blood pressure increases**
- **Digestion slows**
- **Blood flow to muscles increases**
- **Muscles tighten**

RESISTANCE STAGE
- **Pupils constrict**
- **Hearing is normal**
- **Saliva increases**
- **Heart rate decreases**
- **Blood pressure drops**
- **Digestion slows**
- **Blood flow to muscles decreases**
- **Muscles relax**

EXHAUSTION STAGE
- **The body is worn down**
- **Accidents are likely to occur**
- **Diseases might develop**

Stress Management Skills

Stress management skills are techniques to cope with the body changes produced by stress. Practicing these skills helps prevent the exhaustion stage of the GAS. When you experience stress, adrenaline is secreted. Body changes occur. Using the following stress management skills helps your body return to its normal state.

1. Use responsible decision-making skills.

One type of skill focuses on doing something about the cause of stress (the stressor). You can apply the steps in *The Responsible Decision-Making Model™* to a difficult situation. This will help you feel confident instead of anxious and stressed.

2. Get enough rest and sleep.

This helps prevent exhaustion. When you are resting or sleeping, blood pressure decreases, heart rate slows, and muscles relax. Then you have more energy to face difficulties.

3. Participate in physical activities.

Physical activity relieves tension by providing an outlet for the energy that builds up with stress. Physical activity uses up adrenaline.

4. Use a time management plan.

Keeping a daily calendar helps you focus on what you need to do. You can plan your time more effectively. This keeps you from being overwhelmed.

5. Write in a journal.

Writing is a healthful outlet for expressing feelings. It might help you focus more clearly on what is happening. You might choose to share your journal with a trusted family member or friend.

6.

Spend time with close friends.

Friends can listen and offer suggestions without judging you. You will worry less when you have support from friends.

7.

Talk with parents and other trusted adults.

You can benefit from the wisdom of adults. They can provide support, suggestions, and reassurance.

8.

Help others.

Helping people who are less fortunate than yourself can make stressful situations seem less important.

9.

Express affection in appropriate ways.

Expressing affection in appropriate ways provides a feeling of closeness, which in turn relieves stressful feelings.

10.

Care for pets.

Taking care of and holding a pet is comforting and relaxing. The physical contact involved in the care of a pet helps reduce feelings of stress.

11.

Change one's outlook.

Developing a positive attitude is helpful. A difficult situation can be seen as a challenge instead of a problem.

12.

Keep a sense of humor.

A good laugh relaxes you and relieves muscle tension. Laughter helps lower your heart rate and blood pressure.

Depression

Teenage years are filled with ups and downs. At times, you might feel very positive and in control of your life. At other times, you might feel depressed. **Depression** is the feeling of being sad, unhappy, or discouraged. Teens experience depression for some of the following reasons:

- **Disappointment** They expect something and it does not happen. Someone let them down, or they let someone else down.

- **Loss of self-respect** They expect too much of themselves or feel that others expect too much of them.

- **Unfair comparisons** They believe they do not measure up to other teens.

- **Illness** They might have a long-term illness that prevents them from doing what other teens are doing.

- **Broken relationships** They might feel very sad because family members are separated. A friend might have moved. A family member or friend might have died.

Short periods of depression are common during the teenage years. However, prolonged depression is not. Symptoms of teenage depression include:

- **loss of sleep;**
- **loss of interest;**
- **loss of appetite;**
- **loss of energy;**
- **loss of ability to concentrate;**
- **lack of interest in having a neat and clean appearance;**
- **physical ailments, such as headaches, muscle aches, tightening of the chest, dizziness, or difficulty in breathing;**
- **use of alcohol and other drugs;**
- **change in personality;**
- **unusual behavior, such as running away from home.**

Teens who are depressed might begin to withdraw from others. They might drop out of school activities. When around others, they might appear anxious and irritable. They might show signs of sadness. All teens should have a plan for dealing with prolonged depression.

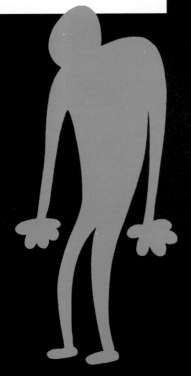

The Teenage Quick-Action Plan for Dealing with Depression

Discuss your feelings with your parents or guardian. They can offer encouragement. They can suggest actions that are healthful. Plan activities with family members. Being involved helps change your mood.

Spend time with other adults who support you. Think of two other adults with whom you spend time. You might have regular contact with a friend's parent, a relative, a teacher, a coach, or a member of the clergy. Adults who you know can support you.

Know places in your community that provide help. Do not wait until you feel depressed. Ask your parents or guardian about places that offer teens help. Professionals can help teens deal with depression.

Practice stress management skills daily. Refer to the list of stress management skills. When you use these skills daily, you are less likely to tire from stress. You are less likely to feel overwhelmed.

Take Charge...Be Resilient

To be **resilient** is to be able to prevent or "bounce back" from misfortune, change, or pressure. Being resilient includes bouncing back from a disappointment. Being resilient includes bouncing back from feeling depressed or feeling stressed. To be resilient, you must feel empowered. To be empowered means to be inspired because you feel some sense of control over your behavior and decisions.

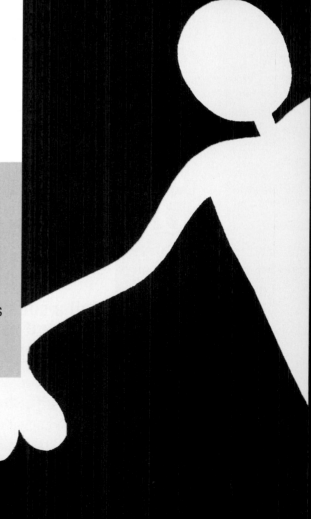

Suicide Prevention Skills

Suicide is the intentional taking of one's own life. The signs of suicide are similar to those for depression. This is why you must always take action when you feel depressed. You also must know what to do when someone close to you is very depressed or mentions suicide.

Suicide prevention skills are steps to take when a person shows signs of suicide.

Recognize the signs of suicide. A person might be very depressed, show changes in behavior, and talk about death.

2. **Do not ignore any signs or take the person lightly.** If someone seems very depressed or mentions suicide, you must take action. It is better to be overly concerned than to pretend nothing is wrong.

3. **Ask a trusted adult for help.** Although you usually keep confidences, this is not the time to do so. This is a serious situation that requires the help of an adult. The adult will know what steps to take. For example, a parent or guardian of the person needs to be contacted.

4. **Call a suicide hotline service or an emergency service if needed.** Call for help if help from a trusted adult is not available.

5. **Stay with the person.** A person who is thinking about suicide should not be left alone. Someone should stay with the person until help arrives.

6. **Show concern for the person.** Never underestimate the importance of showing concern. It is reassuring to know that others care.

Sky Watch

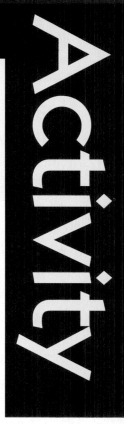

Activity

Life Skill I will follow a plan to manage stress.

Materials: Construction paper, markers, scissors, paper, pen or pencil

Directions: Complete this activity to motivate you to practice stress management skills.

1. **Create a list of actions you can take to manage stress. Make them personal to you.**
You might write:
"Walk 30 minutes every day."
"Play with my dog Ginger."

2. **Design an object that moves in the sky such as a balloon or jet.** Draw and cut it out of the construction paper.

3. **Copy your list of actions onto your design.**

4. **Hang your design from the ceiling.**

Lesson 5

Review

Vocabulary

Write a separate sentence using each of the vocabulary words listed on page 34.

Health Content

Write responses to the following:

1. What are the series of changes that occur in each of the three stages of the general adaptation syndrome? **page 35**

2. What are twelve stress management skills? **pages 36–37**

3. What are five reasons teens might experience depression? **page 38**

4. What are ten signs of teenage depression? **page 38**

5. What are six suicide prevention skills you can use when a person shows signs of suicide? **page 40**

Unit 1 Review

Health Content

Review your answers for each Lesson Review in this unit. Then write answers to each of the following questions.

1. How can practicing life skills help you achieve optimal health? **Lesson 1 page 5**

2. How can a *Health Behavior Inventory* help you gain health awareness? **Lesson 1 page 8**

3. Outline and explain the steps in *The Responsible Decision-Making Model™.* **Lesson 2 page 13**

4. How do positive peer pressure and negative peer pressure influence the decisions you make? **Lesson 2 page 14**

5. What influences your personality? **Lesson 3 page 17**

6. What are reasons teens might practice addictive behavior? **Lesson 3 page 20**

7. How can a mixed message be sent? **Lesson 4 page 29**

8. How can you improve your writing skill? **Lesson 4 page 32**

9. How does the third stage of the general adaptation syndrome affect your health? **Lesson 5 page 35**

10. Why might teens experience depression? **Lesson 5 page 38**

Vocabulary

Number a sheet of paper from 1–10. Select the correct vocabulary word. Write it next to the corresponding number. DO NOT WRITE IN THIS BOOK.

adrenaline	realistic standard
alarm stage	relapse
empowered	resistance skills
eustress	risk behaviors
hidden anger	self-discipline

1. The _____ is the first stage of the GAS in which adrenaline is secreted into the bloodstream. **Lesson 5**

2. A(n) _____ is the return to addictive behavior after a period of having stopped it. **Lesson 3**

3. _____ are skills that are used when a person wants to say NO to an action or to leave a situation. **Lesson 2**

4. To be _____ is to be inspired because one feels some sense of control over behavior and decisions. **Lesson 2**

5. _____ is a healthful response to a stressor. **Lesson 5**

6. A(n) _____ is a requirement a person sets for himself or herself that can reasonably be achieved. **Lesson 3**

7. _____ is a hormone that prepares the body for quick action. **Lesson 5**

8. _____ is the effort or energy with which a person follows through on intentions or promises. **Lesson 1**

9. _____ are voluntary actions that threaten health; increase the likelihood of illness and premature death; and harm the quality of the environment. **Lesson 1**

10. _____ is anger that is not expressed or that is expressed in a harmful way. **Lesson 4**

The Responsible Decision-Making Model™

You have set a standard for yourself that you will make a "100" on every test and assignment in every subject. You feel depressed if you receive a lower grade. You stay up late to study. You are feeling very tired. You know you should get more rest but you feel compelled to do perfect schoolwork. Answer the following questions on a separate sheet of paper. Write "Does not apply" if a question does not apply to you.

1. Is it healthful to be obsessed with doing perfect schoolwork? Why or why not?

2. Is it safe to be obsessed with doing perfect schoolwork? Why or why not?

3. Is it legal to be obsessed with doing perfect schoolwork? Why or why not?

4. Will you show respect for yourself if you are obsessed with doing perfect schoolwork? Why or why not?

5. Will your parents or guardian approve if you are obsessed with doing perfect schoolwork? Why or why not?

6. Will you demonstrate good character if you are obsessed with doing perfect schoolwork? Why or why not?

What is the responsible decision to make in this situation?

Health Literacy

Effective Communication

Write an article on addictive behaviors to submit to your favorite teen magazine. Include information you have learned in this lesson.

Self-Directed Learning

Find the CDC Web site on the Internet (www.cdc.gov). Gather information on the six categories of risk behaviors for teens. Print out this information and share it with your class.

Critical Thinking

Keep a journal in which you write ways your friends have tried to influence you. Write how you responded to the pressure. If you gave in to negative pressure, write how you could use resistance skills the next time.

Responsible Citizenship

Make a list of ways students can improve their self-respect at school. Get permission to post your list in your school.

Multicultural Health

Choose a country different from your own and read about it. Imagine how your personality might be different if you had been raised in that country. Write a paragraph to describe how it might be different.

Family Involvement

Discuss with your family activities you can do together to increase mental alertness.

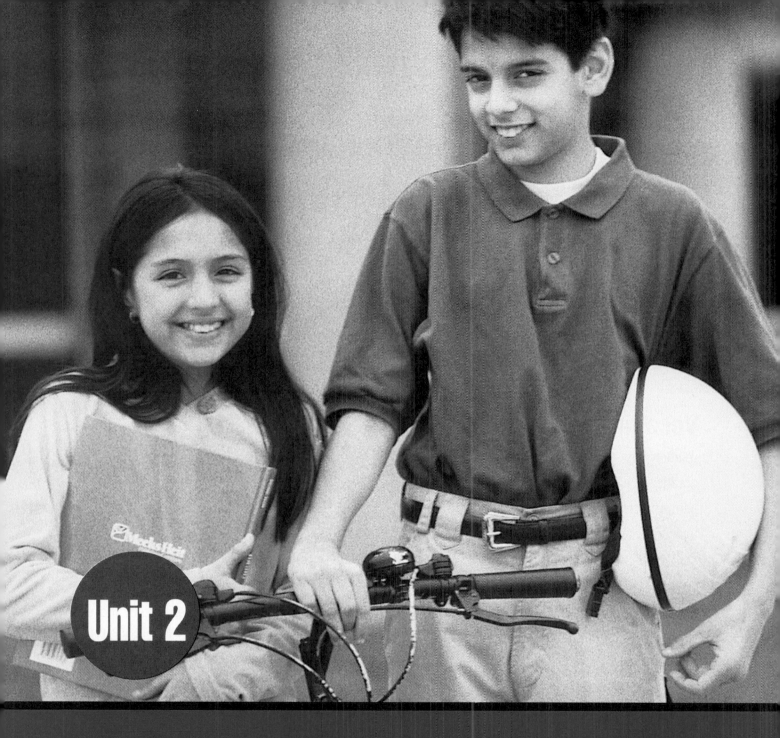

Family and Social Health

Extraordinary Relationships

Vocabulary

relationship

conflict

healthful relationship

loving person

social skills

shyness

empathy

rejection

mental rehearsal

selfish

discriminate

conflict

intrapersonal conflict

interpersonal conflict

intergroup conflict

violence

conflict resolution skills

mediation

mediator

peer

 Life Skill • **I will use conflict resolution skills.**

To be extraordinary is to be very special—to be in a class by yourself. You can have extraordinary relationships. A **relationship** is the connection a person has with others. To have extraordinary relationships requires effort and skills. All relationships involve conflicts. A **conflict** is a disagreement between two or more people or between two or more choices. You need to learn to resolve conflicts in a way that helps maintain healthful relationships.

The Lesson Objectives

- Describe characteristics of a loving person.
- Identify ways you can improve your social skills.
- Discuss behaviors that are roadblocks to healthful relationships.
- Outline ten conflict resolution skills.
- Explain the steps in the mediation process.

Healthful Relationships

A **healthful relationship** is a relationship that promotes mutual respect and responsible behavior. Suppose you find a four-leaf clover in the grass. You might decide to keep it for good luck. You value the four-leaf clover because it is extraordinary.

You will meet many different people throughout your life. Some of these people will be as special as the four-leaf clover. They will be able to love themselves and others easily. There is something extraordinary about a person who is loving. A **loving person** is someone who is respectful, responsible, understanding, and self-disciplined. Look at the four-leaf clover. Review the characteristics that a loving person has. Are you a loving person?

Understanding
You share the feelings of others. You are aware of other people's points of view.

Respectful
You care about the feelings of others as much as you care about your own.

A Loving Person

Self-Disciplined
You control your own actions and make healthful choices instead of harmful ones.

Responsible
You can be depended upon to choose healthful behaviors.

Social Skills

Social skills are skills a person can use to relate well with others. Social skills that improve relationships are listed below.

Using manners Manners make a lasting impression. Saying "Please," "Thank you," "Excuse me," and "Pardon me" shows respect for others. Listening without interrupting is another way to show respect. Writing notes to express sympathy shows thoughtfulness. Carefully selecting a birthday card also shows thoughtfulness.

Dealing with shyness **Shyness** is withdrawing from contact with other people or activities. A person who is shy hesitates to say and do certain things. Teens who are shy might hold back what they are thinking and feeling. They might dislike being forced to participate. They might prefer being gently encouraged to talk or do something. If being shy is troublesome to you, you might want to talk to a trusted adult about these feelings.

Responding to other people's feelings **Empathy** is the ability to share in another person's emotions or feelings. Empathy involves listening and caring. It requires that you respond in a warm and sincere way. Sometimes you might not know what to say. For example, a friend's grandparent might die. You might not know what to say. It is OK to be at a loss for words. This happens to everyone at times. You can simply say, "I do not know what to say right now. I just want you to know I care."

Coping with rejection **Rejection** is the feeling of being unwanted. Being rejected can be painful. If you feel rejected, choose to respond in a healthful way. Do not ignore this feeling of rejection or pretend you do not care. Do not attack or harm people who reject you. Try to learn why you were not included. Brainstorm a list of ways you might deal with your feelings. Discuss your list with a friend or trusted adult.

Coping with stressful conversations or events Be prepared. You might want to have a mental rehearsal when you anticipate a stressful experience. A **mental rehearsal** is a technique that involves imagining a stressful conversation or situation, pretending to say and do specific things, and imagining how the other person will respond. Several mental rehearsals might be needed to reduce your stress level and to prepare for a conversation or event.

Roadblocks to Relationships

Some behaviors are roadblocks to having healthful relationships.

Being selfish To be **selfish** is to care about oneself without thinking about others. Teens who are selfish do not care about other people's feelings. They want things to be exactly as they want them. For example, a teen who is selfish might break plans with a friend if something better comes along.

Talking about others and sharing confidences Some teens enjoy talking behind the backs of others. They say negative and hurtful things. Their friends cannot rely on them to keep secrets. They cannot be trusted.

Being distrustful Trust is very important in relationships. Teens who are distrustful find it difficult to trust others. They question the motives and actions of friends. Teens who are distrustful make it difficult for others to become close to them.

Choosing to discriminate To **discriminate** (dis·KRIM·uh·nayt) is to treat some people or groups of people differently from others. A person who discriminates might believe that some individuals or groups of people are better than others. Calling people names or excluding them because they are different from you is an example of this behavior. Telling jokes or laughing at jokes about people of a different race or religion is another example. This behavior can lead to disagreements and fights. People do not like to be put down because they are different. All people should be treated with respect.

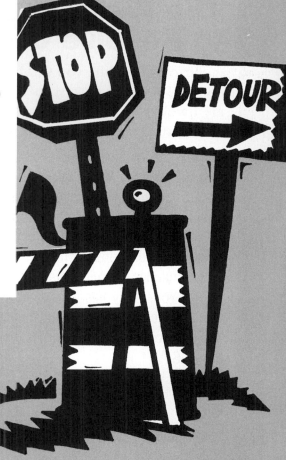

Conflict

Conflict occurs in all relationships. A **conflict** is a disagreement between two or more people or between two or more choices. In general, three kinds of conflicts occur. An **intrapersonal conflict** is a conflict that occurs within a person. Suppose you have a test for which you need to study. A friend asks you to go to the movies. You might struggle to decide which to do. An **interpersonal conflict** is a conflict that involves two or more people. Suppose you are in line to buy a ticket for a movie. Someone cuts in the line and gets ahead of you. A disagreement might begin. An **intergroup conflict** is a conflict that occurs between two or more groups of people. The conflict might involve different families, school groups, gangs, racial groups, religious groups, or nations.

The Risks of Being Unable to Resolve Conflict

Throughout life, you will be faced with different kinds of conflict. Do you have skills to resolve conflict? Three risks are involved with being unable to resolve conflict. Being unable to prevent or resolve conflict:

Harms health. When you stay in a constant state of conflict, changes occur in your body. The changes are the same as those of the alarm stage of the GAS. Heart rate and blood pressure increase. You might have headaches and stomachaches. It might be difficult for you to sleep. Your body becomes tired and run down. You are more at risk for developing diseases or having accidents. Refer to Lesson 5 to review the GAS.

Harms relationships. If you are not able to work out disagreements in relationships, it might be difficult to get close to others. You might feel on edge much of the time. It is difficult to share your true feelings.

Causes violence. Violence is the use of physical force to injure, damage, or destroy oneself, others, or property. Teens who have conflict within themselves and with others are more likely to harm themselves. Teens who cannot resolve conflicts are more likely to get into fights. They might "get even" in other ways, such as by destroying property.

Conflict Resolution Skills

It is important to recognize that every conflict does not have to have a winner and a loser. People can work together to find a solution in which everybody wins. You can use conflict resolution skills. **Conflict resolution skills** are steps that can be used to resolve a disagreement in a healthful, safe, legal, respectful, and nonviolent way. The following list identifies ten steps used to resolve conflict.

1. **Remain calm.**
2. **Set the tone.**
   - Avoid blaming.
   - Avoid interrupting.
   - Affirm others.
   - Be sincere.
   - Avoid put-downs.
   - Reserve judgment.
   - Avoid threats.
   - Separate the person from the problem.
   - Use positive nonverbal messages.
3. **Define the conflict.**
4. **Take responsibility for personal actions.**
5. **Use I-messages to express needs and feelings.**
6. **Listen to the needs and feelings of others.**

7. **List and discuss possible solutions. Evaluate each solution:**
   - Will the solution result in actions that are healthful?
   - Will the solution result in actions that are safe?
   - Will the solution result in actions that are legal?
   - Will the solution result in actions that are respectful of everyone who is involved?
   - Will the solution result in actions that are nonviolent?
8. **Agree on a solution.**
9. **Keep your word and follow the solution upon which you agreed.**
10. **Ask for the assistance of a trusted adult if the conflict cannot be resolved.**

Mediation

Sometimes people in conflict need the help of a third person to reach a solution. **Mediation** is a process in which a third person helps people in conflict reach a solution. A **mediator** is a person who helps people in conflict reach a solution. This person might be a parent, teacher, counselor, or other trusted adult. Sometimes adults recommend that a peer be a part of the mediation process. A **peer** is a person who is similar in age or status. Mediation involves seven steps.

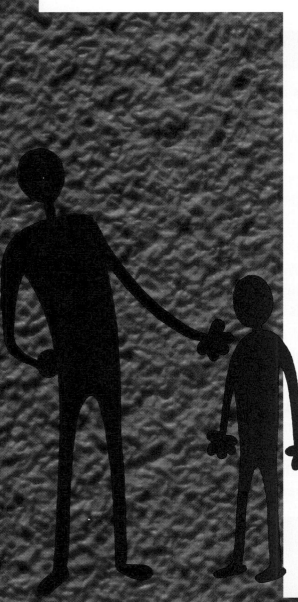

1. **Keep a neutral position.**
   - The mediator listens to both sides.

2. **Set ground rules.**
   - The opposing sides agree to treat each other with respect. Blaming, put-downs, threats, name-calling, hitting, and pushing are not allowed. Each side agrees to listen.

3. **Define the conflict.**
   - Each side clearly identifies and describes the reason for the conflict. Each person shares how (s)he feels about what has happened.

4. **Identify solutions to the conflict.**

5. **Evaluate suggested solutions.**
   - It is important to evaluate each solution. Will the solution result in actions that are healthful? Safe? Legal? Respectful of all people involved? Nonviolent?

6. **Agree to try a solution.**
   - An agreement stating the solution the people will follow is written. The people involved should be sincere about following the agreement. They should sign and date the agreement.

7. **Schedule a follow-up meeting.**
   - Decide when to have a follow-up meeting.
   - Review how well the agreement is working. If the agreement is not working, begin the process again.

Conflict Fix

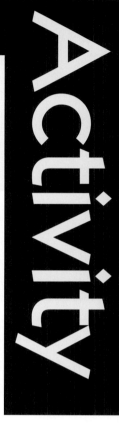

Life Skill
I will use conflict resolution skills.

Materials: Paper, pen or pencil

Directions: Role play a situation that involves conflict to help you gain skill in resolving conflicts.

1. **Work with a partner to write about a situation that involves conflict.** The conflict can be real or one you create. For example, you might write, "My sister (or brother) and I fight all the time. We can't seem to stop."

2. **Use the ten conflict resolution skills to resolve the conflict.** Write down responses for skills 3, 5, 7, and 8 on page 51.

3. **Prepare a two- to three-minute skit in which you role play how you resolved the conflict.** For example, you might play yourself and your partner might play your brother or sister.

4. **Present your skit to your class.**

Lesson 6

Review

Vocabulary

Write a separate sentence using each of the vocabulary words listed on page 46.

Health Content

Write responses to the following:

1. What are four characteristics of a loving person? **page 47**
2. What are five social skills that improve relationships? **page 48**
3. What are four roadblocks to healthful relationships? **page 49**
4. What are ten conflict resolution skills? **page 51**
5. What are seven steps in the mediation process? **page 52**

Fantastic Family Relationships

Vocabulary

family relationship

healthful family relationship

healthful family

couple family

traditional family

foster family

single-parent family

joint-custody family

single-custody family

blended family

extended family

separation

divorce

remarriage

stepfamily

Life Skills

- **I will develop healthful family relationships.**
- **I will make healthful adjustments to family changes.**

A **family relationship** is the connection a person has with family members. A **healthful family relationship** is one in which family members relate well and make necessary adjustments to family changes. Families are similar in many ways. Family members have similar needs and wants. They want the family to provide feelings of closeness and belonging. They need to feel supported and protected during difficult times. In other ways, families differ from one another. They might differ in size and living arrangements. Families can be structured in many different ways.

The Lesson Objectives

- List behaviors adults in healthful families teach their children.
- Identify different kinds of family patterns.
- Discuss changes that might occur in family relationships.
- Describe ways you can adjust to changes in family relationships.

Healthful Family Relationships

A **healthful family** is a family in which members behave in ways that are loving and responsible. Adults in a healthful family teach their children to:

- **Show respect for others.**
- **Trust others.**
- **Follow guidelines for responsible behavior.**
- **Demonstrate self-discipline.**
- **Spend time with family members.**
- **Share feelings in healthful ways.**
- **Practice effective coping skills.**
- **Resolve conflicts in nonviolent ways.**
- **Avoid alcohol and other drugs.**
- **Use kind words and actions.**

In some families, adults do not teach their children these actions. Their children might learn actions that harm relationships. In Lesson 8, you will learn about harmful family relationships.

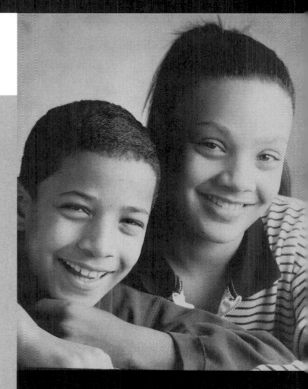

Family Structures

- A **couple family** consists of two adults who do not have children.
- A **traditional family** consists of a husband and wife and their children.
- A **foster family** includes an adult(s) who cares for a child or children who do not live with the birth parents.
- A **single-parent family** consists of one parent and a child or children.

- A **joint-custody family** consists of two parents living apart sharing custody of their children.
- A **single-custody family** consists of two parents living apart and a child or children living with only one parent.
- A **blended family** consists of two adults, one or both of whom has children from a previous relationship.
- An **extended family** consists of family members from three or more generations who live together. Other relatives might live with them.

Family Changes

Family relationships are constantly changing. Family changes can be unexpected and stressful. Making adjustments when changes occur promotes healthful family relationships.

Death of a Family Member

A family member might die unexpectedly. As a result, family members experience stress. Family members can share feelings and support each other. In other cases, a family member might have an illness that cannot be cured. Other family members might have the opportunity to spend time with the family member who is dying. Sharing feelings with this family member is important.

Separation of Parents

Married couples might struggle at times to maintain a meaningful relationship. During such times, some couples live together while others do not. A **separation** is an agreement between a couple to live apart, but remain married. Teens whose parents are separated usually find this situation stressful. At a time when they are dealing with their own relationships, they would prefer to have their parents in a successful relationship. The separation might cause teens to feel insecure. They might have concerns about what will happen in their future. Sharing worries and feelings with parents, a counselor, or other trusted adults is helpful.

Divorce of Parents

A **divorce** is the legal end of a marriage. When parents stay close with their teenage children, the teenage children are more likely to feel secure and loved. When parents do not stay close with their teenage children, teens feel abandoned and unloved. They might have difficulty concentrating in school. They might feel very sad. Talking with parents or a counselor is helpful.

Parental Dating

Teens often have difficulty when their single parents date. When a parent is dating, a teen might have mixed feelings. Dating might reduce the amount of time a parent spends with the teen or it might seem to affect time together. Teens often wonder if they should accept or like someone a parent is dating. They might wonder if this acceptance would be disloyal to the other parent. They might wonder if this person will be a threat to the family. Getting answers to these questions helps teens sort out their confusion.

Remarriage

A **remarriage** is a marriage in which a previously married person has married again. Teens might have mixed feelings about a parent's new spouse. They might feel angry if they believe the new spouse caused the breakup of their parents' marriage. They might still be struggling with the fact that their parents will not get back together. Being patient and sharing feelings eases the adjustment to a remarriage.

Formation of a Stepfamily

A **stepfamily** is a family that is formed as a result of the remarriage of one of the parents. In a stepfamily, the greatest source of conflict often is accepting new family rules. Teens might have difficulty accepting the rules of the stepparent. They might prefer the previous way of living. Teens tend to have an easier time adjusting if their parent spends quality time alone with them.

Birth of a Baby

When a baby is born, everyone in the family has to make adjustments. Parents have many demands. The baby needs to be fed, clothed, cared for, and loved. Teens might have mixed feelings about the baby. They might feel the baby gets too much attention. They might have wanted the family to stay as it was. Teens often want reassurance that they are loved. Sharing concerns and needs makes family members closer.

Lesson 7

Review

Vocabulary

Write a separate sentence using each of the vocabulary words listed on page 54.

Health Content

Write responses to the following:

1. What are ways families are alike and different? **page 54**
2. What are ten behaviors adults in healthful families teach their children? **page 55**
3. What are eight different family structures? **page 55**
4. How can family members adjust to the death of a family member? **page 56**
5. How can family members adjust to separation of parents? **page 56**
6. How can family members adjust to the divorce of parents? **page 56**
7. How can family members adjust to parental dating? **page 56**
8. How can family members adjust to the remarriage of a parent(s)? **page 56**
9. How can family members adjust to the formation of a stepfamily? **page 57**
10. How can family members adjust to the birth of a baby? **page 57**

Strengthening Family Relationships

Vocabulary

harmful relationship

dysfunctional family

drug dependence

codependence

enabler

abuse

child abuse

spouse abuse

parent abuse

elder abuse

physical abuse

emotional abuse

neglect

sexual abuse

violence

domestic violence

juvenile offender

domestic shelter

formal intervention

mentor

Life Skill

- **I will work to improve difficult family relationships.**

A **harmful relationship** is a relationship that harms self-respect and includes harmful behavior. Some teens have harmful family relationships. These teens need to learn facts to recognize the harmful patterns of behaving in their families. These facts also help them examine how family relationships affect their other relationships.

The Lesson Objectives

- Identify three kinds of problems that can occur in dysfunctional families.

- Explain why teens in families with drug dependency have difficulty in relationships.

- Describe why teens who are abused need help sorting out their feelings.

- State actions family members can take when their safety is at risk.

- Discuss intervention and treatment for dysfunctional families.

The Dysfunctional Family

A **dysfunctional family** is a family in which members behave in ways that are not responsible or loving. One or more family members might be affected by drug dependence, abuse, or violence. The health and safety of family members are at risk.

Drug Dependence

One factor in the breakdown of a family is drug dependence. **Drug dependence** is the continued use of a drug even though it harms the body, mind, and relationships. The lives of family members who are drug-dependent become dominated by the need to obtain and use drugs. Drug dependence causes them to do things they normally would not do. They do not think clearly and are unable to make wise decisions. Drug dependence is an illness that requires treatment. This illness is believed to develop in 10 to 20 percent of those who use harmful drugs.

Drug dependence, whether it is related to alcohol, cocaine, marijuana, or other drugs, harms the body. It damages family relationships and is considered a family disease. Family members might ignore their own needs in an effort to cope with the family member who is drug-dependent.

Family members usually try to keep the problem a secret. They often protect the family member who is drug-dependent by making excuses or lying. They deny the problem and stop trusting their own feelings.

I will work to improve difficult family relationships.

Family members might develop codependence. **Codependence** is a mental disorder in which a person denies feelings and copes in harmful ways.

Family members deny feelings by:

- pretending a problem does not exist;
- blaming someone else for what is happening;
- offering excuses;
- attacking others who talk about the problems.

Teens brought up in families in which an adult is drug-dependent or has an addiction often develop codependence. They deny their feelings and have difficulty forming healthful relationships. They might copy the behavior and begin to use drugs. They might put "blinders" on and not recognize harmful behavior in others. Because the family is unhealthy, they often form other relationships that are not healthy. They might try to rescue others who have drug problems. They might allow others to treat them poorly. They might treat others poorly.

Teens who have codependence cannot tell the difference between sick relationships and healthy ones. They are used to sick relationships. They tend to choose sick relationships because they are more comfortable in them. When a person treats them in kind ways, they might think the person is "too nice." They might not respect the person. They see the healthful behavior of this person as being boring.

As a result, teens who have codependence feel alone. They know they lack support but do not know how to get it. The people they ask for support might not be capable of giving it. They do not get into relationships where they can get support.

Teens with Codependence Might Become Enablers

An **enabler** is a person who knowingly or unknowingly supports the harmful behavior of another person. Suppose a teen has drug dependence in the family. Suppose a teen has abuse or violence in the family. The teen is used to pretending a problem does not exist. The teen is used to living with someone who makes excuses. This teen is used to relationships that are sick. The teen might relate with friends in the same way. The teen might have a friend who abuses drugs. The teen ignores the drug use. The teen makes excuses for the friend. In these ways, the teen supports the harmful behavior of the friend.

I will work to improve difficult family relationships.

Abuse

Abuse (uh·BYOOS) is the harmful treatment of another person. **Child abuse** is the harmful treatment of a minor. **Spouse abuse** is the harmful treatment of a husband or wife. **Parent abuse** is the harmful treatment of a parent. **Elder abuse** is the harmful treatment of an aged family member. A family member who abuses another usually has low self-esteem. This person has a need to control others.

Four kinds of abuse can occur in a family.

- **Physical abuse** is harmful treatment that results in physical injury to the victim.

- **Emotional abuse** is "putting down" another person and making the person feel worthless.

- **Neglect** is failure to provide proper care and guidance.

- **Sexual abuse** is sexual contact that is forced on a person.

Teens who have been abused need help sorting out their feelings. Often, an abused teen is told, "I love you" and at the same time is beaten, put down, or sexually abused. The words and actions of the abuser are inconsistent. These mixed messages are confusing. Because teens need to feel loved, they might believe the words used. However, the words do not match the actions. To cope, teens begin to deny their feelings that something is wrong. They might even begin to blame themselves for the way they are treated.

Often, an abusive family member is also drug-dependent. The abusive family member might drink alcohol or use another drug. This changes the mood of the abuser. Teens who live in families with abuse and drug dependence become very distrustful. They know they might be harmed when the mood of the abusive family member changes.

The Dysfunctional Family

Violence

Violence is the use of physical force to injure, damage, or destroy oneself, others, or property. **Domestic violence** is violence that occurs within a family. This includes physical abuse and sexual abuse. In most families, domestic violence and drug dependence are connected.

The family member who begins the violence wants to control others. Violent outbursts become the way to gain control. Family members often respond by giving the violent family member even more control as a way to avoid disagreements. They change their behavior to avoid upsetting the violent family member. They look for reasons for the violent outbursts. They might even begin to blame themselves.

Family members give up control when they begin to make excuses for the violent family member. They might lie to protect the violent family member. For example, a family member who has been hit might cover up a bruise with makeup. Or the person might tell others that (s)he fell. Lying to others might be a substitute for discussing violent behavior within the family.

As with drug dependence and abuse, violence is usually a family secret. Family members deny what is happening. They often do not tell others. When sexual abuse occurs within a family, the abuser usually tells the victim to keep it a secret. A teen who has been sexually abused might feel the family will break up or the family will suffer if anyone knows the truth. Teens who have been abused often wait for years to tell someone why they are troubled.

Teens who live in homes with violence are at special risk. During a violent outburst, they might be harmed. They might copy the behavior they have experienced and try to control others by force. They are at risk for becoming juvenile offenders. A **juvenile offender** is a legal minor who commits a criminal act.

Teens who have been sexually abused are at risk for being sexually active. They might act out and have harmful relationships. They are then at risk for infection with HIV, other sexually transmitted diseases, and unwanted parenthood. These teens also are at risk for using drugs and becoming drug-dependent.

The
Dysfunctional
Family

Intervention and Treatment

It is difficult for a family to overcome problems related to drug dependence, abuse, or violence. Family members are usually hopeful that something will change without any action being needed. The family member who is being abusive might make promises to change. For example, the day after striking or beating someone, an abusive family member might be kind and gentle. This family member might promise never to have another violent outburst. After a drinking binge, a family member with alcoholism might promise never to drink again. However, these promises are usually broken.

What can family members do to change these harmful patterns? Family members must consider the two S's—safety and secrecy. Safety is the first consideration. When family members feel they are in danger, they must take action. They might call for help or leave the situation. Help is available by calling 9-1-1, the operator, the police, or a crisis intervention center. The caller should stay on the line until (s)he is told to hang up the telephone.

To assure safety, family members might need to leave the home. A **domestic shelter** is a place where family members can stay to be safe. These shelters are available in most cities. In a shelter, family members are protected from the abuser. They can make a plan for a healthful way to live.

Secrecy is a second consideration. One or more family members must recognize that secrecy is not in the best interest of the family. They must not be afraid to speak up. They must not feel ashamed. They must trust that help is available. If someone is unwilling to help, they must talk to someone else. Drug dependence, abuse, and violence must be discussed and treated. There are skilled counselors who help families in which there is drug dependence.

The Pain and Joy Connection

There is a saying about emotions. It goes like this, "If you are out of touch with pain, you will not feel joy." This saying has to do with denial. A person who denies the hard times does not allow certain emotions to surface. This person keeps anger, sadness, and fear inside. It takes a lot of energy to hide to keep these emotions inside. It takes a lot of energy to hide these emotions from others. As a result, there is little energy left for joy. This is why young people who live in dysfunctional families have a hard time having fun. They often are very serious. They are not spontaneous. They are afraid to show emotions.

A skilled counselor might suggest a formal intervention. A **formal intervention** is an action by people, such as family members, who want a person to get treatment. During the formal intervention, people share difficult experiences they have had with the abuser. They want the abuser to understand how his or her behavior has affected others. They make it clear that they expect a change. The abusive family member might need to enter a hospital or receive treatment for drug dependence. Other family members might need treatment. Their behavior might have become harmful, too.

Resources for Recovery

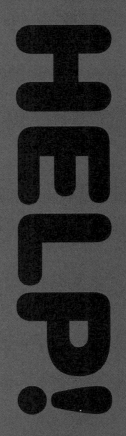

Teens can recover and change behavior in additional ways. Important resources include mentors and support groups. A **mentor** is a responsible, trusted person who guides and helps a younger person. Teens living in families in which adults choose harmful ways of behaving might need mentors. A mentor might be a teacher, coach, friend's parent, religious leader, or other trusted adult. Such teens need to spend quality time with mentors to learn responsible behavior.

Teens also can benefit from attending meetings of support groups for teens who have survived different kinds of abuse. These groups address codependency issues, such as denial. They help teens to stop accepting the harmful behavior of others. Teens are encouraged to know that other teens have been able to change their behavior. They learn that it is possible to change. They have the support and encouragement of others.

Teens also practice showing their emotions. They share anger, sadness, and depression. This releases energy. Then they are able to share feelings of joy and love. The other teens in their group give them feedback. They give them a safe place to learn to express feelings.

Apply...

The Responsible Decision-Making Model™

Your best friend has confided to you that (s)he has been beaten several times recently by his or her stepfather. (S)he shows you the bruises, which (s)he has been covering with long sleeves and pants. Your friend tells you that (s)he must keep this a secret. And (s)he says (s)he will never forgive *you* if you tell anyone.

Answer the following questions on a separate sheet of paper. Write "Does not apply" if a question does not apply to this situation.

1. Is it healthful for your friend to keep the abuse secret? Why or why not?

2. Is it safe for your friend to keep the abuse secret? Why or why not?

3. Is it legal for your friend to keep the abuse secret? Why or why not?

4. Will your friend show respect for herself or himself if (s)he keeps the abuse secret? Why or why not?

5. Will other responsible adults approve if your friend keeps the abuse secret? Why or why not?

6. Will your friend demonstrate good character if (s)he keeps the abuse secret? Why or why not?

What is the responsible decision to make in this situation?

Lesson 8

Review

Vocabulary

Write a separate sentence using each of the vocabulary words listed on page 58.

Health Content

Write responses to the following:

1. What are three kinds of problems that occur in dysfunctional families? **pages 59–62**

2. Why do teens in families with drug dependency have difficulty in relationships? **page 60**

3. What are four kinds of abuse? **page 61**

4. What actions can family members take when their safety is at risk? **pages 63–64**

5. What happens during a formal intervention? **page 64**

Fabulous Friendships

Vocabulary

healthful friendship

peer pressure

people pleaser

Life Skills
- **I will develop healthful relationships.**
- **I will recognize harmful relationships.**

Your friendships affect your health status. Some friendships are healthful and contribute to your well-being. Other friendships are harmful and interfere with your well-being. In this lesson, you will learn to recognize the difference between healthful and harmful friendships.

The Lesson Objectives

- Describe the balance of giving and taking in a healthful friendship.
- List the six criteria to use to evaluate decisions made with friends.
- Explain when and how to end a friendship.

Friendship: A Balancing Act

A **healthful friendship** is a balanced relationship that promotes mutual respect and healthful behavior. To have a healthful friendship, at times, you need to do the giving. Your friend does the taking. For example, your friend might have missed school for several days. You might bring the homework assignments to your friend after school. You might call to see if your friend is feeling better. At other times, you do the taking. Perhaps you are sad because your grandparent has died. You need your friend to do the giving. Your friend listens to you as you express your sadness. Your friend might help you with household chores. You feel comforted when taking or receiving these gifts of friendship.

In a healthful friendship, you benefit from giving and taking. You feel good about yourself when you are able to do the giving. Giving makes you feel helpful and important. You also feel good when you are taking or receiving. It is a good feeling to know that you can count on someone else to meet some of your needs. Being able to give and to take helps you become closer to a friend.

Sometimes friendships are out of balance and need to be re-evaluated. Perhaps you have had a friendship in which you or a friend wanted to do the taking most of the time. A friend who wants to take without ever giving is selfish. This friend likes things to be done for him or her without doing anything in return. This deprives the other friend of a basic need in friendship—the need to receive attention and acts of kindness.

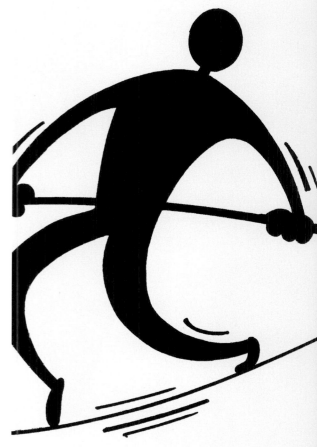

Perhaps you have had a friendship in which you or a friend wanted to give most of the time. When one friend does everything for another friend, the other friend does not have a chance to act in kind ways. This deprives the other friend of a basic need in friendship—the need to do something for someone.

Think about your friendships. Are your friendships balanced? Are you giving and taking? Are your friends giving and taking? If not, you need to work to achieve balanced friendships.

Decision-Making with Friends

During your teen years, you will make many decisions when you are with friends. Because you want to be close to others and feel as if you belong, you will be interested in what friends want you to do. Friends might use peer pressure when they want to influence you. **Peer pressure** is influence that people of similar age or status place on others to encourage them to make certain decisions or to behave in certain ways.

No matter how close you feel to friends, you need to be objective when making decisions. You must recognize the importance of making responsible decisions.

Decisions made with friends should result in actions that:

- are healthful;
- are safe;
- are legal;
- show respect for self and others;
- follow the guidelines of responsible adults, such as your parents or guardian;
- demonstrate good character.

Some teens have difficulty making decisions with friends. A **people pleaser** is a person who is more concerned about having the approval of others than doing what (s)he believes to be best. People pleasers place more emphasis on other people's opinions than their own. The people pleaser is likely to do what other people say. Being a people pleaser has drawbacks. People-pleasing behavior can result in harmful decisions. Doing what others want you to do is not a responsible way to make a decision.

Being a people pleaser is not a guarantee of being liked. Often people who encourage people pleasers to do something harmful or wrong lose respect for them. They know they can "walk all over them" and get their own way. They view the people pleaser as a doormat. Healthful relationships have a balance. Healthful relationships have mutual respect. One person does not do all the giving and the other all the taking.

Teens who are people pleasers need to change their behavior. Trusted adults, such as parents, teachers, and counselors, can help. Teens must be helped to understand why they behave this way. They might have learned this behavior in their family. They might feel neglected and have low self-esteem. They might constantly worry about being liked.

People pleasers also must stop going to extremes to please others. This is often easier said than done. It takes much effort to change people-pleasing behavior. Using the resistance skills in Lesson 2 helps teens learn to stand up to others. They learn to state their opinions and make decisions without backing down. They also learn to resist asking others repeatedly what to do. People pleasers must gain confidence in making decisions and accepting the consequences.

Don't be a doormat for other people to walk on.

Ending Friendships

Your friendships change for many different reasons. A friend might move away and not keep in touch. A friend might break a confidence and the friendship is never the same again. Sometimes your interests change, and new friends replace old ones. At other times, you need to be objective and examine ways that a friendship affects you. A friend might bring out the worst in you. You might treat others poorly when you are with this person. You might be involved in activities that are harmful when you are with this person. You might have friends who use drugs or who are abusive. It is not in your best interest to continue such friendships.

When you end a friendship, avoid gossiping about your former friend. Remember to keep the confidences your former friend shared. If you do not, others will question whether or not you can be trusted. Do not try to get even if you end a friendship because someone has hurt you. Nothing will be gained. Recognize that you cannot control how a former friend will behave when a friendship ends. However, you are in control of your own behavior.

Know that you might feel sad for a period of time. You might feel disappointed. You might feel let down. It is difficult to end a friendship. You have positive memories. But remember why you ended the friendship. You ended the friendship to protect your health. You ended the friendship to keep a good reputation. Your parents might have asked you to end the friendship.

Discuss your feelings with your parents or guardian. They can help you deal with your feelings of loss. Focus on your other friendships. Put time and effort into healthful friendships. Think of ways to begin new friendships. Perhaps there is someone who you would like to know better. Ask this person to do something.

Good-bye

Doormat

Life Skill

I will recognize harmful relationships.

Materials: Paper, pen or pencil

Directions: The chart below contains situations and responses of a teen who is a people pleaser (doormat). On a separate sheet of paper, write a way that a teen who makes his or her own decisions might respond to each situation.

Situation	Response of a Doormat
1. Your best friend did not make the soccer team. Other teens are putting him or her down.	1. You say nothing because you are afraid you might appear uncool.
2. A teen you are attracted to asks you to do his or her homework.	2. You do the homework, hoping the teen will like you.
3. Some teens at a party are smoking a joint and laugh at you when you decide to leave.	3. You smoke the joint because you do not want their disapproval.
4. You are trying to decide how to wear your hair.	4. You repeatedly ask your friends what you should do because you cannot make a decision.

Lesson 9

Review

Vocabulary

Write a separate sentence using each of the vocabulary words listed on page 66.

Health Content

Write responses to the following:

1. What are ways you and your friends give and take in a healthful friendship? **page 67**
2. What are the six criteria you can use to evaluate decisions made with friends? **page 68**
3. How does a people pleaser behave? **page 69**
4. What are reasons to end a friendship? **page 70**
5. What should you do and not do when you end a friendship? **page 70**

Preparing for Future Relationships

Vocabulary

sex role

affection

abstinence

resistance skills

commitment

prenatal care

premature delivery

- **I will develop skills to prepare for dating.**
- **I will practice abstinence.**
- **I will develop skills to prepare for marriage.**
- **I will develop skills to prepare for parenthood.**

Think about your future for a moment. Do you feel prepared to enter high school? What will you do when you graduate from high school? Will you continue to go to school? Will you prepare for a career? Have you thought about relationship choices? Will you have a committed relationship? Will you marry someday? Will you bring up children? During your teen years, you can develop skills to prepare for future relationship choices.

The Lesson Objectives

- Explain how a person develops attitudes about sex roles.
- List the ten questions included on *The Respect Checklist*.
- State why it is important to set limits for affection.
- Give reasons for choosing abstinence.
- Identify ten choices that support abstinence.
- Outline responsibilities of adulthood for which married teens are not prepared.
- Discuss reasons teen parenthood is risky.

Your Sex Role

In Lesson 9, you learned skills to practice that promote friendship. These skills help you have better relationships with members of both sexes. Other factors also promote healthful relationships.

Let's begin by examining the importance of attitudes about being male and female. **Sex role** is the way a person acts and the feelings and attitudes (s)he has about being a male or a female. Your attitudes about male and female sex roles were shaped by the important adults in your life. You observed their attitudes and drew certain conclusions. Suppose the important adults in your life enjoyed being male or female. They also respected members of the opposite sex. If so, you probably feel good about being male or female. And you probably respect members of the opposite sex.

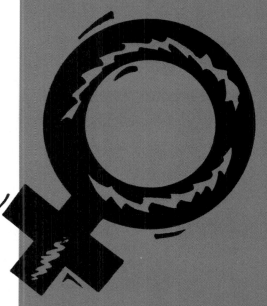

Suppose you grew up in a home where the adult female was very angry and bitter about a relationship she had with a male. Suppose you grew up in a home where the adult male put down females and believed they were not as important as males. These attitudes might have influenced you. You might then behave in ways that reflect these attitudes. To have healthful opposite sex relationships, you must respect both sexes.

You might want to check your beliefs about sex roles. Make a list of your beliefs about males. Then make a list of your beliefs about females. Examine your lists. Discuss what you have listed with an adult who respects both sexes.

Make certain you show respect for both sexes. Do not tell jokes in which you make fun of males or females. Suppose someone you know tells such a joke. Do not laugh or show support. If you do, you are showing disrespect. You might begin to believe what you hear even though it is wrong. Turn the situation around. Explain to the person that members of both sexes deserve respect. Tell reasons why.

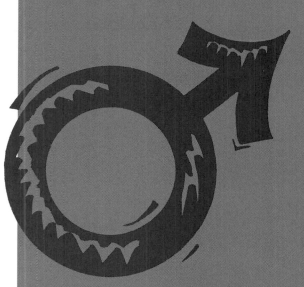

Dating

Teens might have an interest in dating, or going out. Parents and guardians have different viewpoints about the appropriate age for dating. Some parents and guardians allow teens to date at an earlier age than do other parents and guardians. Some allow their teens to attend school functions or other parties, but do not allow individual dating. They might approve of their teens going out in groups. Teens might choose to share social activities with several people of both sexes.

Discuss dating guidelines with your parents or guardian. Follow their dating guidelines to avoid conflicts. Do not begin to date until you have their approval. When you begin to date, discuss plans with them. Tell them where you plan to go and with whom. Have them meet and talk with people you date. Make certain they approve of people you date.

Expect a date to treat you with respect at all times. Use *The Respect Checklist* to examine how you are treated. Each YES response shows that you are treated with respect. A NO response to any of the questions is a warning signal. The signal should flash in your mind: I am not being treated with respect. I should not be treated this way!

Use *The Respect Checklist* in another way. Reword each question to examine how you treat others. For example, ask yourself, "Do I put down this person?" or "Am I interested in what this person says and does?" Remember, you must always treat others with respect.

Set high standards for your relationships. Do not settle for less. Suppose someone puts you down. Do not ignore this person's behavior. Do not say to yourself, "He or she really does not mean it." Suppose you walk all over someone. You always get your way. Do not accept this behavior in yourself. Be honest with the other person. Say you need to change your behavior and make an effort to do so. Ask the other person to call you on it if you continue to be disrespectful.

The Respect Checklist

Does this person avoid put-downs?

Is this person interested in what I say and do?

Does this person make responsible decisions that are healthful, are safe, are legal, are respectful of self and others, follow the guidelines of trusted adults, and demonstrate character?

Is this person drug-free?

Is this person nonviolent, never harming me or other people in any way?

Is this person willing to say NO to sexual activity?

Does this person encourage me to do my best in school?

Does this person choose friends who are responsible?

Does this person have a healthful attitude about members of both sexes?

Expressing Affection

Your sexuality includes everything that makes you male or female. It includes your sex role and your feelings. It includes the attitude you have about your body. Your sexuality also includes how you express affection toward others.

In Unit 3, you will learn ways in which your body changes as you grow. Your body is becoming that of an adult male or female. As your body matures, you experience new feelings. You will experience an attraction to certain people. You might notice an attraction to a specific male or female. This attraction is a warm feeling. It is a special "chemistry" that is difficult to explain.

When this special chemistry occurs between two people, they are drawn to each other. They enjoy being together. They might want to express affection. **Affection** is a warm feeling. Holding hands and hugging are ways to show affection. It is normal to want to express affection. However, you must make decisions about how and when to express affection.

How might a teen express warm feelings for another person? When is it appropriate for you to hold hands? Hug? Kiss? These are important questions to discuss with your parents, guardian, or other trusted adult. They can provide you with guidelines for expressing affection. They can help you set limits for expressing warm feelings because warm feelings can be very powerful.

Part of being responsible is setting limits and sticking to them. Being responsible includes understanding the need to set limits. As you express affection, warm feelings might become more intense. They cause changes to occur in your body. Controlling your expression of feelings might become more difficult. This is why it is important to set limits.

Remember: Set Limits and Do Not Become Sexually Active.

Setting limits and sticking to these limits keeps you from becoming sexually active. You stick to your values. You obey your parents or guardian. You keep a good reputation. You do not feel guilty or regret your actions. When you practice your values, you keep your self-respect. Other people respect you for practicing your values. And if they do not, they are not the right people with whom you should spend time.

You protect your health when you set limits and stick to them. Being sexually active can result in pregnancy and unwanted parenthood. If you are female, you are not ready to have a baby. Your body is still growing. You need to get your education. If you are male, you are not ready to give a pregnant female the love and understanding she needs. You need to get your education.

You also are not ready for parenthood. Parenthood is a demanding job. Parents must make the needs of their children a top priority. A baby is dependent upon its parents. You are not ready to drop what you are doing and take care of a baby. You need more time to clarify your values. You need time to learn about the growth and development of infants.

You do not want to become infected with STDs or HIV. By setting limits and sticking to them you do not have to worry about having these infections.

Choosing Abstinence

You are a very special person. When you respect yourself, you show that you believe you are worthwhile. An important aspect of self-respect involves choosing sexual behaviors that show you value yourself and others. Choosing behaviors that follow the beliefs of your family is important. Placing limits on sexual behaviors promotes self-respect. You can decide to avoid behaviors that might arouse strong sexual feelings. You can decide to avoid situations that might make it more difficult to use self-discipline. You can make responsible decisions about your sexual behavior. Responsible decisions promote your health and improve your self-respect.

Abstinence is a responsible decision.

Abstinence is choosing not to be sexually active. Setting limits and practicing abstinence provide you with several advantages. Apply the guidelines to the right for making responsible decisions to the question, "Why should I choose abstinence?"

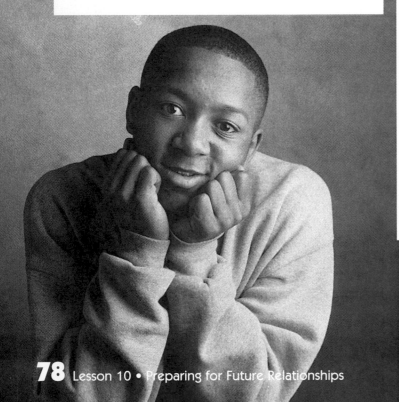

Abstinence is healthful and safe.

Being sexually active is associated with many health risks. Over one million unwanted pregnancies occur among teen females. Four out of ten females become pregnant before their twentieth birthday. Babies born to teens are much more likely to have birth defects.

Being sexually active increases the risk of becoming infected with sexually transmitted diseases, including HIV. Some of these diseases are curable but can result in serious complications. There are no known cures for genital herpes and HIV. To date, AIDS is a fatal disease.

Being sexually active can affect your mental health. Stress can result from guilt that is associated with being sexually active. Stress might occur because of fear of unwanted pregnancy.

Abstinence is legal.

Sexual involvement with a person before the legal age of consent is considered corruption of a minor. The legal age of consent is that age when a person is considered legally responsible for his or her actions. The parents of a person under the legal age of consent can take legal action against an older sexual partner. This situation can be avoided by not being sexually active.

Abstinence demonstrates good character.

You have good character when your actions are consistent with your value system. Practicing abstinence is consistent with the values you learned from your family. You show good character when you use self-discipline and put values into practice in daily living.

Abstinence shows respect for yourself and others.

Having clear values and behaving in ways to support your values promote self-respect. You feel good about yourself when you use self-control and say NO to being sexually active. When you think highly of yourself, others will, too. When you choose abstinence, you do not regret your actions. You do not get a reputation for being sexually active.

When you do not pressure someone else to be sexually active, you show respect for that person. You want the other person to live by his or her values. You are a positive influence.

I will practice abstinence.

I will practice abstinence.

I will practice abstinence.

I will practice abstinence.

I will practice abstinence.

I will practice abstinence.

Abstinence follows family guidelines.

Most parents and guardians do not want their teens to be sexually active. They want to protect their teens. Disregarding family guidelines for sexual behavior causes stress in family relationships. You show respect for your parents or guardian when you say NO to being sexually active.

Resisting Pressure to Become Sexually Active

You can use resistance skills if someone pressures you to become sexually active. **Resistance skills** are skills that are used when a person wants to say NO to an action or to leave a situation. Resisting Pressure to Become Sexually Active is a list of suggested ways to resist pressure to become sexually active.

1. **Be confident and say, "NO, I do not want to be sexually active."**
   - Look directly at the person to whom you are speaking.
   - Say NO in a firm and confident voice.
   - Discuss your limits and talk about appropriate ways to express affection.

2. **Give reasons you practice abstinence.**
   - I want to follow family guidelines.
   - I want to respect myself.
   - I want to respect others.
   - I want to have a good reputation.
   - I do not want to feel guilty.
   - I am not ready for marriage.
   - I do not want to risk pregnancy.
   - I am not ready to be a parent.
   - I do not want to be infected with an STD.
   - I do not want to be infected with HIV.

3. **Repeat your reasons for practicing abstinence.**
   - Give the same responses to convince the person who is pressuring you.

4. **Do not send a mixed message.**
   - Use nonverbal behavior to match verbal behavior.
   - Do not get involved in behaviors that result in strong sexual feelings.
   - Do not lead someone on.

5. **Avoid situations in which there might be pressure to be sexually active.**
   - Do not go to parties that are not supervised by adults.
   - Do not spend time alone with someone in places such as a bedroom.
   - Do not go to parties where teens are using drugs. Drugs change the ability to make responsible decisions.

6. **Break off a relationship when someone does not respect your limits.**
   - Avoid being with teens who pressure you to be sexually active.

Remember, a person who does not respect your limits cares more about himself or herself than about you.

7. **Influence others to choose abstinence.**
   - Share your decision to choose abstinence with your friends.
   - Set a good example for others.
   - Be proud that you have chosen abstinence.

"Stuck in a Groove" Technique

Suppose you are playing a cassette tape. The tape gets stuck and you keep hearing the same music lyrics over and over. Each time it replays you are more likely to remember the line you heard. Now suppose someone pressures you to be sexually active. Say NO and give your reason. Your reason might be, "I want to have a good reputation." If the person continues to pressure you, repeat what you said. Get "Stuck in a Groove."

Soon the person will give up. The person will be convinced you are not changing your mind. Soon the person will give up. The person will be convinced you are not changing your mind.

Ten Choices That Support Abstinence

You need to be armored with personal strength to resist pressure to be sexually active. You can prepare for pressure that you might receive to be sexually active. Here are some suggestions for you.

1. **Be involved in activities that promote self-respect.** Feeling good about yourself is important in developing the self-confidence to resist peer pressure.

2. **Establish goals.** Clear goals help you focus on what you need to do. They help you examine how teen marriage or pregnancy might interfere with reaching your goals.

3. **Develop loving family relationships.** Your family can provide a sense of belonging and reinforce your values. You are less likely to become sexually active when your needs for belonging are met by your family.

4. **Be assertive and use decision-making skills.** Think ahead about situations in which there might be pressure to be sexually active. Rehearse saying NO in an assertive manner to such pressures.

5. **Establish relationships with trusted adults.** Your parents or guardian and other adults can help you focus on your future. They can help you make wise decisions.

6. **Select friends who choose abstinence.** Having friends who are sexually active adds additional temptation. Select friends who help you have the self-discipline to say NO.

7. **Date other teens who choose abstinence.** This will relieve the pressure to be sexually active.

8. **Avoid situations that tempt you to be sexually active.** Certain situations are too tempting. For example, lying in bed listening to music with someone is not a wise choice. There are many other situations that must be avoided.

9. **Do not use alcohol or other drugs.** Alcohol and other drugs depress the part of the brain used for reasoning and judgment. It is more difficult to say NO when you do not think clearly.

10. **Select entertainment that promotes sex within a monogamus traditional marriage.** Some movies, soap operas, videos, compact discs, and magazines highlight people in casual sexual relationships. The consequences of casual sexual relationships are often not expressed. You might get the wrong idea if you fill your mind in this way. Remember, there are serious consequences to being sexually active.

It's Never Too Late to Choose Abstinence

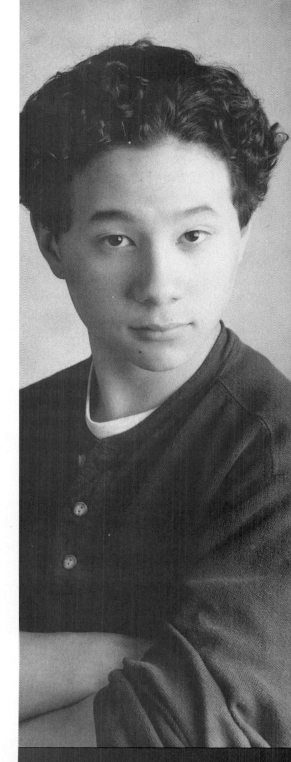

Suppose you have been sexually active in the past. It is never too late to change this behavior. Talk to your parents or guardian. They probably will be upset that you were sexually active. But they will be glad that you regret your past behavior. They can give you support and courage to change your behavior. They can help you sort through your feelings. They can advise you about your relationship. They might think it is best for you to stay away from the person with whom you were involved. Respect their wishes. Remember, they want the best for you. With their support, you might continue to see someone with whom you were involved. If so, here are some suggestions.

Talk to the person with whom you were sexually active.

Give reasons why you want to change your behavior and practice abstinence:

- I do not want to hide wrong actions from my parent or guardian.
- I do not like feeling guilty.
- I do not want to worry about a pregnancy anymore.
- I do not want to risk infection with STDs and HIV.
- I want to get back my self-respect.
- I do not want a relationship based on sex.

Ask the person to agree to practice abstinence.

- Be firm that this is the only way you can continue to spend time together.
- Do not accept pressure to change your mind.

Set new rules for your relationship.

- Set new limits for expressing affection.
- Avoid situations and places that led to sexual involvement.
- Avoid spending time alone for several weeks.
- Spend more time with other teens rather than being alone.

End the relationship if you and the other person do not follow the new rules.

Follow a...

Health Behavior Contract

Copy the health behavior contract on a separate sheet of paper.

DO NOT WRITE IN THIS BOOK.

Name: _____ **Date:** _____

Life Skill: I will practice abstinence.

Effect On My Health: If I practice abstinence, I will respect myself and others. I will have a good reputation. I will not feel guilty. I will not risk pregnancy or infection with HIV or other STDs. I will be able to prepare for the responsibilities of adulthood. I will be able to finish school and pursue my career goals.

My Plan: I will be involved in activities that promote my self-respect. I will select entertainment that promotes sex within marriage. In my journal, I will list activities and entertainment that support my choice to practice abstinence. I will keep my journal for two weeks. I will evaluate the activities and entertainment I chose. I will put a check beside my choices that support my decision to practice abstinence. I will put an X beside ones that encourage being sexually active or that present casual sex as acceptable.

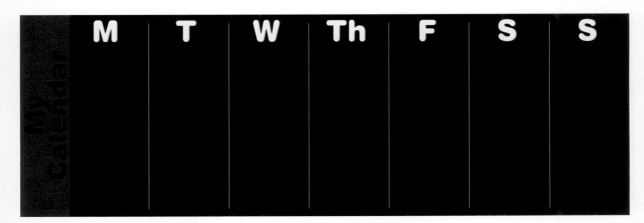

	M	T	W	Th	F	S	S
My Calendar							

How My Plan Worked: (Complete after two weeks.) I will review the activities and entertainment I checked. I will make a commitment to avoid those activities and entertainment that do not support my decision to choose abstinence.

Apply...

The Responsible Decision-Making Model™

Your sister is almost 16. She says, "I can't wait to turn 16. I'm going to drop out of school and get married. When I get married, I'll be an adult." You are trying to decide what to say to your sister.

Answer the following questions on a separate sheet of paper. Write "Does not apply" if a question does not apply to this situation.

1. Is it healthful for your sister to marry while she is a teen? Why or why not?

2. Is it safe for your sister to marry while she is a teen? Why or why not?

3. Is it legal for your sister to marry while she is a teen? Why or why not?

4. Will your sister show respect for herself and others if she marries while she is a teen? Why or why not?

5. Will your parents or guardian approve if your sister marries while she is a teen? Why or why not?

6. Will your sister demonstrate good character if she marries while she is a teen? Why or why not?

What is the responsible decision to make in this situation?

What would you say to your sister?

What's Awesome/What's Not

Life Skill

I will practice abstinence.

Materials: Paper, pen or pencil

Directions: The beginning of a What's Awesome/What's Not chart appears below. Copy the chart on a separate sheet of paper. Add four more items to each column that show why it's awesome to be abstinent.

What's Awesome	What's Not
Being free of STDs	Having herpes for life
Having a clear conscience	Feeling guilty
Not worrying about pregnancy	Risking pregnancy

Activity

Preparing for Marriage

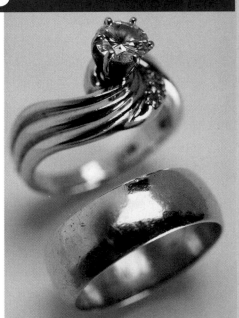

In the future, the choice of whether or not to marry will be yours. You can prepare yourself to make this important decision. Begin by taking notice of the importance of commitment in relationships. A **commitment** is a pledge or promise to do something. Avoid making any commitment if you do not intend to do what you say. If you promise someone you will be somewhere at a set time, be there at that time. If you agree to help someone with a task, help the person.

Another way to prepare for a committed relationship is to choose friends carefully. Look for traits that you and your family value. Use *The Respect Checklist* to make certain that you are treated with respect. Be aware of the Traits to Consider When Choosing a Marriage Partner.

Traits to Consider When Choosing a Marriage Partner

Personality Traits People with similar personality traits are more likely to have a stable marriage.

Interests People who share common interests and enjoy similar activities are more likely to enjoy each other's company.

Intelligence People with similar intelligence can learn together and grow closer.

Health Choices People who do not use drugs and are not abusive or violent show respect for each other.

Physical Attraction People are closer when they have warm feelings for each other.

Age People who marry after age 22 are three times more likely to have a successful marriage than those who marry during the teenage years. When teens marry, they have had fewer learning experiences and less time to set goals.

Financial Resources People who have financial resources and who agree on money matters are more likely to have a successful marriage.

Family Background People from families with similar beliefs and values are more likely to agree on their choices.

Teen Marriage

Suppose you rent a movie to watch. You place the movie in your VCR and it gets stuck on fast forward. The tape is played so fast that you miss the best parts of the movie. You did not get what you bargained for!

Teen marriage is much the same way. When teens marry, their lives are placed on fast-forward. They quickly move from the teen years to the responsibilities of adulthood. Married teens miss many opportunities. This is why three out of four teen marriages fail.

Teen Marriage: Fast-Forward into Adulthood

Married teens are fast-forwarded into adulthood without having enough time to:

1. gain a sense of who they are;
2. develop friendships with several people of the opposite sex;
3. form a support network of mature friends to help them during the early years of marriage;
4. participate in a variety of social activities;
5. understand the emotions of adolescence;
6. understand the difference between strong physical attraction and love;
7. develop a value system;
8. achieve emotional and financial independence from parents;
9. prepare for a career;
10. earn enough money to support a family.

Preparing for Parenthood

Being a parent also requires making a commitment. Consider The Parent Pledge to a Child. This pledge lists actions parents can take. Each action requires some skill. A person must be ready for these actions. Consider the responsibility that accompanies each promise. "I will provide food, shelter, and clothing." To fulfill this promise, a parent or parents should have an education and a job. "I will bring you up in a family that is free from drug dependency, abuse, and violence." To fulfill this promise, a parent should value his or her own health. By reviewing the parent pledge, you can learn ways you can prepare for parenthood now.

The Parent Pledge to a Child

1. "I will treat you with respect."
2. "I will teach you rules to keep you healthy and safe."
3. "I will teach you self-discipline."
4. "I will learn how you will grow and change."
5. "I will set aside time to spend with you."
6. "I will provide food, clothing, and shelter for you."
7. "I will give you love and affection."
8. "I will bring you up in a family that is free from drug dependency, abuse, and violence."
9. "I will teach you how to communicate without using put-downs."
10. "I will teach you clear values."

Teen Parenthood

Being a teen parent is very risky. The lives of the mother, father, and baby are affected.

Health risks to the pregnant female During pregnancy, teens are at much higher risk for having health problems. Teens often do not get good prenatal care. **Prenatal care** is the care given to both the mother-to-be and her unborn baby. Pregnant teens might develop anemia. They might develop high blood pressure during the pregnancy. They are more likely to have a premature delivery. A **premature delivery** is the birth of a baby before the 37th week of the pregnancy.

I will practice abstinence.

Health risks to the baby of a teen mother Babies who have a premature delivery have more health problems. Their organs have not developed as fully as they should have before birth. They usually have a low birth weight. They are more likely to have long-lasting illnesses.

School and job risks for teen parents Teen parents are not as likely to complete school as are their peers. A female who becomes a teen parent earns half the lifetime wages of a female who waits until she is at least 20 to have her first child. Teen fathers are much more likely to be high school dropouts than are their peers. They also earn less money than do their peers.

Emotional risks to children brought up by teen parents Most children born to a teen mother are brought up by the mother. The father does not live with the mother. After one year, fewer than one-third of the fathers see their children once a week. This is difficult for the mother, father, and baby.

Remember: Set Limits and Do Not Become Sexually Active.

Abstinence is choosing not to be sexually active. Abstinence is the only 100 percent safe way to avoid being a teen parent. A pregnancy can occur the first time a couple has sex.

Lesson 10

Review

Vocabulary

Write a separate sentence using each of the vocabulary words listed on page 72.

Health Content

Write responses to the following:

1. How does a person develop attitudes about the male and female sex roles? **page 73**

2. What topics should you include when discussing dating with your parents or guardian? **page 74**

3. What are the ten questions included on *The Respect Checklist?* **page 75**

4. What are three health risks associated with being sexually active? **page 78**

5. What are ten reasons for saying NO to being sexually active? **page 80**

6. What are ten choices that support abstinence? **page 82**

7. What are eight traits to consider when choosing a marriage partner? **page 86**

8. What are ten responsibilities of adulthood for which married teens might not have enough time to prepare? **page 87**

9. What are ten actions parents should be able to pledge or promise their children they will do? **page 88**

10. What are four reasons teen parenthood is risky? **pages 88–89**

Unit 2 Review

Health Content

Review your answers for each Lesson Review in this unit. Then write answers to each of the following questions.

1. What are the differences between intrapersonal, interpersonal, and intergroup conflict? **Lesson 6 page 50**

2. What are three risks involved with being unable to resolve conflict? **Lesson 6 page 50**

3. How can you distinguish different family structures? **Lesson 7 page 55**

4. What are ways family members can adjust to the divorce of parents? **Lesson 7 page 56**

5. What are two actions family members should take to change harmful patterns? **Lesson 8 pages 63–64**

6. What are ways a domestic shelter provides safety? **Lesson 8 page 63**

7. What are guidelines to evaluate decisions made with friends? **Lesson 9 page 68**

8. Why might you end a friendship? **Lesson 9 page 70**

9. What questions should you use to examine how you are treated by a date? **Lesson 10 page 75**

10. How are the lives of teens fast-forwarded when they marry? **Lesson 10 page 87**

Vocabulary

Number a sheet of paper from 1–10. Select the correct vocabulary word. Write it next to the corresponding number. DO NOT WRITE IN THIS BOOK.

child abuse	intrapersonal conflict
commitment	loving person
elder abuse	prenatal care
foster family	social skills
healthful friendship	traditional family

1. _____ is the care given to both the mother-to-be and her unborn baby. **Lesson 10**

2. A(n) _____ consists of a husband and wife and their children. **Lesson 7**

3. _____ is the harmful treatment of a minor. **Lesson 8**

4. A(n) _____ is a conflict that occurs within a person. **Lesson 6**

5. _____ is the harmful treatment of an aged family member. **Lesson 8**

6. A(n) _____ is a balanced relationship that promotes mutual respect and healthful behavior. **Lesson 9**

7. _____ are skills a person can use to relate well with others. **Lesson 6**

8. A(n) _____ includes an adult(s) who cares for a child or children who do not live with their birth parents. **Lesson 7**

9. A(n) _____ is a pledge or promise to do something. **Lesson 10**

10. A(n) _____ is someone who is respectful, responsible, understanding, and self-disciplined. **Lesson 6**

The Responsible Decision-Making Model™

You have plans to go to the movies with a friend. Another friend invites you to a party the same evening. You really want to go to the party. You consider how your friendship with the first friend will be affected if you go to the party. Answer the following questions on a separate sheet of paper. Write "Does not apply" if a question does not apply to this situation.

1. Is it healthful for you to break the first plans you made? Why or why not?

2. Is it safe for you to break the first plans you made? Why or why not?

3. Is it legal for you to break the first plans you made? Why or why not?

4. Will you show respect for yourself and others if you break the first plans you made? Why or why not?

5. Will your parents or guardian approve if you break the first plans you made? Why or why not?

6. Will you demonstrate good character if you break the first plans you made? Why or why not?

What is the responsible decision to make in this situation?

Health Literacy

Effective Communication

Create a visual—computer graphic, poster, chart, painting, or sculpture—to illustrate friendship as a balancing act involving giving and taking.

Self-Directed Learning

Find five credible sources of information on teen pregnancy or teen parenthood. Write a three-page paper.

Critical Thinking

On average, people who graduate from high school earn more money in their lifetimes than do people who did not graduate from high school. What do you think are reasons for this difference?

Responsible Citizenship

Hold a contest for your classmates to think of a slogan to promote abstinence. Decide a prize for the winner. Display your slogans in your school.

Multicultural Health

Visit your library to find books on manners in cultures different from yours. Research differences. For example, in some cultures, it is polite to look someone in the eye when you are talking to them. In other cultures, this is a sign of disrespect.

Family Involvement

Ask your parents or guardian to form a weekly family meeting. At this meeting, each family member thinks of one action he or she can take that is loving and responsible. Each family member takes that action toward another family member during that week.

Lesson 11
The Amazing Body

Lesson 12
Moving Toward Maturity

Lesson 13
Learning About Pregnancy and Childbirth

Lesson 14
Understanding the Stages in the Life Cycle

Lesson 15
Aging, Dying, and Death

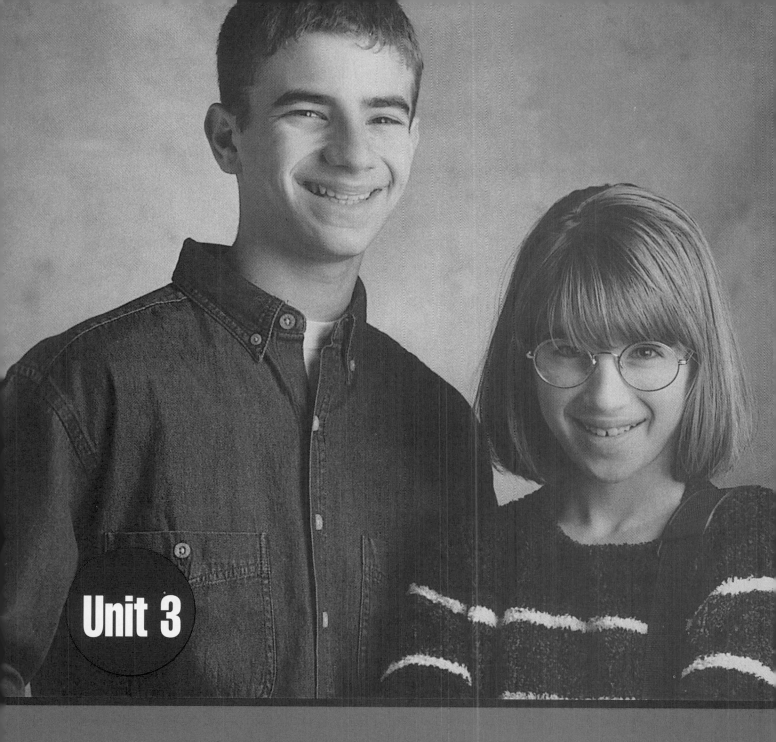

Unit 3

Growth and Development

The Amazing Body

Vocabulary*

body system

nervous system

circulatory system

respiratory system

skeletal system

muscular system

integumentary system

digestive system

urinary system

*A complete listing of vocabulary words appears at the end of the lesson.

Life Skill • **I will keep my body systems healthy.**

You have an amazing body that performs many tasks. Your body has four levels of organization: cells, tissues, organs, and body systems. A **cell** is the smallest living part of the body. A **tissue** is a group of cells that are similar in form or function. An **organ** is a body part consisting of several kinds of tissues that do a particular job. A **body system** is a group of organs that work together to perform a main body function. In this lesson, you will learn about eight body systems. In the next lesson, you will learn about two more body systems.

The Lesson Objectives

• Compare cells, tissues, organs, and body systems.

• Describe the functions of eight body systems.

• Explain ways to care for eight body systems.

The Nervous System

The **nervous system** is the body system that carries messages to and from the brain and spinal cord and all other parts of the body. The nervous system consists of the brain, the spinal cord, and branching nerves. It is divided into the central nervous system (CNS) and the peripheral (puh·RIF·uh·rul) nervous system (PNS).

The Central Nervous System

The **central nervous system (CNS)** is the part of the nervous system that consists of the brain and spinal cord. The brain is a mass of nerve tissue. It has three major parts. The **cerebrum** (suh·REE·bruhm) is the part of the brain that controls the ability to memorize, think, and learn. The **cerebellum** (ser·uh·BEL·uhm) is the part of the brain that controls the coordination of muscle activity. The **brain stem** is the lowest section of the brain. It includes the **medulla** (muh·DUH·luh), the part of the brain that controls involuntary actions, such as heart rate and breathing.

The **spinal cord** is a thick band of nerve cells that extends through the backbone. Thirty-one pairs of spinal nerves branch out from the spinal cord. These nerves branch out between the bones of the spine.

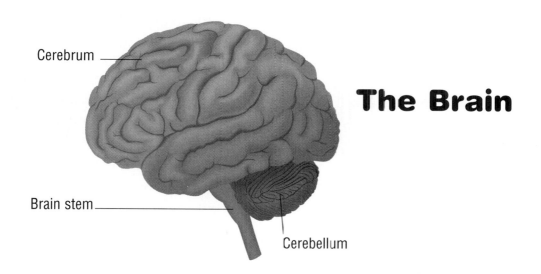

Cerebrum

The Brain

Brain stem

Cerebellum

The Nervous System

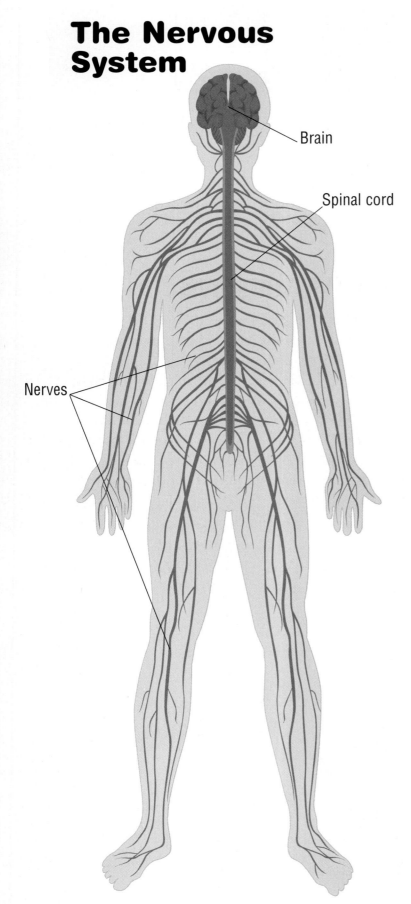

Brain

Spinal cord

Nerves

The Peripheral Nervous System

The **peripheral** (puh·RIF·uh·rul) **nervous system (PNS)** is the part of the CNS that consists of all of the nerves that branch out from the CNS to the muscles, skin, internal organs, and glands. The PNS includes cranial nerves and spinal nerves. The cranial nerves are nerves that control the senses and motor activity. They control muscles in the face and neck. Twelve pairs of cranial nerves branch out from the brain. Thirty-one pairs of spinal nerves branch out from the spine. Spinal nerves transmit information to and from all other parts of the body.

Neurons (NOO·rahnz) are nerve cells. Sensory and motor neurons in the PNS work together to help you respond to your environment. Sensory neurons carry messages from the sense organs to the spinal cord and brain. Motor neurons carry messages from the brain and spinal cord to the muscles and glands. They tell muscles and glands what to do.

Suppose you touch a hot object. Sensory neurons carry a message to the spinal cord and brain. The brain interprets this message—This object is too hot to touch! Motor neurons carry the message back to your muscles. You respond quickly and move your hand. A **reflex action** is an involuntary action in which a message is sent to the spinal cord where it is interpreted and responded to immediately. Reflex actions help keep you safe.

The PNS also helps with body actions over which you have no control. The PNS regulates heart rate and body temperature.

Five Ways to Care for Your Nervous System

1. **Use a safety belt when riding in a car.** Use both your lap belt and shoulder belt to prevent injury to your brain and spinal cord.

2. **Wear a safety helmet for sports.** Wear a helmet to prevent head injuries when playing contact sports, such as boxing or football, or when rollerblading, skating, skateboarding, or playing baseball.

3. **Follow safety rules.** Follow safety rules to protect yourself and others from injury when participating in sports. Avoid horsing around, pushing, and shoving. Many injuries of the brain and spinal cord are permanent.

4. **Avoid alcohol, other drugs, and poisons.** These substances interfere with the way you think and feel. They can kill brain and nerve cells. They can interrupt the body functions that are normally automatic.

5. **Get plenty of rest and sleep.** Your brain cells and nerve cells need rest for you to think clearly and to remember what you learn.

The Circulatory System

The **circulatory system** is the body system that transports nutrients, oxygen, and cellular waste products throughout the body. The circulatory system consists of the blood, blood vessels, and heart.

The Blood

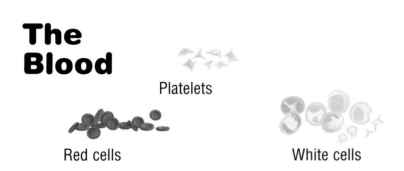

Platelets

Red cells

White cells

Blood is composed of plasma and blood cells. **Plasma** is the liquid component of blood. It is about 95 percent water. Plasma contains blood cells. Two major types of blood cells are red cells and white cells. **Red blood cells** are cells that carry oxygen. They are the most numerous type of blood cells. They live about 100 days. **White blood cells** are cells that attack, surround, and destroy pathogens that enter the body and prevent them from causing infection. If an infection occurs, the number of white blood cells increases. White blood cells live from three months to ten years. **Platelets** are the smallest parts of blood that help blood clot. When you get a cut, platelets help form the scab.

Your body has three major kinds of blood vessels. **Arteries** (AR·tuh·reez) are blood vessels that carry blood away from the heart. **Veins** (VAYNZ) are blood vessels that return blood to the heart. **Capillaries** are tiny blood vessels that connect arteries and veins. When blood flows through the capillaries, nutrients and oxygen are delivered to body cells, and cell waste products are picked up.

The Heart

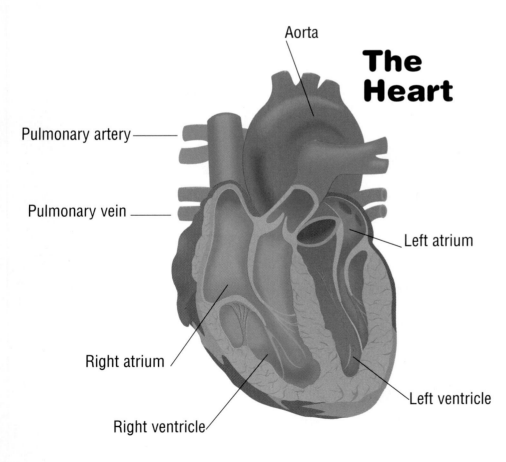

Aorta

Pulmonary artery

Pulmonary vein

Left atrium

Right atrium

Left ventricle

Right ventricle

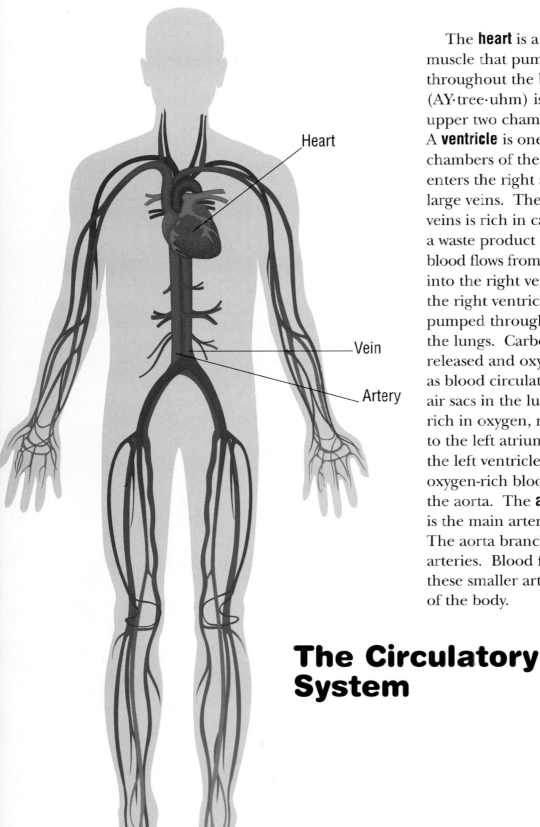

Heart

Vein

Artery

The **heart** is a four-chambered muscle that pumps blood throughout the body. An **atrium** (AY·tree·uhm) is one of the upper two chambers of the heart. A **ventricle** is one of the lower two chambers of the heart. Blood enters the right atrium from two large veins. The blood in these veins is rich in carbon dioxide, a waste product of cells. This blood flows from the right atrium into the right ventricle. From the right ventricle, blood is pumped through arteries to the lungs. Carbon dioxide is released and oxygen is absorbed as blood circulates around the air sacs in the lungs. This blood, rich in oxygen, returns in veins to the left atrium. It flows into the left ventricle from which oxygen-rich blood flows through the aorta. The **aorta** (ay·OR·tuh) is the main artery in the body. The aorta branches into smaller arteries. Blood flows through these smaller arteries to all parts of the body.

The Circulatory System

Understanding Blood Pressure

Blood pressure is the force of blood against the artery walls. Two kinds of blood pressure are routinely measured. The **systolic** (si·STAH·lik) **blood pressure** is the force of blood against the artery walls when the heart is beating. The **diastolic** (dy·uh·STAH·lik) **blood pressure** is the force of blood against the artery walls between heart beats. When you have normal blood pressure, you keep your heart from working too hard. This reduces wear and tear on your arteries.

Understanding Blood Transfusions

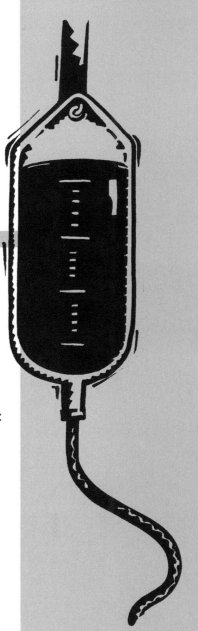

A **transfusion** is the transfer of blood from one person to another. You might need blood from another person if you are in an accident or have surgery. Not all blood is the same. **Blood type** is the kind of red blood cells a person has: A, B, AB, or O. If you need a transfusion, you will need a blood type that will match or mix well with yours. Certain blood types do not mix. You can die if you are transfused with the wrong blood type.

You also need to know your Rh factor. The **Rh factor** is the presence (Rh positive) or absence (Rh negative) of a special substance in the blood.

People with Rh-positive blood can receive blood from those with Rh-positive or Rh-negative blood. People with Rh-negative blood can receive blood only from others with Rh-negative blood.

When people give blood, they are asked questions about their behavior. The blood is checked for the presence of viruses, including HIV. This helps protect you and others who might need a transfusion. You cannot become infected with HIV or other viruses when giving blood. A sterile needle for collecting blood is used for each donor.

Six Ways to Care for Your Circulatory System

1.

Reduce the amount of fat in your diet. When you eat a high-fat diet, fat can deposit on the walls of your arteries. These deposits make arteries narrower and cause blood pressure to increase. Your heart works harder to circulate blood.

2.

Exercise regularly. Regular exercise strengthens your heart muscle. A strong heart muscle pumps more blood with each beat. Your heart beats less often at rest.

3.

Avoid tobacco products. Tobacco products, such as cigarettes and snuff, contain nicotine. Nicotine is a drug that narrows arteries. Blood pressure must increase to circulate blood.

4.

Maintain a healthful weight. If you are overweight, your heart must work extra hard to circulate blood.

5.

Practice stress management skills. When you are under stress, your body secretes adrenaline. This increases blood pressure.

6.

Spend time with loving friends and family members. Contact with people and pets can reduce both stress and blood pressure.

The Respiratory System

The **respiratory system** is the body system that provides body cells with oxygen and removes the carbon dioxide that cells produce as waste.

As you inhale, blood near the surface of the nose and throat warms the air, and mucous linings add moisture. The air moves through the mouth or nose to the trachea. The **trachea** (TRAY·kee·uh) is the windpipe through which air travels to the lungs. **Cilia** (SIH·lee·uh) are hair-like structures in the respiratory tract that trap dust and other particles and remove them.

The **epiglottis** (e·puh·GLAH·tis) is a flap that covers the entrance to the trachea. The epiglottis closes over the trachea when you swallow. This prevents food or liquid from entering the trachea. From the trachea, air enters the bronchi. The **bronchi** are two short tubes through which air enters the lungs. The bronchi enter each lung where they branch into thousands of smaller tubes. The **bronchioles** are small tubes that lead into the alveoli. The **alveoli** (al·vee·OH·ly) are small air sacs at the ends of the bronchioles.

The Respiratory System

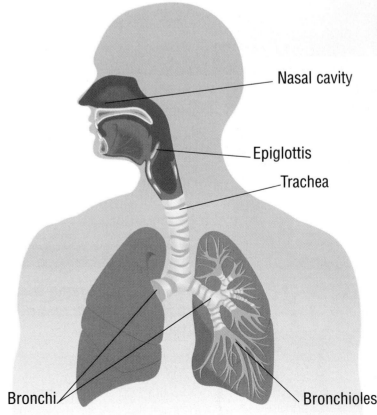

Nasal cavity

Epiglottis

Trachea

Bronchi

Bronchioles

Five Ways to Care for Your Respiratory System

1. **Exercise regularly.** Exercise strengthens the diaphragm muscle and makes it easier for you to inhale air.

2. **Avoid polluted air.** When you breathe air that is polluted, you do not get as much oxygen with each breath. Particles and gases in polluted air can collect in the alveoli and make the exchange of air more difficult.

3. **Avoid tobacco smoke.** Avoid smoke from cigarettes, cigars, and pipes. If you inhale smoke, harmful chemicals and other substances enter and damage your lungs. You are at increased risk for lung cancer and other respiratory diseases.

4. **Seek medical help for respiratory infections.** Infections of the nose, throat, and lungs can be serious. Your body can become weakened, making it easier for other infections to enter your body. Lung damage can occur.

5. **Sit, stand, and walk with correct posture.** Correct posture allows you to breathe easily.

The Skeletal System

The **skeletal system** is the body system that serves as a support framework, protects vital organs, works with muscles to produce movement, and produces blood cells. The skeletal system has 206 bones.

Most bones have cartilage and ligament tissues attached to them and a layer of periosteum. **Cartilage** (KAR·tuhl·ij) is a soft material that is on the ends of some bones. It acts as a cushion where bones come together. **Ligaments** are the fibers that connect bones together. Perhaps you have suffered a sprained ankle at some time. A sprained ankle is caused by ligaments being stretched or torn. The **periosteum** (per·ee·AHS·tee·um) is a thin sheet of outer tissue that covers bone. It contains nerves and blood vessels. The periosteum causes you to feel pain when you suffer a blow to the bone.

A **joint** is the point at which two bones meet. The bones in the human body are connected by several different kinds of joints. A **hinge joint** is a joint that allows bones to move back and forth. The knee and elbow are examples of hinge joints. A **ball and socket joint** is a joint that allows movement in a full circle. The shoulder joint is an example of a ball and socket joint. A **fixed joint** is a joint that does not move. Bones in the cranium come together to form fixed joints.

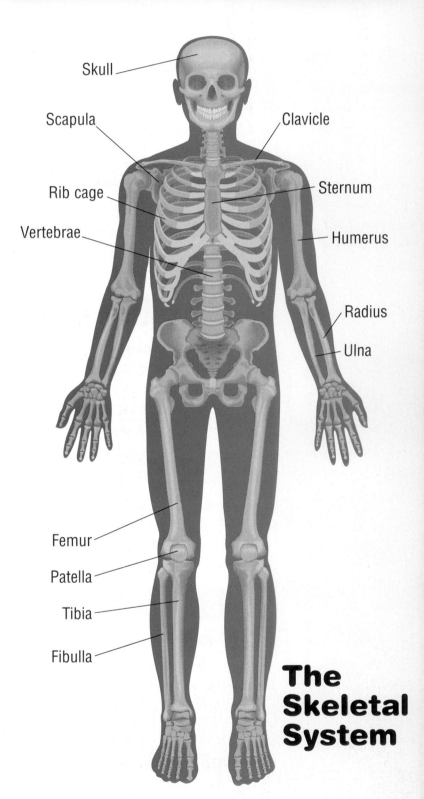

Skull
Scapula
Clavicle
Rib cage
Sternum
Vertebrae
Humerus
Radius
Ulna
Femur
Patella
Tibia
Fibulla

The Skeletal System

Understanding Scoliosis

Scoliosis (skoh·lee·OH·sis) is a deformity of the spine in which the spine develops an S-shaped curve. This condition is more common in females than males. It often becomes apparent in young people ages 10 to 16. If it is not treated, scoliosis can lead to permanent disfigurement.

Many schools do screenings to check for scoliosis. If the spine has a curvature, professional help is recommended. An X-ray is taken. Treatment might involve wearing an upper body cast to reduce the curvature.

Five Ways to Care for Your Skeletal System

1. **Exercise regularly.** The movement of muscles creates stress on the bones. When bones are properly stressed, they become stronger. Walking and jogging strengthen the weight-bearing bones in your legs.

2. **Wear properly-fitting shoes.** The shoes you wear should allow for the movement of your toes and should support the arches in your feet.

3. **Select foods and beverages rich in calcium, phosphorus, and vitamin D.** Proper nutrition strengthens the bones.

4. **Sit, stand, and walk with correct posture.** Erect posture allows the vertebrae to protect the spinal cord.

5. **Participate in screening for scoliosis.** When detected early, treatment can be provided.

The Muscular System

The **muscular** (MUHS·kyuh·ler) **system** is the body system that consists of muscles that provide motion and maintain posture. Your body has more than 600 muscles.

Muscles can be divided into two major groups. **Voluntary muscles** are muscles that a person can control. The muscles in your legs that help you walk are voluntary. **Involuntary muscles** are muscles that function without a person's control. Muscles in your stomach are involuntary because you do not control your stomach's churning action.

Your body has three types of muscles. A smooth muscle is an involuntary muscle that is found in many internal body organs. A skeletal muscle is muscle that is attached to bone. It is under voluntary control.

Cardiac muscle is unique from either of the other types of muscles, as it does not need outside stimulation. Contractions are generated from within.

Tendons are tough tissue fibers that connect muscles to bones. Movement occurs when a muscle shortens. The type of movement that occurs depends on the location of the muscle.

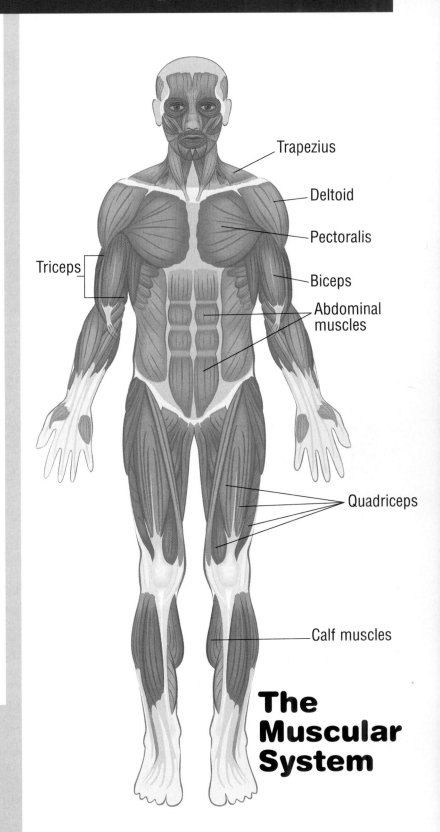

Trapezius

Deltoid

Pectoralis

Triceps

Biceps

Abdominal muscles

Quadriceps

Calf muscles

The Muscular System

Low Back Pain

Muscles can become strained and injured. One type of muscle strain affects the muscles in the back. Low back pain, also called LBP, is one of the most common complaints of adults. LBP usually results from poor health habits that have been practiced during the teen years. Poor posture is a risk factor for LBP. If you slouch when you sit and walk as a teen, you are at risk for having LBP as an adult. Lack of exercise can result in weak abdominal muscles. These weak muscles can put you at risk for low back pain. They can cause the back to lose its correct position.

To reduce the risk of LBP, sleep on a firm mattress. Try not to sleep on your stomach. Instead, sleep in a fetal position as much as possible. In a fetal position, you lie on your side and your knees are slightly drawn up to your stomach. This position keeps your back muscles from becoming strained. Do not become overweight. Extra weight causes the muscles in the back to become strained.

Always lift an object by bending your knees and keeping your back straight. Try to hold the object as close to you as possible. This procedure allows your leg muscles, rather than your back muscles, to provide the necessary force for lifting.

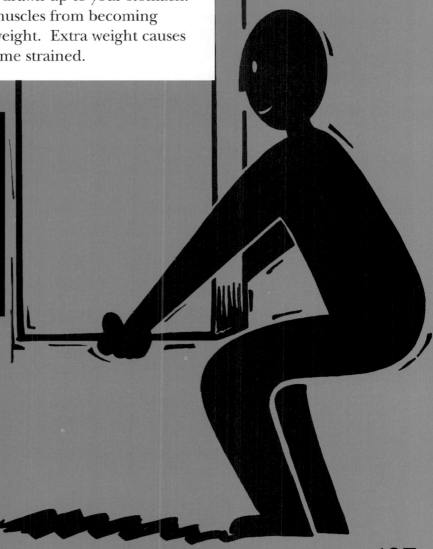

Six Ways to Care for Your Muscular System

1. **Exercise regularly.** Choose exercises for different muscle groups to maintain muscle tone.

2. **Warm up before exercising.** Light exercising and stretching prepare your muscles for more difficult exercise. This warm-up routine helps prevent muscle injury.

3. **Select foods containing carbohydrates and protein.** Carbohydrates are a main source of energy. Protein is needed for the growth of muscle cells.

4. **Sleep in the fetal position on a firm mattress.** A firm mattress gives your back more support. Sleeping in the fetal position keeps your back muscles from becoming strained.

5. **Practice weight management.** Extra weight causes the muscles in the back to become strained.

6. **Lift objects correctly.** Lift an object by bending your knees and keeping your back straight.

The Integumentary System

The **integumentary** (in·TEH·gyuh·ment·tuh·ree) **system** is the body system composed of parts that cover and protect the body. This body system consists of the skin, hair, nails, and glands associated with the skin.

The skin is the largest and most visible organ of the body. The **epidermis** is the outer layer of dead cells of the skin. The **dermis** is the thick layer of living cells below the epidermis. The **subcutaneous** (suhb·kyoo·TAY·nee·uhs) **layer** is a layer of fatty tissue located below the dermis. Your skin has different kinds of nerve cells that help you detect pain, pressure, touch, heat, and cold.

Cross Section of Layers of Skin

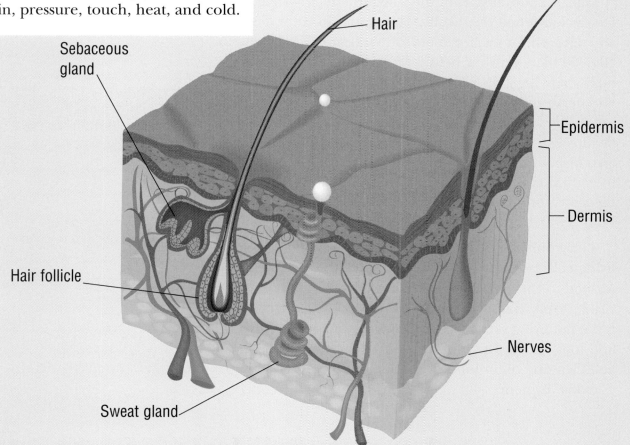

Hair

Sebaceous gland

Epidermis

Dermis

Hair follicle

Nerves

Sweat gland

Important Functions of the Skin

- The skin protects other body parts from injury and helps keep microorganisms from entering the body. In this way, the skin provides a natural defense against infection.

- The skin helps maintain body temperature and helps rid the body of waste. If your body produces excess heat during exercise, sweat glands in the skin will produce perspiration. The water in perspiration evaporates from the surface of your skin and cools you.

- The skin contains melanin. **Melanin** (MEL·uh·nin) is a pigment that gives the skin its color and provides protection from the ultraviolet rays of the sun. Freckles on the skin are a collection of pigment cells.

- The skin contains oil glands that release a substance that helps keep hair from drying and becoming brittle. Gland secretions form a film on the skin that slows evaporation and keeps the skin soft.

Hair is another part of the integumentary system. Hair is hardened dead cells. Hair varies in color, texture, and amount for each person. You might have 100,000 to 200,000 hairs on your head. The roots of your hair are made of living cells. These cells are supplied with blood and nerve cells. As new hair cells are made, old hair cells are pushed up through the scalp. These hairs are the dead cells. Each person has inherited an individual pattern of hair growth. Your hair might grow a length of six to eight inches each year. Your hair functions to protect the skin from harmful sun rays and to help maintain body temperature.

Like your hair, nails are made up of dead cells. As living cells below the skin are replaced, the dead cells are pushed to the surface of the skin where they become visible. Your nails are surrounded by cuticles. A cuticle is the nonliving skin that surrounds the nails of the fingers and toes. Proper care of the nails includes trimming and cleaning them for a neat appearance and good personal hygiene.

Seven Ways to Care for Your Integumentary System

1. **Clean your skin and scalp.** Daily cleaning keeps germs, dirt, and oil off the skin and scalp.

2. **Treat dandruff.** Dandruff is flakes of dead skin cells on the scalp. If normal washing does not control dandruff, use a medicated shampoo.

3. **Select foods containing vitamin A.** Whole milk products and yellow and orange vegetables contain vitamin A, which keeps skin and hair healthy.

4. **Wear a sunscreen containing a sun protection factor (SPF) of at least 15, and wear protective clothing.** Exposure to the sun's harmful rays increases the risk of developing skin cancer and wrinkled skin.

5. **Read directions when using makeup.** Ingredients in makeup might cause skin rashes. Read labels and discontinue use if side effects occur.

6. **Seek proper medical care for skin rashes.** A skin rash might be a sign of a more serious condition.

7. **Check moles, warts, and freckles regularly.** Changes in any of these might be a sign of skin cancer.

The Digestive System and Urinary System

The **digestive** (dy·JES·tiv) **system** is the body system that breaks down food so that nutrients can be used by the body. The digestive system allows nutrients to be absorbed and eliminates waste from the body.

The Digestive System

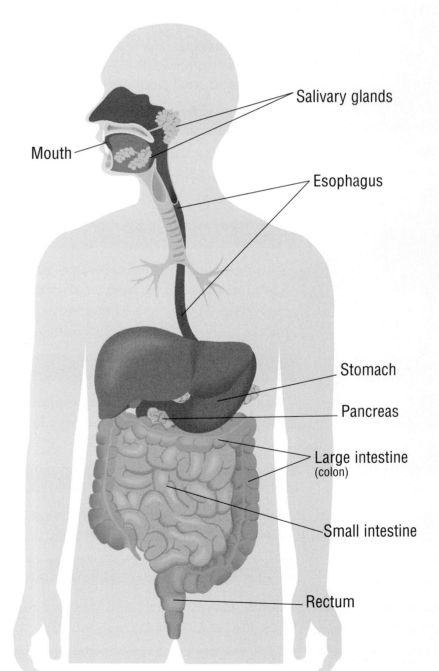

Salivary glands

Mouth

Esophagus

Stomach

Pancreas

Large intestine
(colon)

Small intestine

Rectum

Digestion is the process by which food is broken down so that it can be used by the body's cells. Digestion begins in the mouth. The teeth tear, cut, and grind food. The **salivary** (SA·luh·vehr·ee) **glands** are glands that produce saliva. Saliva is a fluid that helps soften food so that it can be swallowed.

When you swallow, food moves to the esophagus. The **esophagus** (i·SAH·fuh·guhs) is a tube through which food passes to the stomach. The **stomach** is an organ that releases acids and juices that mix with the food and produces a thick paste called chyme (KYM). After about four hours, muscles in the stomach push the food into the small intestine.

The **small intestine** is a coiled tube in which the greatest amount of digestion and absorption take place. Other body organs help digest food while it is in the small intestine. The **pancreas** (PAN·kree·uhs) is a gland that produces digestive enzymes and chemicals that control blood sugar levels. The **liver** is a gland that produces and releases bile to help break down fats; maintains blood sugar levels; and filters poisonous wastes. Bile is a liquid that helps in the digestion of fats. The **gallbladder** is an organ that stores bile.

From the small intestine, undigested food moves to the large intestine. The **large intestine,** or colon, is a tube extending below the small intestine where undigested food is prepared for elimination from the body.

When the large intestine is full, the lower part contracts and solid waste leaves the body as a bowel movement.

The Urinary System

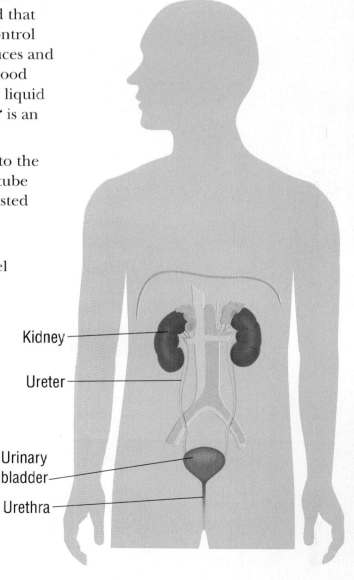

Kidney

Ureter

Urinary bladder

Urethra

The **urinary system** is the body system that removes liquid wastes from the body. The **kidney** is an organ through which blood circulates as wastes are filtered. The body has two kidneys. Urine is formed as liquid and waste products are filtered from the blood. **Urine** is a pale yellow liquid composed of water, salts, and other waste substances. As urine forms, it flows from the kidneys through the ureters to the bladder. The **ureter** (YU·ruh·ter) is a narrow tube that connects the kidney to the bladder. As the bladder fills with urine, it expands. When it is full, the bladder releases urine into the urethra. The **urethra** (yu·REE·thruh) is the tube leading from the bladder and through which urine passes out of the body.

Four Ways to Care for Your Digestive System and Your Urinary System

1. **Drink the equivalent of at least six to eight glasses of water each day.** This amount of water is needed to help the kidneys function properly. It also helps your body maintain the proper balance between water and salt.

2. **Maintain healthful blood pressure.** Blood pressure is the force of blood against the interior walls of the arteries. High blood pressure damages the kidneys.

3. **Eat food slowly.** When you eat slowly and chew food thoroughly, the organs in the digestive system function at their best.

4. **Eat plenty of fiber.** Fiber is the part of grains and plant foods that cannot be digested. Fiber helps you have a bowel movement. Fruits, vegetables, and grains are good sources of fiber.

Review

Vocabulary

Write separate sentences using twenty of the vocabulary words listed below.

cell
tissue
organ
body system
nervous system
central nervous system
cerebrum
cerebellum
brain stem
medulla
spinal cord
peripheral nervous system
neurons
reflex action
circulatory system
plasma
red blood cells
white blood cells
platelets
arteries
veins
capillaries
heart
atrium
ventricle
aorta
blood pressure
systolic blood pressure
diastolic blood pressure
transfusion
blood type
Rh factor
respiratory system
trachea
cilia

epiglottis
bronchi
bronchioles
alveoli
skeletal system
cartilage
ligaments
periosteum
joint
hinge joint
ball and socket joint
fixed joint
scoliosis
muscular system
voluntary muscles
involuntary muscles
tendons
integumentary system
epidermis
dermis
subcutaneous layer
melanin
dandruff
digestive system
digestion
salivary glands
esophagus
stomach
small intestine
pancreas
liver
gallbladder
large intestine
urinary system
kidney
urine
ureter
urethra

Health Content

Write responses to the following:

1. What are the four levels of organization in the body? **page 94**

2. What is the function of the nervous system? **page 95**
What are ways to care for the nervous system? **page 97**

3. What is the function of the circulatory system? **page 98**
What are ways to care for the circulatory system? **page 101**

4. Describe the flow of blood through the heart. **page 99**

5. What is blood pressure? **page 100**

6. Why must blood type and Rh factor be known when having a blood transfusion? **page 100**

7. Why are you protected from infection with HIV when giving blood? **page 100**

8. What is the function of the respiratory system? What are ways to care for the respiratory system? **pages 102–103**

9. What are the functions of the skeletal system? Ways to care for the skeletal system? **pages 104–105**

10. What are three kinds of joints and examples of each? **page 104**

11. What is scoliosis? **page 105**

12. What is the function of the muscular system? **page 106**
What are ways to care for the muscular system? **page 108**

13. How can you reduce the risk of low back pain? **page 107**

14. What is the function of the integumentary system? **page 109** What are ways to care for the integumentary system? **page 111**

15. What are four functions of skin? **page 110**

16. What is the function of the digestive system? **page 112**

17. Describe the path of food through the digestive system. **page 112**

18. What is the function of the urinary system? **page 114**

19. Describe the path of liquid waste through the urinary system. **page 113**

20. What are ways to care for the digestive system and the urinary system? **page 114**

Moving Toward Maturity

Vocabulary*

endocrine system

reproductive system

*A complete listing of vocabulary words appears at the end of the lesson.

Life Skills

- **I will recognize habits that protect female reproductive health.**
- **I will recognize habits that protect male reproductive health.**

To **mature** is to become fully grown or developed. You are maturing in many ways. Your endocrine and reproductive systems help you move toward maturity. You recognize changes in your body and in the ways you think and feel. Your relationships with others have new meaning because of these two body systems.

The Lesson Objectives

- Describe the functions of the endocrine and reproductive systems.
- Explain ways to care for your endocrine and reproductive systems.
- Identify physical changes that occur in puberty.
- Trace the path of an unfertilized egg through the female reproductive organs.
- Trace the path of a sperm cell through the male reproductive organs.
- Discuss how your body and your sex role can help you feel good about yourself.

The Endocrine System

The **endocrine** (EN·duh·krin) **system** is the body system that consists of glands that produce hormones. A **hormone** is a chemical messenger that is released into the bloodstream. Hormones control many of your body's activities. A **gland** is a group of cells or an organ that secretes hormones.

The **pituitary** (pi·TOO·i·tehr·ree) **gland** is a gland that produces hormones that control other glands. It also produces hormones that control the growth of bones and the movement of smooth muscles.

The Endocrine System

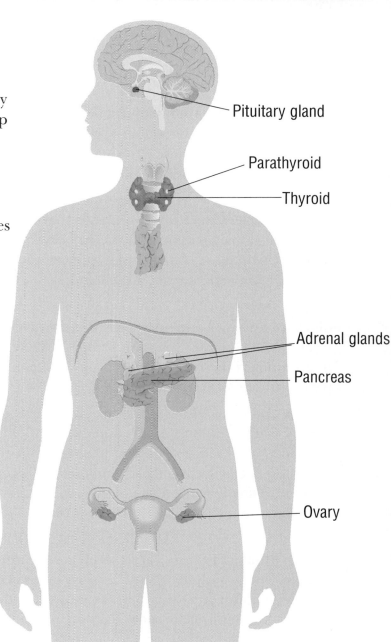

Pituitary gland

Parathyroid

Thyroid

Adrenal glands

Pancreas

Ovary

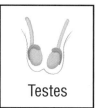

Testes

The **thyroid gland** is a gland that produces thyroxin. **Thyroxin** (thy·RAHK·sin) is a hormone that controls metabolism. **Metabolism** (muh·TA·buh·li·zuhm) is the rate at which food is converted to energy in the cells. Too much thyroxin can result in high metabolism. A person might feel restless and lose weight. Too little thyroxin can result in low metabolism. A person might feel tired and gain weight.

The **parathyroid** (pehr·uh·THY·royd) **glands** are four glands that control the amount of calcium and phosphorus in the body. When these glands are overactive, calcium leaves the bones and enters the blood. This causes muscle weakness.

The **adrenal glands** are two glands that control the body's water balance, help in the digestive process, and secrete adrenaline. Adrenaline prepares the body to react quickly during stress or in an emergency.

The **pancreas** (PAN·kree·uhs) is a gland that produces digestive enzymes and chemicals that control blood sugar levels. The pancreas releases insulin. **Insulin** is a hormone that regulates the blood sugar level. The pancreas is also part of the digestive system.

The **ovaries** (OH·vuh·reez) are two female reproductive glands that produce egg cells and estrogen. **Estrogen** (ES·truh·juhn) is a female sex hormone that controls the development of secondary sex characteristics during puberty. **Puberty** is the stage of growth and development when secondary sex characteristics appear. Puberty occurs in females usually between the ages of 8 and 15.

The **testes** (TES·teez) are two male reproductive glands that produce sperm cells and testosterone. **Testosterone** (te·STAH·stuh·rohn) is a male sex hormone that controls the development of the secondary sex characteristics during puberty. Puberty occurs in males usually between the ages of 12 and 15.

Both males and females might experience changes in mood during puberty. This is due to changing levels of male and female hormones. Slight changes in mood are normal. If changes in your body or your feelings bother you, discuss them with your parents, guardian, or physician.

Physical Changes During Puberty

Males

- **Increase in height of 4–12 inches**
- **Deepening of voice**
- **Increase in perspiration**
- **Growth of facial hair**
- **Growth of underarm hair**
- **Growth of pubic hair**
- **Broadening of shoulders**
- **Increase in muscle mass**
- **Enlargement of reproductive organs**
- **Onset of sperm development**

Females

- **Increase in height of 2–8 inches**
- **Increase in perspiration**
- **Growth of underarm hair**
- **Growth of pubic hair**
- **Enlargement of breasts**
- **Widening of hips**
- **Enlargement of reproductive organs**
- **Onset of menstruation**
- **Formation of mature eggs**

Two Ways to Care for Your Endocrine System

1. **Have regular medical checkups.** Your physician will check the progress of your growth and development.

2. **Keep a list of questions to ask your physician.** You might ask your physician about the changes in your body and changes in your feelings. You might ask your physician for ways to care for your body during puberty and adulthood. Your physician can explain the effects of hormones on your body. Your physician can reassure you about the changes that occur as you grow and develop.

The Female Reproductive System

The **reproductive system** is the body system that consists of the organs involved in producing offspring. In this lesson, you will learn about the organs in this system, how they function, and ways to care for them. In the next lesson, you will learn about conception, pregnancy, and childbirth.

The **female reproductive system** is the body system that consists of the female organs involved in producing offspring. The female reproductive organs include the ovaries, Fallopian tubes, uterus, and vagina. The **ovaries** (OH·vuh·reez) are two female reproductive glands that produce egg cells and estrogen. **Egg cells**, or **ova**, are female reproductive cells. A female is born with 200,000 to 250,000 immature egg cells in her ovaries. About 400 of these egg cells will mature in her lifetime. Each egg is enclosed in a small, hollow ball called a follicle. The follicles form a layer of the ovary.

During puberty, the egg cells begin to develop. Each month, one egg matures and is released from its follicle. One egg will be released by one of the ovaries each month. **Ovulation** (ahv·yuh·LAY·shun) is the release of a mature egg from an ovary and is part of the menstrual cycle. The **menstrual cycle** is the monthly series of changes that take place in the female reproductive system. The cycle is associated with hormone production and ovulation. The menstrual cycle and timing of ovulation vary from one female to another. The length of the cycle also may vary. Some females have a very regular menstrual cycle; others do not.

A mature egg that is released from an ovary and is not fertilized will leave the body during the menstrual flow. Once an egg is released from an ovary, it enters a Fallopian tube. A **Fallopian tube** is a four-inch-long tube that extends from the ovary to the uterus. A female has two Fallopian tubes. The unfertilized egg moves through the Fallopian tube to the uterus. The **uterus** is a muscular organ that supports the fertilized egg during pregnancy. The egg either disintegrates or leaves the body through the vagina as part of the menstrual flow. The **vagina** is a muscular tube that connects the uterus to the outside of the body.

If sperm are present when an egg is moving through a Fallopian tube, a sperm might penetrate the egg. **Conception,** or **fertilization,** is the union of an egg and a sperm. This usually occurs in the upper third of a Fallopian tube. Conception will be discussed in the next lesson.

The Female Reproductive System

Front View

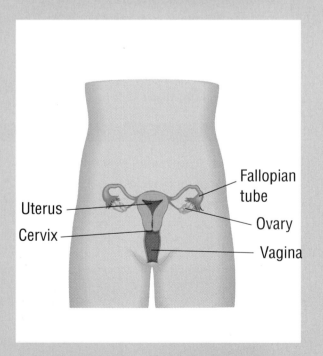

Side View

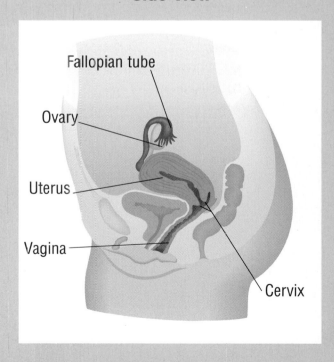

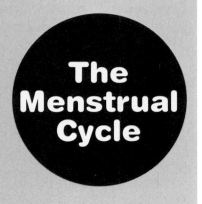

The Menstrual Cycle

The onset of the menstrual cycle usually occurs between the ages of 8 and 13. During the menstrual cycle:

- **one ovary produces a mature egg cell;**
- **the lining of the uterus prepares for a fertilized egg;**
- **the lining breaks down and leaves the body if an egg is not fertilized.**

Menstruation is the part of the menstrual cycle in which an unfertilized egg and the inner lining of the uterus leave the body. It is also called the menstrual flow. **Menarche** (MEN·are·kee) is the first menstrual cycle.

Days 1–4 The menstrual flow occurs. About two ounces (50 to 60 ml) of blood are lost. An egg in the ovary begins to mature.

Days 5–12 After the menstrual flow stops, the lining of the uterus starts to thicken again. The mature egg gets ready to be released.

Days 13–14 Ovulation occurs. The egg is released into the Fallopian tube.

Days 15–20 Progesterone is secreted. Progesterone is a hormone that thickens the lining of the uterus. The thickened lining of the uterus is prepared to support a fertilized egg. If conception occurs, progesterone continues to be produced during pregnancy.

Days 21–28 If conception does not occur, no more progesterone is made. The cells in the lining of the uterus die without the progesterone. The unfertilized egg becomes part of the menstrual flow.

Days 1–4 The cycle begins again. The menstrual flow occurs. About two ounces (50 to 60 ml) of blood are lost. An egg in the ovary begins to mature.

Female Reproductive Health

To work toward good health, a female must understand how her body works. She needs to know what she can do to keep herself healthy. She must learn and practice ways that she can care for her body.

Menstrual Protection

Several products that absorb the menstrual flow are available. External methods of protection include pads and panty shields. These products should be changed every four to six hours. A tampon is used to provide internal protection during menstruation. A tampon is a small, tube-shaped product that absorbs the menstrual flow. It is inserted into the vagina. Tampons should be changed every four to six hours. Pads, panty shields, and tampons should be wrapped in tissue and disposed of in a closed container. They should not be flushed down the toilet.

Toxic Shock Syndrome (TSS)

Toxic shock syndrome (TSS) is an illness caused by the presence of harmful bacteria in the body. TSS occurs most often in females who use tampons during menstruation. TSS is more likely to occur when tampons are not changed regularly. It also is more likely to occur when super-absorbent tampons are used. Females who use tampons should be aware of the symptoms of TSS. Symptoms include a sudden high fever, headache, diarrhea, rash, vomiting, dizziness, and fainting. Prompt medical care is needed if these occur.

Menstrual Cramps

Some females have cramps during their periods. Painful cramps usually are caused by contractions of the uterus. They might be relieved by exercise and relaxation. Sometimes, taking a warm bath might help. Medication might relieve the pain.

Premenstrual Syndrome (PMS)

Premenstrual syndrome (PMS) is a group of changes that can affect a female before her menstrual period. Some of these changes include headache, backache, tenderness of the breasts, a bloated feeling, weight gain, quick mood changes, and depression. The exact cause of PMS is unknown, but it is believed to result from hormonal changes. A female can reduce the symptoms of PMS. She can decrease or eliminate caffeine in her diet. She can reduce the amount of salt in her diet. This will help lower the amount of water her body retains. A physician might recommend medication to relieve symptoms.

Seven Ways to Care for the Female Reproductive System

1. **Choose abstinence.** Abstinence is choosing not to be sexually active. Choosing abstinence prevents unwanted pregnancy and infection with sexually transmitted diseases.

2. **Have regular medical checkups.** Your physician can examine you and discuss the many changes in your body.

3. **Keep track of your menstrual periods.** Record the first and last day of the menstrual flow each month. This record helps a physician know if your menstrual period is regular. You might want to discuss the amount of blood flow and any cramps with your physician.

4. **Practice good health habits during your menstrual flow.** Change your pad or tampon every four to six hours. Consider wearing a pad instead of a tampon at night to reduce the risk of TSS. Wrap used pads and tampons in tissue and dispose of them in a closed container. Never flush them down the toilet.

5. **Exercise regularly and reduce caffeine and salt in the diet.** These healthful habits will reduce menstrual cramping.

6. **Perform regular breast self-examinations.** Check your breasts for lumps and changes. A self-examination should be performed after your menstrual period. This is an important habit to develop now and practice for a lifetime.

7. **Discuss any concerns you have with your parents or guardian.** You might have questions about body changes. Discuss your concerns with your parents or guardian.

The Male Reproductive System

The **male reproductive system** is the body system that consists of the male organs involved in producing offspring. The external male organs include the penis and scrotum. The **penis** is the male sex organ for reproduction and urination. The reproductive function of the penis is to deposit sperm in the vagina. **Sperm** are the male reproductive cells.

The **scrotum** is a sac-like pouch that holds each testis and helps regulate temperature for sperm production. The scrotum hangs from the body so that the testes have a lower temperature than the rest of the body. This allows the testes to produce sperm.

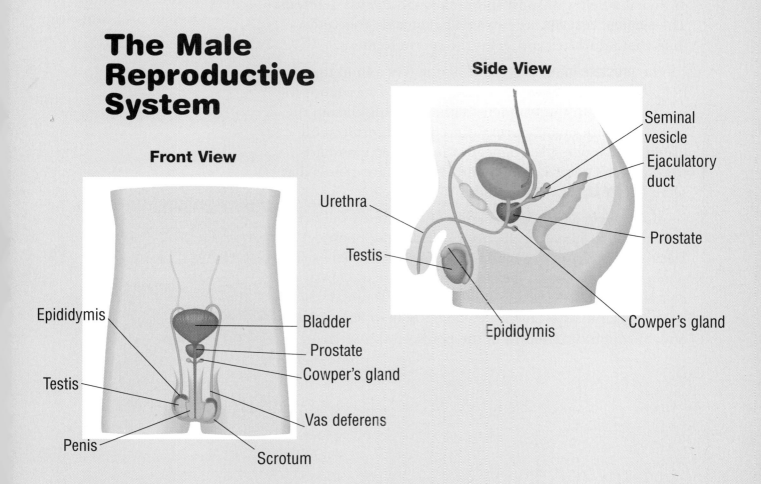

The Male Reproductive System

Front View

Epididymis

Testis

Penis

Bladder

Prostate

Cowper's gland

Vas deferens

Scrotum

Side View

Seminal vesicle

Ejaculatory duct

Urethra

Prostate

Testis

Epididymis

Cowper's gland

Males have several internal reproductive organs. The testes are two male reproductive glands that produce sperm cells and testosterone. The testes contain a network of coiled tubes. The **seminiferous** (se·muh·NI·fuh·ruhs) **tubules** are a network of coiled tubes in which sperm are produced.

After sperm are produced, they pass into the epididymis. The **epididymis** (e·puh·DI·duh·mus) is a comma-shaped structure on the rear upper surface of each testis where sperm are stored.

The epididymis leads into the vas deferens. The **vas deferens** are two long, thin tubes that function as a passageway for sperm and as a place for sperm storage. The vas deferens wind upward in the scrotum to the abdominal cavity. They circle the bladder and connect with the urethra. The urethra serves as a passageway for sperm to leave the body. The walls of the vas deferens are lined with cilia. The contraction of the vas deferens and the action of the cilia help transport sperm through the vas deferens. The **seminal vesicles** are two small glands that secrete a fluid that nourishes and helps the sperm to move.

The **prostate gland** is a gland that makes a fluid that helps keep sperm alive. The prostate gland surrounds the urethra beneath the bladder. Without the fluid from the prostate gland, many sperm would die and fertilization would not be possible. Beneath the prostate gland are the Cowper's glands. The **Cowper's glands** are glands that secrete a clear, lubricating fluid.

After sperm are produced, one of two events will occur. Sperm will be stored in the body or leave the body. **Ejaculation** is a series of muscular contractions that expel semen from the penis. **Semen** is the fluid that consists of a combination of sperm and fluids from the seminal vesicles, prostate gland, and Cowper's glands. Semen leaves the body through the urethra in the penis.

Male Reproductive Health

The male reproductive system requires care. At birth, the end of the penis is covered by a loosely fitting skin called the foreskin. **Circumcision** is the surgical removal of the foreskin. This procedure is usually done within several days after birth. It might reduce the risk of urinary infections and cancer of the penis. Males who are not circumcised should pull the foreskin back and clean the penis regularly.

Six Ways to Care for the Male Reproductive System

1. **Choose abstinence.** Choosing abstinence prevents infection with sexually transmitted diseases. It also keeps you from becoming a teen father.

2. **Have regular medical checkups.** Your physician can examine you and discuss body changes.

3. **Bathe or shower daily.** Keep your external reproductive organs clean.

4. **Wear protective clothing and equipment when playing sports.** Some shorts contain an athletic supporter that provides support for the penis and scrotum. Protective equipment, such as a cup, helps prevent injury to these organs.

5. **Perform regular testicular examinations.** Check for lumps and changes. This is an important habit to develop now and practice for a lifetime.

6. **Discuss any concerns you have with your parents or guardian.** You might have questions about body changes or erections. Discuss your concerns with your parents or guardian.

Physical Uniqueness

It is helpful to feel good about your changing body during puberty. Remember, no one is exactly like you. Your appearance is unique. You might be shorter or taller than your classmates. You might begin to mature earlier or later than others. Heredity and diet, along with your exercise plan, influence your appearance.

You might have a slim body build or be muscular. You might have a more rounded appearance. **Body image** is the perception a person has of his or her body's appearance. Body image is often influenced by how well you accept the physical changes that occur during puberty. When you like and accept your body, it is easier to like and accept yourself. It is helpful to speak with a trusted adult about your feelings if you have concerns about your appearance.

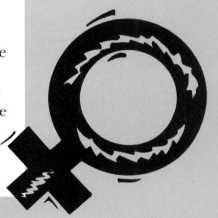

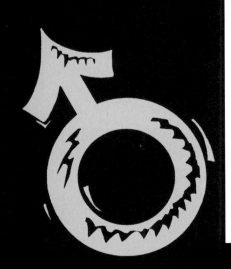

Maleness and Femaleness

Sexuality includes the feelings and attitudes a person has about his or her body, sex role, and relationships. It is important to have good feelings about your body. It is also important to feel good about the body changes that accompany puberty.

A **sex role** is the way a person acts and the feelings and attitudes (s)he has about being a male or a female. Your sex role also includes the expectations you have for the ways males and females behave. The adults who brought you up helped form your sex role. You learned from their attitudes and feelings about males and females. It is important to feel good about being a male or a female. You should not feel limited by your sex role.

Lesson 12

Review

Vocabulary

Write a separate sentence using each of the vocabulary words listed below.

mature
endocrine system
hormone
gland
pituitary gland
thyroid gland
thyroxin
metabolism
parathyroid glands
adrenal glands
pancreas
insulin
ovaries
estrogen
puberty
testes
testosterone
reproductive
 system
female reproduc-
 tive system
ovaries
egg cells
ova
ovulation
menstrual cycle
Fallopian tube
uterus

vagina
conception or
 fertilization
menstruation
menarche
toxic shock
 syndrome (TSS)
premenstrual
 syndrome (PMS)
male reproductive
 system
penis
sperm
scrotum
seminiferous
 tubules
epididymis
vas deferens
seminal vesicles
prostate gland
Cowper's glands
ejaculation
semen
circumcision
body image
sexuality
sex role

Health Content

Write responses to the following:

1. What is the function of the endocrine system? **page 117**
 What are ways to care for the endocrine system? **page 119**

2. What are ten physical changes that occur in males during puberty? In females during puberty? **page 119**

3. Compare the functions of the female and the male reproductive systems. **pages 120–121 and 125–126**

4. Describe the path of an unfertilized egg through the female reproductive system. **page 121**

5. What happens during a 28-day menstrual cycle? **page 122**

6. What are ways a female can care for her body before and during menstruation? **page 123**

7. What are seven ways to care for the female reproductive system? **page 124**

8. Describe the path of a sperm cell through the male reproductive system. **page 126**

9. What are six ways to care for the male reproductive system? **page 127**

10. How do your body image and your sex role help you feel good about yourself? **page 128**

Learning About Pregnancy and Childbirth

Vocabulary

conception
fertilization
uterus
placenta
umbilical cord
amniotic sac
zygote
embryo
fetus
pregnancy
prenatal care
obstetrician
fetal alcohol syndrome
   (FAS)
miscarriage
toxemia
premature birth
childbirth
labor
effacement
afterbirth
cesarean section
Apgar score
postpartum period
prolactin

Life Skills

- **I will learn about pregnancy and childbirth.**
- **I will practice abstinence to avoid teen pregnancy and parenthood.**

You have been learning about ways in which you are moving toward maturity. Your body is changing as you grow. You are learning to accept your body, which is becoming more like an adult body, and to understand changing feelings. You are exploring what it means to be male or female. As you prepare for adulthood, it is important to learn about conception, pregnancy, and childbirth.

The Lesson Objectives

- Explain the process of conception.
- List the signs of pregnancy.
- Describe the development of a baby from conception through birth.
- Discuss the importance of prenatal care.
- Identify problems that can occur during pregnancy.
- Outline the stages of labor.
- State why abstinence is the best choice for teens.

Conception

As a part of a female's normal menstrual cycle, one of the ovaries releases a mature egg each month. The mature egg moves through a Fallopian tube toward the uterus. Conception might take place in the Fallopian tube. **Conception,** or **fertilization,** is the union of an egg and a sperm. Once an egg has been fertilized, it undergoes cell division and moves to the uterus. The **uterus** is a muscular organ that supports the fertilized egg during pregnancy.

By the end of the first week, these dividing cells become implanted in the inner wall of the uterus. The outer cells of the fertilized egg form the placenta. The **placenta** is an organ that attaches the egg to the inner wall of the uterus. The umbilical cord attaches to the placenta and the developing baby's navel. The **umbilical cord** is a ropelike structure through which the mother and developing baby exchange oxygen, nutrients, and waste. It contains two arteries and one vein.

A thin membrane surrounds the baby throughout its growth. The **amniotic sac** is a thin membrane filled with fluid in which the developing baby floats. This fluid helps maintain a constant temperature for the developing baby. The fluid also serves as a cushion to help protect the baby from injury.

A **zygote** is the single cell that is formed from the union of the sperm and egg. The zygote divides to form two cells, then four cells, then eight cells, and so on. Finally, it becomes an embryo. The **embryo** is the mass of cells during the first eight weeks after conception. The **fetus** is the developing of cells from the eighth week of conception until birth.

Sperm Count and Conception

Conception is the union of one egg and one sperm. But many sperm are needed for conception to take place. As the sperm approach the egg, they release an enzyme. The enzyme works on the egg so that one sperm can enter.

Pregnancy

Pregnancy is the time period from conception to birth. When a female becomes pregnant, hormones change how her body works. These changes include the absence of menstruation, enlarged or tender breasts, frequent urination, fatigue, and morning sickness. Morning sickness is the nausea that can occur any time of the day during pregnancy.

These physical changes alone do not always indicate that a female is pregnant. To make a definite diagnosis, a female should have a pregnancy test. Pregnancy tests determine if HCG is present in the urine. HCG is a hormone produced during pregnancy. A physician can give this test and have the results analyzed in a laboratory. Most drugstores sell pregnancy test kits that can be used at home. However, these home pregnancy tests might not be as accurate as the tests sent to a laboratory.

An early pregnancy test is very important. During the first trimester of pregnancy, the embryo grows rapidly. The first trimester of pregnancy is the first three months of pregnancy. The embryo is the name given to the fertilized egg. A female who does not know she is pregnant might choose harmful behavior. She might harm the embryo because she does not know she is pregnant.

For example, she might skip meals because she is busy. She should not skip meals even if she is not pregnant. But there is even more reason not to skip meals if she is. If she knows she is pregnant, she probably would not skip meals. She would want to give the embryo the best nutrition possible.

Development of the Baby

The growth of an embryo and fetus is described in trimesters, or three month periods. The developing baby changes in many ways during each trimester.

Development of the Baby— Conception Through Birth

First Trimester

End of 1st month

- Heart, brain, nerves, and lungs form.
- Digestive system forms.
- Eyes and ears can be seen.
- Length is 1/3 inch.
- The baby is called an embryo.

End of 2nd month

- Arms, fingers, legs, and toes form.
- Heart becomes four chambers.
- Head becomes larger.
- Facial characteristics appear.
- Length is 1 inch.
- The baby is called a fetus.

End of 3rd month

- First external signs of sex appear.
- Some movement begins.
- Weight is about 1.5 ounces.
- Length is about 1.5 inches.

Second Trimester

End of 4th month

- Skin is developing.
- Fetus kicks its legs and moves its arms.
- Weight is about 6–7 ounces.
- Length is about 4–5 inches.

End of 5th month

- Fine hair develops.
- Eyelashes and nails appear.
- Rate of growth slows.
- Weight is about 1 pound.
- Length is about 9–10 inches.

End of 6th month

- Fetus responds to noise and pressure with movement.
- Heartbeat increases.
- Fetus moves vigorously.
- Weight is about 1.5 pounds.
- Length is about 11.5 –12.5 inches.

Third Trimester

End of 7th month

- Eyes open.
- Legs and arms move often.
- Weight is about 3 pounds.
- Length is about 15 inches.

End of 8th month

- Almost all organs are complete.
- Weight is about 4 pounds.
- Length is about 18 inches.

End of 9th month

- Skin is smooth and polished.
- Eyes are slate-colored.
- Birth weight is about 6–9 pounds.
- Birth length is about 19–21 inches.

Prenatal Care

Pregnancy is a responsibility for both parents-to-be. The mother-to-be must care for her health because her behavior and choices also affect her baby's health. The parents need to provide a healthful environment as the baby develops before and after birth.

A female should begin having regular medical checkups as soon as a pregnancy is determined. Early prenatal care promotes the health of the mother-to-be and her baby. **Prenatal care** is the care given to both the mother-to-be and her unborn baby. An **obstetrician** (ahb·stuh·TRI·shun) is a physician who specializes in the care of a mother-to-be and her developing baby.

An obstetrician will examine the pregnant female to determine her health status. The physician will discuss healthful behaviors the mother-to-be should follow. She must take responsibility for choosing behaviors that promote a healthful pregnancy. She should eat a healthful diet. She should discuss how much weight to gain with her physician.

A pregnant female should avoid harmful drugs during pregnancy. She should take only those medications pre-scribed by her physician. She should not drink alcohol at any time. **Fetal alcohol syndrome (FAS)** is the presence of severe birth defects in babies born to mothers who drink alcohol during pregnancy. Babies with FAS suffer from mental retardation, central nervous system disorders, heart and muscular problems, and defects of joints and limbs.

Smoking should be avoided during pregnancy. Smoking increases the developing baby's risk of having physical problems. Nicotine and other toxic substances in cigarette smoke reduce the amount of oxygen the baby receives. Nicotine decreases appetite. As a result, the mother-to-be might not eat as much as she should. Babies born to females who smoke weigh less than babies born to nonsmokers.

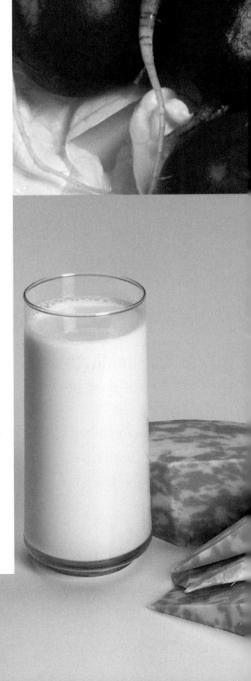

Problems During Pregnancy

About one in ten pregnancies ends in miscarriage. A **miscarriage** is a natural ending of a pregnancy before a baby is developed enough to survive on its own. Most miscarriages occur before the twelfth week of pregnancy. In some cases, the uterine lining might not have grown properly. In other cases, the baby might have had a health problem.

Some pregnant females develop toxemia. **Toxemia** is a condition in which high blood pressure, sudden weight gain, blurred vision, headaches, and swelling of the hands and feet occur. These symptoms usually appear after the twenty-fourth week of pregnancy. Toxemia can harm the mother-to-be and baby. Toxemia might be caused by heredity and poor nutrition.

Another problem that can result during pregnancy is premature birth. **Premature birth** is the birth of a baby before it is fully developed. A baby is premature if it is born less than 38 weeks from time of conception. Premature babies have low birth weight. The lower the birth weight of a premature infant, the less chance of survival. Fortunately, new medical methods can help reduce the risk of premature birth. New methods also help premature babies survive.

Most females have healthful pregnancies. They check with their physician and continue the activities they enjoy. Their physician approves their plan for safe and healthful workouts. They continue to work and enjoy social activities. They do not have problems with miscarriage, toxemia, or premature birth.

They take actions to prevent problems in their pregnancy. For example, they talk to their physician about travel plans. They know ahead of time where they will be. They check out the location of a hospital and physician if they will be out of town. They choose safe forms of transportation. They do not make foolish choices, such as getting on an amusement ride that shakes them back and forth.

Labor and Delivery

Childbirth is the process by which a baby moves from the uterus to the outside world. As the baby is about to be born, some or all of the following might occur. The mother will experience severe cramps. A discharge of blood will come from the cervix. The amniotic sac will break and cause water to flow out.

Labor is a series of three stages that result in the birth of the baby. The first stage of labor is called effacement and dilation. **Effacement** is the thinning and shortening of the cervix. Contractions of the uterus cause the cervix and the cervical opening to dilate or stretch. This allows the baby's head to enter the vagina, or birth canal. Near the end of this stage, contractions can last as long as a minute and a half. This stage can last from one hour to fifteen hours or more.

The second stage of labor is the delivery of the baby. The baby moves out of the uterus and into the birth canal. The mother pushes during uterine contractions to move the baby through the birth canal. When the baby's head is seen at the opening of the vagina, the baby will soon be delivered. This second stage lasts about thirty minutes to one and one-half hours.

Positioning of the Baby During the Birth Process

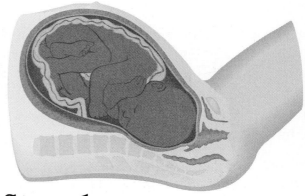

Stage 1:
Dilation of the Cervix

The third stage of labor is delivery of the placenta. The afterbirth is expelled during this stage. The **afterbirth** is the placenta and other membranes that support the fetus. This stage lasts about ten to thirty minutes.

Cesarean section is a surgical procedure in which the baby and the placenta are delivered through an incision in the abdominal wall and uterus. This procedure is used when the baby cannot be delivered through the vagina.

One minute after delivery, the baby's health is rated. The **Apgar score** is a scoring system to rate the health of a newborn baby. It grades heart rate, breathing rate, muscle tone, reflexes, and skin color.

The **postpartum period** is the six- to eight-week period after the birth of a baby. During this time, the mother's body releases a hormone. **Prolactin** is a hormone that causes the mammary glands in the mother's breasts to produce milk. The mother can nurse her baby. Breast-feeding gives the baby antibodies to fight infections. It helps the mother form a close emotional bond with her baby. A mother should not use any drugs, including alcohol and tobacco, while breast-feeding. Drugs can pass from the mother's breast milk to the infant. A mother infected with HIV should not breast-feed. HIV can pass to the baby in breast milk.

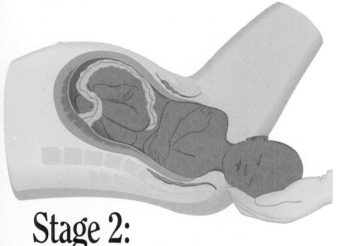

Stage 2:
Delivery of the Baby

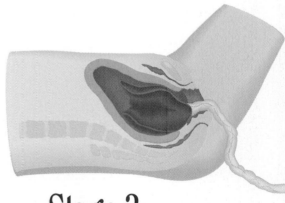

Stage 3:
Delivery of the Placenta

Practice Abstinence to Avoid Teen Pregnancy and Parenthood

Being physically able to reproduce does not mean a person is ready for parenthood. Teens who are sexually active risk becoming parents. Being a parent is an important and serious responsibility. Teens are not prepared to be responsible parents. It is important that you wisely consider the time you choose to become a parent. Become a parent only when you can healthfully meet the needs of a child. Parenthood can be very rewarding at the right time. Think about your behavior. You are not ready for parenthood.

Abstinence is the best choice for teens. Choosing not to be sexually active is the ONLY sure way not to become a parent.

Say NO!

Apply...
The Responsible Decision-Making Model™

You are at a football game with a person to whom you are attracted. (S)he tells you his or her older brother said both of you could use his or her car "for whatever you wanted" during the game. The car is parked far away from the football field in an unlighted area.

Answer the following questions on a separate sheet of paper. Write "Does not apply" if a question does not apply to this situation.

1. Is it healthful to go to the car with your friend? Why or why not?

2. Is it safe to go to the car with your friend? Why or why not?

3. Is it legal to go to the car with your friend? Why or why not?

4. Will you show respect for yourself and others if you go to the car with your friend? Why or why not?

5. Will your parents or guardian approve if you go to the car with your friend? Why or why not?

6. Will you demonstrate good character if you go to the car with your friend? Why or why not?

What is the responsible decision to make in this situation?

Lesson 13

Review

Vocabulary

Write a separate sentence using each of the vocabulary words listed on page 130.

Health Content

Write responses to the following:

1. Explain the process of conception. **page 131**

2. What is the function of the amniotic sac? **page 131**

3. What are signs of pregnancy? **page 132**

4. In what ways does a baby develop during the first, second, and third trimester of pregnancy? **page 133**

5. Why is prenatal care important? **page 134**

6. Why should a mother-to-be avoid alcohol during pregnancy? Avoid smoking? Limit caffeine consumption? **page 134**

7. What are three problems that can occur during pregnancy? **page 135**

8. What are the three stages of labor? **pages 136–137**

9. Describe the postpartum period. **page 137**

10. Why is abstinence the best choice for teens? **page 138**

Understanding the Stages in the Life Cycle

Vocabulary

adolescence

identity

developmental tasks

learning style

learning disability

Life Skills

- **I will provide responsible care for infants and children.**
- **I will achieve the developmental tasks of adolescence.**
- **I will develop my learning style.**

You have learned about the birth process and developed an appreciation that the baby will need care to grow and develop. What happens in each stage of development? What is happening at your stage of development? This lesson will help you understand the stages in the life cycle.

The Lesson Objectives

- Describe characteristics of each of the nine stages in the life cycle.
- State the most important challenge of adolescence.
- Identify the eight developmental tasks of adolescence.
- List six suggestions to improve learning.
- Discuss difficulties teens with learning disabilities might experience.

Stages in the Life Cycle

The life cycle has nine stages. At each stage, your experiences prepare you for the next stage. Knowledge and experience build from one stage to the next. You must master the challenges of the earlier stages before you are ready to deal with the challenges of the later stages.

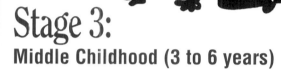

Stage 1:
Infancy (birth to 1 year)

The most rapid period of growth occurs in infancy. Infants grow rapidly and usually triple their birth weight. Other people must meet the needs of an infant. The infant depends on adults for food, clothing, and shelter. The infant learns adults are reliable if needs are met. The challenge of infancy is to learn to trust other people. Infants whose needs are not met are distrustful of others.

Stage 2:
Early Childhood (1 to 3 years)

The rate of growth is slower than in infancy. Children explore the environment with the help of adults. Adults teach them to stay safe. For example, adults teach children to keep their fingers away from electrical sockets. Children begin to mimic adults and say NO. They learn the importance of self-control. Children are toilet trained during early childhood. When they accomplish this task, they feel good about their efforts to gain self-control. The challenge of early childhood is to develop self-control. Children who do not master this challenge have self-doubts.

Stage 3:
Middle Childhood (3 to 6 years)

Children are very imaginative during middle childhood. They might pretend to read to a doll or to put out a fire with a toy fire truck. They act out their impressions of the adult world. Children also learn that they must make choices. Adults help them learn that some choices are better than others. Children learn best when adults impose appropriate consequences for misbehavior. The challenge of middle childhood is to develop a conscience. Children who do not master this challenge do not learn the difference between right and wrong.

Stage 4:
Late Childhood (6 to 12 years)

Children in late childhood have a great deal of physical and mental energy. They ask endless questions: "Why?" "How does this work?" "When can I do this?" Adults encourage mental growth when they are patient and answer questions. Children at this age explore their surroundings. They run, jump, and climb. They develop many new skills—reading, writing, and math at school; chores at home. Adults help children by giving them tasks to do their best. The challenge of late childhood is to feel capable. Children who do not master this challenge have negative self-esteem.

Stage 5:
Adolescence (12 to 18 years)

Adolescence is a physical, emotional, and social transition from childhood to adulthood. Adolescence is a period of rapid physical and emotional growth. Striking differences in growth and development occur among adolescents. Adolescents are aware of their maleness and femaleness. They gain reasoning skills. Adolescents experience different feelings about this period of rapid change. They attempt to accept their changing body and their sexuality. Adults can help adolescents by reassuring them. The challenge of adolescence is to develop identity. **Identity** is a sense of who one is. Adolescents who do not develop identity experience confusion.

Stage 6:
Transition to Adulthood (18 to 30 years)

Young adults strive to become independent of parents. The process of breaking away from parents has been prolonged by many young adults in recent years. One out of four young adults still lives with his or her parents. Young adults must develop skills needed to earn enough money to live on their own. During this stage, they seek a significant relationship with another young adult. This relationship is intended to be one that will provide for emotional needs. This is another move toward being more independent from parents. The challenge during the transition to adulthood is to leave home, support oneself, and form a significant relationship. Young adults who do not master this challenge continue to be dependent.

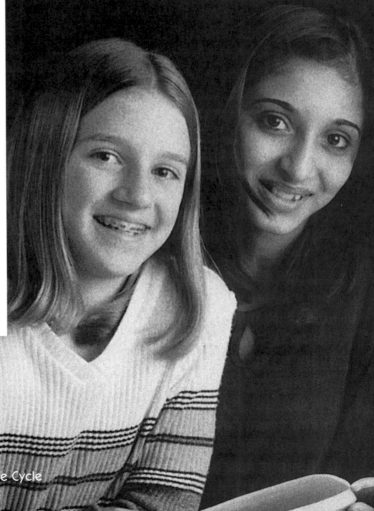

Stage 7:
First Adulthood (30 to 45 years)

Adults in first adulthood are very busy with family life and careers. Much energy is devoted to bringing up children. Decisions must be made about children's education. Organizing children's activities requires much effort and planning. Adults without children also spend time nurturing important relationships. Work is demanding during first adulthood. Adults set financial and achievement goals and work to reach them. The challenge of first adulthood is to balance the demands of relationships and family life with work. Adults who do not master this challenge feel frustrated.

Stage 8:
Second Adulthood (45 to 70 years)

Adults in second adulthood pause to review first adulthood and make adjustments. Family life changes as children mature and prepare to leave home. Adults examine the goals that were set for work. Some adults do not reach their goals. They must make adjustments to feel satisfied. Other adults reach their goals and ask, "What next?" In second adulthood, adults prepare for the years when they will retire or a spouse will retire. They become more interested in developing relationships with others. They also have an interest in the community. Adults often ponder: "What gives my life meaning?" "How will I be remembered by family and friends when I am gone?" "How can I make the world a better place for my grandchildren or for others who will survive me?" They strive to "give back" to others. The challenge of second adulthood for those with children is to focus energy in another direction. The challenge for those with and without children is to show a renewed interest in relationship to self, others, and community. Adults who do not master this challenge feel an emptiness.

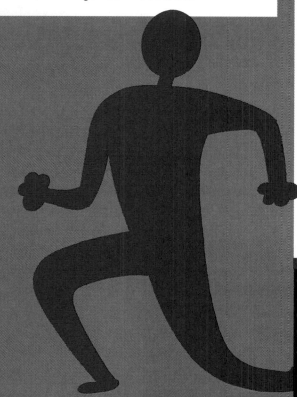

I will achieve the developmental tasks of adolescence.

I will achieve the developmental tasks of adolescence.

Stage 9:
Late Adulthood (70+ years)

It is difficult to state an age range for late adulthood. Several years ago, age 65 was the magic age when adults retired and eased into the golden years. Now some adults take early retirement and might leave the workplace as early as age 50. Others continue to work well into their seventies or beyond. The health status of family members, type of job, and amount of savings influence decision-making at this stage of life. Adults in late adulthood often make plans in case assistance is needed. They must address issues: "Will I (we) live with family?" "Will I (we) live in a nursing home?" "How might I care for a spouse?" Most adults care for themselves, but many become dependent on their children. Adult children might help their parents with decisions and provide care. Adults in late adulthood must come to terms with death. They grieve the loss of friends and loved ones who die. They grieve the eventual loss of their own lives. It is healthful for adults at this stage to share their feelings about death with family members. It also is healthful for family members to share feelings with older adults. The challenge of late adulthood is to feel satisfied with the way life has been lived and to accept death. Adults who do not master this challenge feel despair.

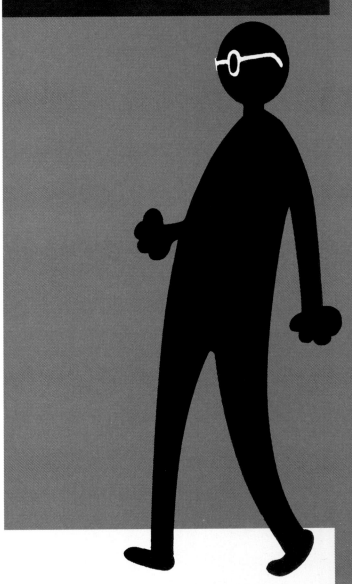

I will achieve the developmental tasks of adolescence.

The Gift of Good Health

Do you have something in your future to which you look forward? Perhaps you look forward to a ball game? Perhaps you look forward to a social event? Did you know that older people stay healthier if they look forward to something? Suppose you have grandparents who are living. Suppose you have a family friend who is in late adulthood. Give him or her a special gift. Think of something you can share that will happen in the future. You might ask the person to go somewhere with you. Suppose you have a grandparent who cannot go places. Talk about something you will do in the future. Explain that you want to take pictures and share them.

Developmental Tasks of Adolescence

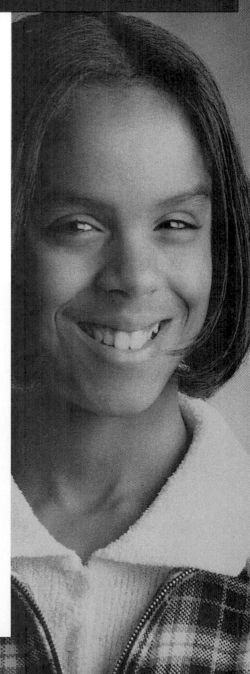

You just learned about the challenges of each of the different stages in the life cycle. Your energy must be focused on meeting the challenges of the stage you are in right now. The challenge of adolescence is to develop identity. Certain tasks must be accomplished to have a sense of who you are. **Developmental tasks** are achievements that need to be mastered as a person grows toward maturity. Eight developmental tasks for adolescence have been identified.

Give thought to each of these important tasks. Are you working on each of the eight tasks? Are some of these tasks more difficult for you than others? Who are the caring adults who might help you achieve these tasks?

Task 1: Having healthful friendships with members of both sexes

Task 2: Being comfortable with your maleness and femaleness

Task 3: Being comfortable with your body

Task 4: Gaining skills that will help you be independent from your parents and other adults

Task 5: Learning skills that you can use later if you marry and become a parent

Task 6: Learning skills that help you get a job and earn money

Task 7: Having a clear set of values to guide your behavior

Task 8: Developing a social conscience

Follow a...

Health Behavior Contract

Copy the health behavior contract on a separate sheet of paper.

DO NOT WRITE IN THIS BOOK.

Name: _____ **Date:** _____

Life Skill: I will develop my learning style.

Effect On My Health: **Learning style** is the way a person acquires basic skills. During adolescence, I need to develop my learning style so that I can learn new skills. Learning new skills will help me achieve the developmental tasks of adolescence.

My Plan: I will keep a journal in which I list tips to help me study and learn.

1. I will choose a quiet place to study.
2. I will set aside time each day to study.
3. I will keep a dictionary, thesaurus, and other reference tools nearby.
4. I will make a checklist of my homework assignments and check off each assignment I complete.
5. I will rewrite class notes.
6. I will ask for help when I do not understand something.

I will complete the calendar to show when and for how long I study each day for a week.

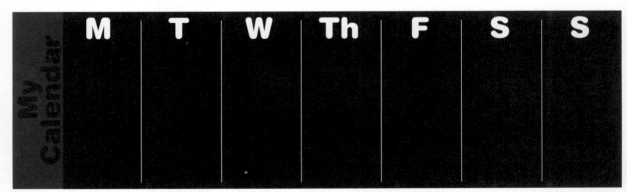

	M	T	W	Th	F	S	S
My Calendar							

How My Plan Worked: (Complete after one week.) I will ask myself, "Did I feel more prepared for my classes?" And "Did I see an improvement in my grades?" If the answers are yes, I will continue my plan. If one or both answers are no, I will ask my parents or guardian to help me follow my plan more effectively.

Learning Styles

Learning style involves your ability to perceive and process sights and sounds, to concentrate, and to remember. Some people need extra help with learning. A **learning disability** is a disorder that causes a person to have difficulty learning. The disorder might be due to physical or psychological causes. Some people cannot understand time and sequence. They have difficulty following directions.

Others change the order of letters and numbers. They have difficulty working math problems and reading. Still other people have difficulty with their attention span. They have difficulty concentrating. Help is available for people who struggle to learn. Tutors are available to help with class assignments and homework. Schools might have special classes for students with learning needs. Classmates and friends can be sensitive and patient. Having a plan for learning and helping others learn is part of being mature.

Lesson 14

Review

Vocabulary

Write a separate sentence using each of the vocabulary words listed on page 140.

Health Content

Write responses to the following:

1. What are characteristics of each of the nine stages in the life cycle? **pages 141–144**

2. What is the most important challenge of adolescence? **page 145**

3. What are the eight developmental tasks of adolescence? **page 145**

4. What are six suggestions to improve learning? **page 146**

5. What are difficulties teens with learning disabilities might experience? **page 147**

Aging, Dying, and Death

Vocabulary

chronological age

biological age

social age

chronic disease

dementia

Alzheimer's disease

terminal illness

five stages of dying

grief

Life Skills

- **I will develop habits that promote healthful aging.**
- **I will share with my family my feelings about dying and death.**

People are living longer and healthier lives today. The average female who is 50, and who does not develop cancer or heart disease, can expect to live to the age of 92. The average healthy male who is 65, and who does not develop cancer or heart disease, can expect to live until the age of 81. Eight in ten people will be healthy past their sixty-fifth birthday. Heredity, the quality of medical care, and health habits influence the aging process.

The Lesson Objectives

- Explain how practicing healthful habits now will help you age in a healthful way.
- List the ten secrets of healthful aging.
- Discuss physical changes, mental conditions, and social needs of people as they age.
- Describe the five stages of dying.
- Identify ways you can comfort someone who is grieving.

Aging

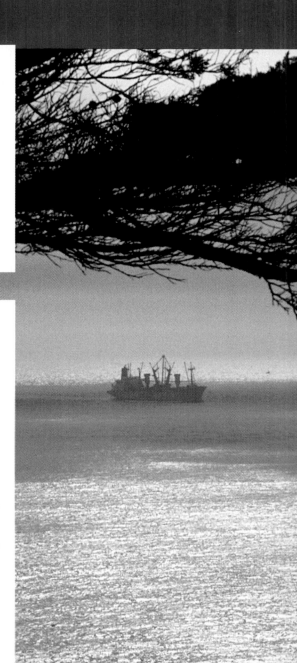

People might use several measures to determine age. **Chronological age** is the number of years a person has lived. **Biological age** is a measure of how well a person's body parts are functioning. Heredity and health habits, such as diet and exercise, influence biological age. The quality of health care a person has received also influences biological age. **Social age** is a measure of a person's involvement in leisure activities. Health habits influence social age. Spending time with others and participating in different activities help a person stay young.

Aging in a Healthful Way

Heredity, the quality of medical care, and health habits influence the aging process. You cannot control or change your heredity. However, you can make some choices with regard to medical care. You do have control over your health habits.

The health habits you practice today will influence how well you age in later years. Teens who practice healthful behaviors most likely will continue these behaviors in adulthood. Teens who practice risk behaviors might continue risk behaviors into adulthood. These teens might intend to stop risk behaviors, but they might have difficulty. They also might harm their health during the teen years. For example, suppose you know a teen who smokes cigarettes. This teen might say, "I'll quit smoking later." The nicotine in cigarette smoke is highly addictive. The younger a person is when he or she begins smoking, the more likely the person will not quit. This teen also harms his or her health right away. Smoking cigarettes during the teen years increases heart rate and blood pressure. It stains teeth and causes bad breath. Take care of your health now and plan to age in a healthful way. Practice the Ten Secrets of Healthful Aging.

Ten Secrets of Healthful Aging

1. Eat a healthful, balanced breakfast each day.

2. Follow the Dietary Guidelines.

3. Exercise regularly.

4. Do not smoke or use other tobacco products.

5. Get plenty of rest and sleep.

6. Have regular medical checkups.

7. Balance work with play.

8. Choose activities to keep your mind alert.

9. Develop healthful relationships with family and friends.

10. Manage your stress.

Physical and Mental Aging

Many physical changes can be seen as a person ages. Some of these changes begin as early as the twenties or thirties. Wrinkled skin might appear. Hair might become gray.

Not all signs of physical aging can be seen. Changes that take place inside a person's body are called internal changes. The heart, blood vessels, and lungs change. The heart does not pump as efficiently when a person reaches late adulthood. The lungs do not hold the same volume of air as in earlier years. A person's reaction time is slower. The body's sense organs become less sensitive with age.

Chronic diseases are more common as a person ages. A **chronic disease** is an illness that develops and lasts over a long period of time. Some chronic diseases that affect people as they age are heart disease, cancer, arthritis, and high blood pressure. Often, these diseases are present because of health habits in the earlier years rather than the aging process. Practice healthful habits right now.

Most people remain mentally alert as they age. This is especially true if they are active—reading books, working crossword puzzles, solving problems. Some people have problems with the thinking process as they age.

Dementia is a condition in which thinking and memory are not sharp. Signs of dementia include a short attention span, memory loss, inability to solve math problems, and difficulty with time and place. Dementia can cause personality changes. People with this condition might be irritated easily and confused.

Alzheimer's disease is a disease characterized by progressive loss of memory and mental function. A person with this disease will lose control of body functions over time. Alzheimer's disease is fatal. The exact cause is unknown but might be related to a person's genetic background.

Vitamin E and Alzheimer's Disease

Health experts continue to do research on Alzheimer's disease. They are studying ways to improve memory and mental function as people age. They are studying ways to slow the progression of the disease. Some health experts have suggested that vitamin E offers some benefits. Studies are being conducted in which family members of people with Alzheimer's disease take 400 I.U. of vitamin E.

Social Aging

People need to remain socially active as they age. Spending time with others helps improve physical and mental aging. Older people need friends with whom to talk; someone to give them love; someone to listen to them; someone with whom to do things; someone with whom to go places; time to be alone; and opportunities to make decisions.

Older people who do not have these needs fulfilled might experience sadness. Sadness and depression can occur when a spouse or aging friends die. New friends and social relationships are needed.

Having a pet also can provide companionship for an older person. Suppose an older person had been a caregiver. This person might have cared for a spouse. If the spouse dies, the caregiver has a void. A puppy or kitten can fill this void. The older person must care for the puppy or kitten.

Dying and Death

Dying and death are a natural part of the life cycle. Perhaps you have already experienced the death of a loved one. You might have had many different feelings. Someone you know might have died unexpectedly. Or someone you know might have had an illness, and you might have known that the person was dying.

A **terminal illness** is an illness that is incurable and will cause death. People who have a terminal illness have many feelings as they face death. Dr. Elisabeth Kübler-Ross, a psychiatrist, identified five stages of dying. The **five stages of dying** are stages of dying that include denial, anger, bargaining, depression, and acceptance. People do not always go through the five stages in the same order. Some might skip a stage, return to a stage, or remain stuck in a stage.

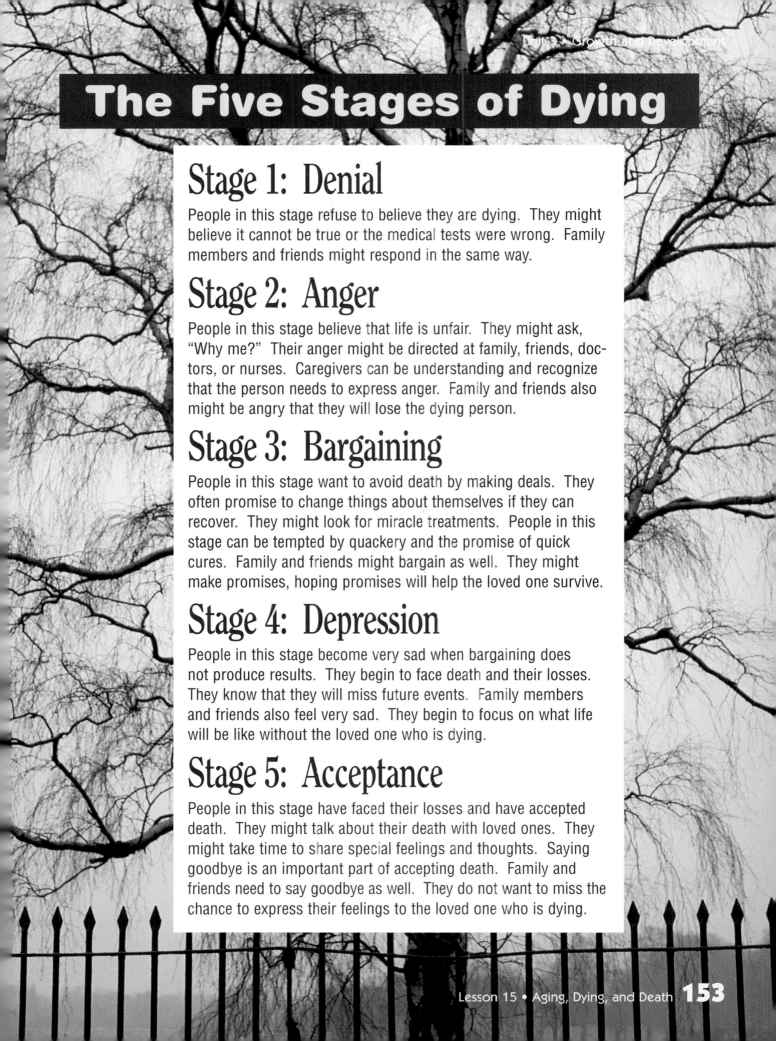

The Five Stages of Dying

Stage 1: Denial

People in this stage refuse to believe they are dying. They might believe it cannot be true or the medical tests were wrong. Family members and friends might respond in the same way.

Stage 2: Anger

People in this stage believe that life is unfair. They might ask, "Why me?" Their anger might be directed at family, friends, doctors, or nurses. Caregivers can be understanding and recognize that the person needs to express anger. Family and friends also might be angry that they will lose the dying person.

Stage 3: Bargaining

People in this stage want to avoid death by making deals. They often promise to change things about themselves if they can recover. They might look for miracle treatments. People in this stage can be tempted by quackery and the promise of quick cures. Family and friends might bargain as well. They might make promises, hoping promises will help the loved one survive.

Stage 4: Depression

People in this stage become very sad when bargaining does not produce results. They begin to face death and their losses. They know that they will miss future events. Family members and friends also feel very sad. They begin to focus on what life will be like without the loved one who is dying.

Stage 5: Acceptance

People in this stage have faced their losses and have accepted death. They might talk about their death with loved ones. They might take time to share special feelings and thoughts. Saying goodbye is an important part of accepting death. Family and friends need to say goodbye as well. They do not want to miss the chance to express their feelings to the loved one who is dying.

Expressing Grief

You might experience grief after the death of someone. **Grief** is the discomfort caused by the death of another person. Grief is a normal reaction to a death. You might have had time to prepare for the death. Yet you still feel a deep sense of loss and sadness. Talking about these feelings with caring adults, such as your parents or guardian, is helpful.

An unexpected death can be more difficult. The stages discussed might be experienced. You might feel very numb and be in a state of denial. You might feel very angry. Why would someone you care about die? You might feel very depressed. Working through your feelings with adults to gain acceptance is helpful. Suppose you have a friend who is grieving. You might want to comfort your friend.

Four Ways to Comfort Someone Who Is Grieving

1. Do something thoughtful for the person. Make a phone call, send a card, or offer help, such as doing errands.

2. Be a good listener. Make yourself available to talk. Simply being a good friend is important.

3. Do not try to lessen the loss. Avoid saying things such as, "Time heals all wounds." Instead, say, "I am sorry that you feel sad."

4. Allow the person to express feelings.

Memories

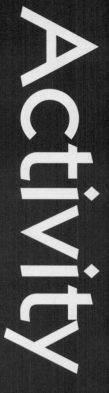

Life Skill

I will share with my family my feelings about dying and death.

Materials: Paper, pen or pencil

Directions: A good philosophy to live by is to live each day as if it were your last. In this activity, you will write a poem to express how you can make each day count.

1. **Suppose tomorrow is the last day you will live.** How would you want people to think of you after you are gone? List five to ten things you would want people to remember about you. You might write, "I let my parents know I appreciated them," or "I was kind to my friend when he or she was down."

2. **Compose a poem titled "I'll Make This Day Count."** Write it yourself or work with a partner. Include actions you can take now that would cause your family and friends to have loving memories of you.

3. **Share the poem with your family.**

Lesson 15

Review

Vocabulary

Write a separate sentence using each of the vocabulary words listed on page 148.

Health Content

Write responses to the following:

1. What are three factors that influence the aging process? **page 148**

2. What are three measures people might use to determine age? **page 149**

3. How can health habits teens practice influence how they age in later years? **page 149**

4. What are the Ten Secrets of Healthful Aging? **page 150**

5. What are signs of physical aging? **page 151**

6. What are four chronic diseases that might affect people as they age? **page 151**

7. What are two conditions that might affect the thinking process in older people? **page 151**

8. What are seven social needs of older people? **page 152**

9. What are the five stages of dying? **page 153**

10. What are four ways to comfort someone who is grieving? **page 154**

Unit 3 Review

Health Content

Review your answers for each Lesson Review in this unit. Then write answers to each of the following questions.

1. Why can you not get HIV or other viruses when you give blood? **Lesson 11 page 100**

2. What actions can you take to prevent low back pain? **Lesson 11 page 107**

3. How would you describe the path of an unfertilized egg through the female reproductive system? **Lesson 12 page 121**

4. How can a male take care of his reproductive system? **Lesson 12 page 127**

5. How might a female know she is pregnant? **Lesson 13 page 132**

6. What happens during the postpartum period? **Lesson 13 page 137**

7. What kinds of behaviors are shown by children ages three to six years? **Lesson 14 page 141**

8. What are characteristics of adolescence? **Lesson 14 page 142**

9. How are the three measures of aging different? **Lesson 15 page 149**

10. What are some ways people physically age? **Lesson 15 page 151**

Vocabulary

Number a sheet of paper from 1–10. Select the correct vocabulary word. Write it next to the corresponding number. DO NOT WRITE IN THIS BOOK.

amniotic sac	learning disability
cerebrum	pituitary gland
Cowper's glands	placenta
digestive system	terminal illness
endocrine system	ureter

1. The _____ is a gland that produces hormones that control other glands. **Lesson 12**

2. The _____ is an organ that attaches the egg to the inner wall of the uterus. **Lesson 13**

3. _____ are glands that secrete a clear, lubricating fluid. **Lesson 12**

4. The _____ is the body system that breaks down food so that nutrients can be used by the body. **Lesson 11**

5. A(n) _____ is a disorder that causes a person to have difficulty learning. **Lesson 14**

6. The _____ is the body system that consists of glands that produce hormones. **Lesson 12**

7. A(n) _____ is an illness that is incurable and will cause death. **Lesson 15**

8. The _____ is a thin membrane filled with fluid in which the developing baby floats. **Lesson 13**

9. The _____ is a narrow tube that connects the kidney to the bladder. **Lesson 11**

10. The _____ is the part of the brain that controls the ability to memorize, think, and learn. **Lesson 11**

The Responsible Decision-Making Model™

One of the students in your learning group of four students has a learning disability. This student has difficulty completing some of the tasks your group was assigned. Another student is annoyed and tries to persuade everyone else in the group to ignore this student.

1. Is it healthful to ignore the student with the learning disability? Why or why not?

2. Is it safe to ignore the student with the learning disability? Why or why not?

3. Is it legal to ignore the student with the learning disability? Why or why not?

4. Will you show respect for yourself and others if you ignore the student with the learning disability? Why or why not?

5. Will your parents or guardian approve if you ignore the student with the learning disability? Why or why not?

6. Will you demonstrate good character if you ignore the student with the learning disability? Why or why not?

What is the responsible decision to make in this situation?

Health Literacy

Effective Communication

Write a short article for your school newspaper about the importance of being screened for scoliosis. Use sources of information from this textbook and from additional sources in the library.

Self-Directed Learning

Select ten vocabulary words from this unit. Search for each of the vocabulary words online in a medical dictionary.

Critical Thinking

Rank order the eight developmental tasks of adolescence. Begin with the one you believe to be most important.

Responsible Citizenship

Volunteer to help a student with a learning disability in your classroom. Help this person with homework or to study for a test.

Multicultural Health

In some cultures, physicians assist in the majority of births. In other cultures, midwives are more common. Research birthing practices in your own and another culture. How are they alike and different?

Family Involvement

Share the list of the Ten Secrets of Healthful Aging with your family. Ask your parents or guardian for additional items to add to this list.

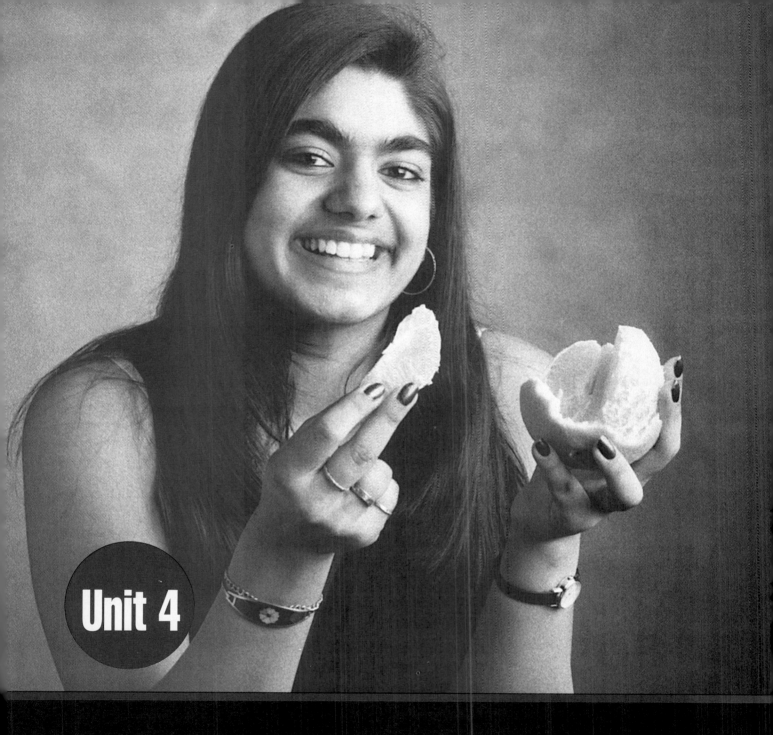

Nutrition

Power Eating

Vocabulary

power eating
nutrient
calorie
protein
amino acids
essential amino acids
complete proteins
incomplete proteins
carbohydrates
simple carbohydrates
complex carbohydrates
fiber
fats
saturated fats
cholesterol
unsaturated fats
water
vitamins
fat-soluble vitamins
water-soluble vitamins
minerals
Food Guide Pyramid

Life Skills

- **I will select foods that contain nutrients.**
- **I will eat the recommended number of servings from the Food Guide Pyramid.**

There is much truth to the saying "You are what you eat." You are at your best when you choose power eating. **Power eating** is eating the appropriate number of servings of food needed for optimal health.

The Lesson Objectives

- Identify the functions of each of the six basic classes of nutrients.
- Give examples of foods that contain each of the six basic classes of nutrients.
- Illustrate the Food Guide Pyramid showing the five basic food groups and the number of servings needed each day.
- Identify examples of foods and the nutrients that can be obtained from each of the five basic food groups.

The Six Basic Classes of Nutrients

Proteins   **Carbohydrates**

Fats   **Water**

Vitamins   **Minerals**

A **nutrient** (NOO·tree·ent) is a chemical substance in foods that:

- **builds, repairs, and maintains body tissues;**
- **regulates body processes;**
- **and provides energy (measured in calories).**

A **calorie** is a unit of measure for both the energy supplied by food and the energy used by the body. The six basic classes of nutrients are: proteins, carbohydrates, fats, water, vitamins, and minerals.

In this lesson, you will learn why you need each of the six nutrients for optimal health. You will learn the function of each of the six nutrients. Then you will learn which foods and beverages contain each of the six nutrients.

Most foods and beverages contain more than one kind of nutrient. For example, milk is a power beverage. A power food or beverage contains several nutrients that are needed for good health. Milk has protein and fat in it. Milk also contains vitamins and minerals. This lesson will give you facts that help you choose power foods and beverages.

Proteins

A **protein** is a nutrient needed to build, repair, and maintain body tissues. Proteins form parts of muscles, bones, blood, cell membranes, and hormones. Proteins are needed to maintain strength and resist infection. They also provide energy. Each gram of protein provides four calories.

Amino acids are the building blocks that make up proteins. The body needs 20 different amino acids. Body cells can produce 11 amino acids. **Essential amino acids** are the nine amino acids the body cannot produce. You can get these amino acids only from the foods you eat. **Complete proteins** are proteins from animal sources that contain all of the essential amino acids. Meat, fish, chicken, turkey, milk, yogurt, and eggs are examples of sources of complete proteins. **Incomplete proteins** are proteins from plant sources that do not contain all of the essential amino acids. Nuts, seeds, and beans are examples of sources of incomplete proteins. Incomplete proteins contain different amino acids. By eating certain combinations of incomplete protein sources, it is possible to get all of the essential amino acids you need for good health.

Carbohydrates

Carbohydrates are nutrients that provide energy to the body. Each gram of carbohydrate provides four calories. **Simple carbohydrates** are sugars that enter the bloodstream rapidly and provide quick energy. Fruits and honey are sources of simple carbohydrates. **Complex carbohydrates** are starches. Starches provide long-lasting energy. Plant foods, such as rice, wheat, and oats, are good sources of complex carbohydrates.

Fiber is the part of grains and plant foods that cannot be digested. Wheat, bran, cereals, fruits, and vegetables are good sources of fiber. Fiber provides no calories because it is undigested. However, fiber helps move waste products through the digestive tract. When you have a bowel movement, you rid your digestive system of solid wastes.

Fats

Fats are nutrients that are a source of energy and make certain vitamins available for use in the body. Fats are stored as fat tissue that surrounds and cushions internal organs such as the heart and kidneys. Each gram of fat provides nine calories.

Two types of fats are saturated fats and unsaturated fats. **Saturated fats** are fats from dairy products, solid vegetable fats, and animal products. Saturated fats contribute to your blood cholesterol level. **Cholesterol** (kuh·LES·tuh·rawl) is a fat-like substance made by the body and found in many foods. Meat, milk products, and egg yolks are sources of cholesterol. While your body needs a certain amount of cholesterol, a high blood cholesterol level is a risk factor for heart disease.

Unsaturated fats are fats from fish and plant products. Some unsaturated fats, such as corn oil, are liquid at room temperature. Unsaturated fats do not pose the same risk for heart disease as do saturated fats.

Water

Water is a nutrient that:

- **makes up a part of blood;**
- **helps the process of digestion;**
- **helps remove body wastes;**
- **regulates body temperature;**
- **and cushions the spinal cord and joints.**

You need about two liters (six to eight glasses) of water each day. You can get this amount from drinking water and other liquids, and from eating a variety of foods. Your body loses water in the form of perspiration and urine.

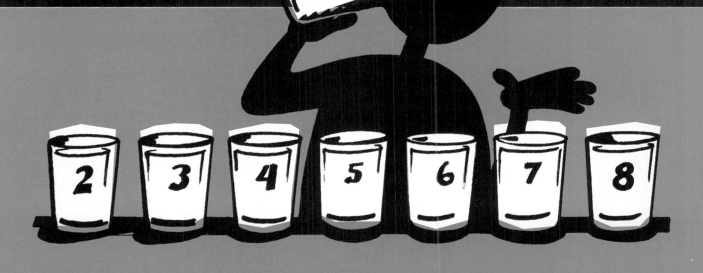

Vitamins

Vitamins are nutrients that help chemical reactions take place in the body. Vitamins do not supply energy (calories), but they are needed to release the energy from fats and carbohydrates. **Fat-soluble vitamins** are vitamins that can be stored in the body. They include vitamins A, D, E, and K. **Water-soluble vitamins** are vitamins that cannot be stored by the body in significant amounts. They are found in the watery parts of foods. Vitamin B_1 and vitamin C are examples of water-soluble vitamins. You need a source of these vitamins each day.

Today there is much interest in vitamins. *The Recommended Dietary Allowances* gives the amounts of vitamins you need for good health. You can find a copy of this chart in a nutrition book. Your physician and school nurse have a copy. The chart is a general guide. If you have a special condition, your physician might change the amounts you take.

You might read articles or listen to news reports on the benefits of a specific vitamin. The results of a study might be mentioned. The study might say that a vitamin helps prevent heart disease. It might say that the vitamin helps with memory. People in the study might have taken large amounts of a vitamin. They took more than the amount normally recommended. Be careful. Talk with your physician before taking large amounts of a vitamin.

Vitamins

Vitamin	Functions	Sources	Deficiencies
A **Retinol**	Helps skin form mucus Helps night vision	Carrots, sweet potatoes, yams, green leafy vegetables	Dry mucous membranes Night blindness
C **Ascorbic Acid**	Forms a substance that holds cells together Strengthens blood vessels Helps resist infection	Broccoli, oranges, grapefruit, tomatoes, strawberries	Frequent bruising Loose teeth Gum disease
B₁ **Thiamine**	Helps body use carbohydrates Promotes healthy nervous system	Lean pork, nuts, fortified cereals, peas, beans, rice, pasta	Muscle weakness Leg cramps Mental confusion
B₂ **Riboflavin**	Helps release energy from foods Promotes healthy nervous system	Liver, milk, yogurt, cottage cheese	Vision problems Skin problems Sore red tongue
B₃ **Niacin**	Helps the body use energy Promotes healthy skin and nerves	Liver, meat, poultry, fish, peanuts, fortified cereal	Abnormal liver function High blood sugar
B₆ **Pyridoxine**	Helps the body absorb protein Helps body use fats Helps form blood cells	Whole-grain cereals, red meats, liver, legumes	Poor growth Anemia Convulsions Kidney, liver, skin damage
B₁₂ **Cobalamin**	Helps form red blood cells Helps nervous system	Liver, meat, fish, eggs, milk, oysters	Anemia Nerve damage
D **Calciferol**	Helps the body use calcium and phosphorus for healthy bones and teeth	Fortified dairy products, fish liver oils, egg yolks, salmon	Rickets (bowed legs) Poor teeth Soft bones
E	Helps maintain normal cell structure Helps form red blood cells	Vegetable oils, almonds, eggs, whole-grain cereals, green leafy vegetables	Destruction of red blood cells Anemia

Minerals

Minerals are nutrients that regulate many chemical reactions in the body. Major minerals are found in the body in amounts larger than five grams. Trace minerals are minerals found in the body in amounts less than five grams. Five percent of your body weight is made up of minerals. You need a small amount of many minerals in your diet each day.

Minerals

Mineral	Functions	Sources	Deficiencies
Calcium	Strengthens teeth and bones Helps blood clot Helps muscles contract and relax Helps nerves send signals	Milk, yogurt, cheese, collards, kale, turnip, mustard greens	Rickets (bowed legs) Osteoporosis (thin bones)
Iron	Helps body use energy Forms part of red blood cells	Prune juice, liver, dried beans, peas, red meat	Fatigue Anemia Poor concentration
Magnesium	Helps fight depression Helps prevent heart attack Promotes healthy teeth and bones	Grapefruit, lemons, nuts, seeds, apples, dark green vegetables	Nervousness Depression Unable to sleep Sensitive to noise Nerve and muscle damage
Phosphorus	Promotes growth and repair of cells Helps use starches Promotes healthy gums and teeth	Eggs, nuts, fish, poultry, meat, whole grains	Rickets (bowed legs)
Potassium	Reduces blood pressure Maintains heart rhythm Helps in waste removal	Orange juice, citrus fruits, green leafy vegetables, bananas	Low blood sugar Edema (retaining water) Abnormal heartbeat Muscle weakness
Sodium	Prevents heat exhaustion Aids in proper nerve and muscle function	Table salt, shellfish, meats, eggs, poultry	Difficulty in digestion of carbohydrates Muscle weakness

The Food Guide Pyramid

Foods that contain the same nutrients belong to a food group. The **Food Guide Pyramid** is daily guidelines for the number of servings of each major food group. The number of servings that are best for you depends upon your age, sex, size, and level of activity.

Examine the Food Guide Pyramid. A balanced diet includes foods from the five basic food groups. Each of these food groups provides some of the nutrients you should have each day. The foods that should be eaten in the largest amounts are at the bottom of the pyramid. Foods that should be eaten in lesser amounts are at the top of the pyramid.

The Food Guide Pyramid

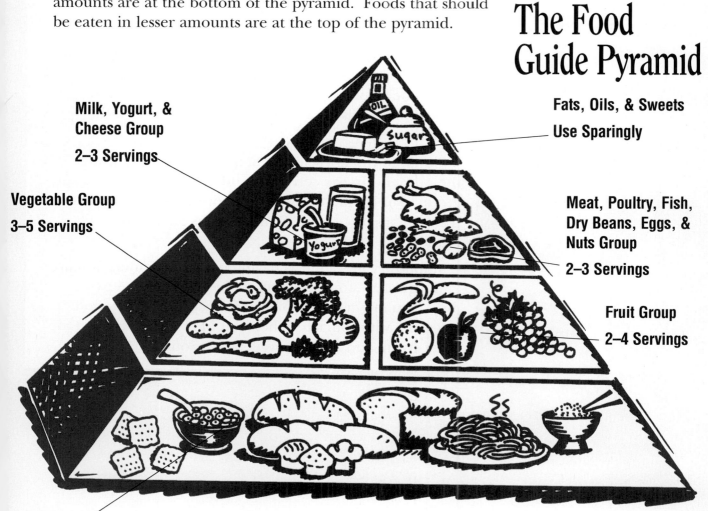

Milk, Yogurt, & Cheese Group

2–3 Servings

Vegetable Group

3–5 Servings

Fats, Oils, & Sweets

Use Sparingly

Meat, Poultry, Fish, Dry Beans, Eggs, & Nuts Group

2–3 Servings

Fruit Group

2–4 Servings

Bread, Cereal, Rice, & Pasta Group

6–11 Servings

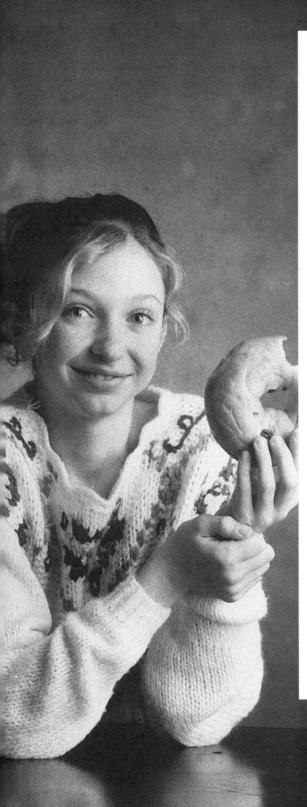

Bread, Cereal, Rice, and Pasta Group

The bread, cereal, rice, and pasta group contains grain products. This food group provides complex carbohydrates, vitamins, and minerals. You need 6 to 11 servings from this food group each day. One serving might include one of the following:

- **1 slice of bread**
- **1 ounce of ready-to-eat cereal**
- **1/2 cup of rice or pasta**

Select power foods as choices for servings from this food group. Remember, a power food has several nutrients in it. You get added benefits. For example, suppose you eat at a fast food restaurant. You order a chicken sandwich. The sandwich comes on a white bun or a whole wheat bun. Select the whole wheat bun. This bun contains more B vitamins. It also is a better source of fiber than the white bun.

Suppose you are selecting a box of cereal. Consider the nutrients in the cereal that do not belong to the grain group. For example, granola has dried fruits in it. The fruits are a source of vitamins. Raisins have vitamin C in them.

Suppose your family is having pasta for dinner. You are at the grocery store selecting the noodles for the pasta dish. You might select spinach fettuccini. These noodles are made with spinach. Then you have nutrients from the pasta group and from the vegetable group.

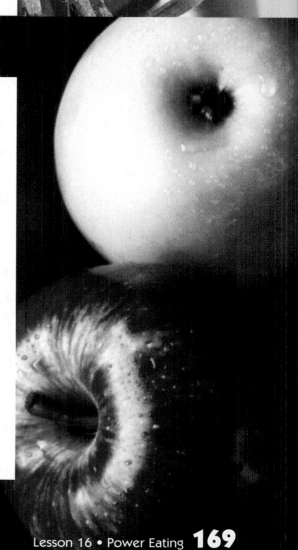

Vegetable Group

The vegetable group provides carbohydrates, vitamins and minerals. This group is low in fat and provides fiber. Vegetables differ in the amount of nutrients they provide, so it is important to eat a variety. You need three to five servings of vegetables each day. One serving might include one of the following:

- **1 cup of raw leafy vegetables**
- **1/2 cup of cooked or raw vegetables**
- **3/4 cup of vegetable juice**

To protect vitamins and minerals in fresh vegetables, eat the vegetables soon after buying them. Do not overcook them. Eating them raw or lightly steamed can help protect the vitamin and mineral content.

Fruit Group

The fruit group provides carbohydrates. It also provides important amounts of vitamins A and C, as well as the mineral potassium. Fruits are low in fat and sodium. You need two to four servings of fruits each day. One serving might include one of the following:

- **1 medium apple**
- **1 banana or orange**
- **1/2 cup of chopped, cooked, or canned fruit**
- **3/4 cup of 100 percent fruit juice**

Only fruit juices that are 100 percent fruit should be counted as a serving. Other fruit drinks, "ades," and punches contain very little fruit juice. They are mostly water and sugar. Use caution when eating canned and frozen fruits. Avoid those that are packed in heavy sauces or syrups that are high in sugar.

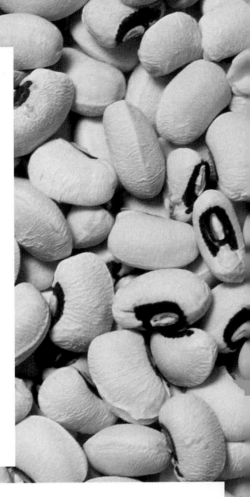

Meat, Poultry, Fish, Dry Beans, Eggs, and Nuts Group

This food group provides protein, B vitamins, and the minerals iron and zinc. You need two to three servings from this food group each day. One serving might include one of the following:

- **2 to 3 ounces of cooked lean meat, poultry, or fish**
- **1/2 cup of cooked dry beans**
- **1 egg**
- **2 tablespoons of peanut butter**

Use caution when making choices from this food group. To lower fat intake, choose lean meat, poultry without skin, fish, and dry beans and peas. Broil, roast, or boil foods rather than frying them. Limit egg yolks to no more than four per week because they are high in cholesterol. Limit nuts and seeds because they have a high fat content.

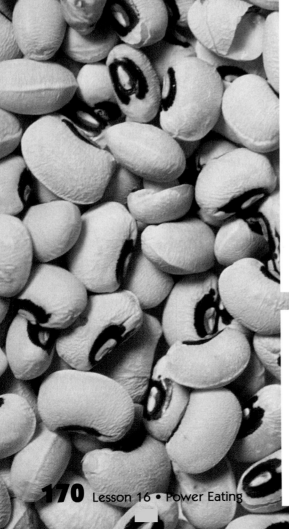

Milk, Yogurt, and Cheese Group

Milk products provide protein, vitamins, and minerals such as calcium. You need two to three servings from this food group each day. One serving might include one of the following:

- **1 cup of milk**
- **1 1/2 ounces of natural cheese**
- **2 ounces of processed cheese**

Choose milk products that provide calcium yet limit fat. Drink skim or nonfat milk, eat low-fat cheese, and use low-fat or nonfat yogurt.

Fats, Oils, and Sweets

This food group includes foods such as salad dressings and oils, cream, butter, margarine, sugars, soft drinks, candies, and sweet desserts. These foods provide few vitamins and minerals. They are high in fats and sugars that contribute to weight gain. For good health, you should limit the amounts of fats, oils, and sweets you eat.

Food Facts for You

Pyramid Food Group	Servings/Day	Sources	Nutrients
Milk, Yogurt, and Cheese	**2–3**	1 cup milk 1 cup yogurt 2 oz. cheese	Protein Calcium Vitamins A&D
Meat, Poultry, Fish, Dry Beans, Eggs, and Nuts	**2–3**	2–3 oz. lean meat 2–3 oz. fish 2–3 oz. poultry	Protein Zinc Iron B vitamins
Fruit	**2–4**	1 piece of fruit 1/2 cup canned fruit 3/4 cup juice	Carbohydrates Vitamins A&C Potassium
Vegetables	**3–5**	1 cup raw vegetables 1/2 cup raw vegetables 1 medium potato	Carbohydrates Fiber, iron Beta-carotene Vitamin A B vitamins Magnesium
Bread, Cereal, Rice and Pasta	**6–11**	1 slice bread 1 oz. cereal 1/2 cup rice or pasta	Carbohydrates B vitamins Iron, zinc, fiber

Follow a...
Health Behavior Contract

Copy the health behavior contract on a separate sheet of paper.

DO NOT WRITE IN THIS BOOK.

Name: _____ Date: _____

Life Skill: I will eat the recommended number of servings from the Food Guide Pyramid.

Effect On My Health: I will get energy, vitamins, and minerals by eating 6–11 servings per day from the bread, cereal, rice, and pasta group. I will get energy, vitamins, minerals, and fiber by eating 3–5 servings per day from the vegetable group and 2–4 servings per day from the fruit group. I will get protein, vitamins, and minerals by eating 2–3 servings per day from the meat, poultry, fish, dry beans, eggs, and nuts group and from the milk, yogurt, and cheese group.

My Plan: I will eat a variety of foods from each of the five food groups. In my journal, I will list foods from each group. I will write those foods on my calendar when I eat them. I will keep a calendar for a week.

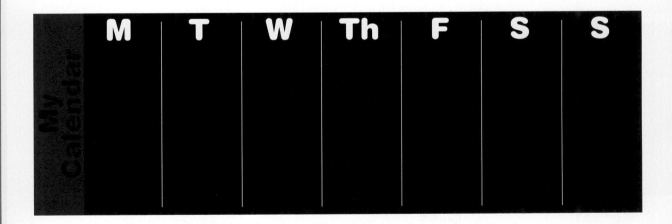

My Calendar	M	T	W	Th	F	S	S

How My Plan Worked: (Complete after one week.) I will ask myself if I ate the foods and number of servings recommended on the Food Guide Pyramid.

Lesson 16

Review

Vocabulary

Write a separate sentence using each of the vocabulary words listed on page 160.

Health Content

Write responses to the following:

1. What are the functions of each of the six basic classes of nutrients? **pages 162–166**

2. What are foods that contain each of the six basic classes of nutrients? **pages 162–166**

3. What is the difference between complete proteins and incomplete proteins? **page 162**

4. What are foods that contain proteins? **page 162**

5. How are simple carbohydrates different from complex carbohydrates? **page 162**

6. What are foods that contain carbohydrates? **page 162**

7. Why is fiber needed for optimal health? **page 162**

8. What are foods that contain fiber? **page 162**

9. How are saturated fats different from unsaturated fats? **page 163**

10. What are foods that contain fats? **page 163**

11. What are foods that are high in cholesterol? **page 163**

12. What are sources of water? **page 163**

13. How are water-soluble vitamins different from fat-soluble vitamins? **page 164**

14. What are the functions, sources, and deficiencies for vitamins A, C, B_1, B_2, B_3, B_6, B_{12}, D and E? **page 165**

15. What are the functions, sources, and deficiencies for calcium, iron, magnesium, phosphorus, potassium, and sodium? **page 166**

16. Explain how to use the Food Guide Pyramid. **page 167**

17. Illustrate the Food Guide Pyramid showing the five basic food groups, examples of foods in each, and the number of servings needed each day. **page 167**

18. What are ways to protect vitamins and minerals in fresh vegetables? **page 169**

19. What are guidelines for choosing foods from the fruit group? **page 169**

20. What are nutrients that can be obtained from eating foods from each of the five basic food groups? **page 172**

Eating for Health

Vocabulary

Dietary Guidelines

desirable weight

calorie

cholesterol

plaque

atherosclerosis

lipoproteins

high density lipoproteins
(HDLs)

low density lipoproteins
(LDLs)

antioxidants

diabetes

insulin

hypoglycemia

Life Skills

- **I will follow the Dietary Guidelines.**
- **I will plan a healthful diet that reduces the risk of disease.**

Your diet consists of what you eat and drink each day. You can improve the likelihood of having better health and reduce the likelihood of getting certain diseases by following dietary guidelines. The **Dietary Guidelines** are recommendations for diet choices for healthy Americans who are two years of age or more. The guidelines are the result of research by the United States Department of Agriculture and the Department of Health and Human Services.

The Lesson Objectives

- Name the Dietary Guidelines and explain why you should follow them.
- Discuss how to choose foods that help reduce your risk of heart disease and cancer.
- Identify healthful dietary choices for people with diabetes and hypoglycemia.

The Dietary Guidelines

1. **Eat a variety of foods.** No single food can provide you with all the nutrients you need. This is the reason it is important to use the Food Guide Pyramid when planning your diet. Get the correct number of servings from the five food groups each day.

   - Bread, cereal, rice, and pasta group (six to eleven servings)
   - Vegetable group (three to five servings)
   - Fruit group (two to four servings)
   - Meat, poultry, fish, dry beans, eggs, and nuts group (two to three servings)
   - Milk, yogurt, and cheese group (two to three servings)
   - Fats, oils, and sweets (eat sparingly)

2. **Balance the food you eat with physical activity— maintain or improve your weight.** Desirable weight is the weight that is recommended for a person's age, height, sex, and body frame. If you are overweight, you have an increased risk of high blood pressure, heart disease, and diabetes. If you are underweight, you might not have the nutrients your body needs for growth. Lesson 19 provides information on how you can maintain a healthful weight.

3. **Choose a diet low in fat, saturated fat, and cholesterol.** A **calorie** is a unit of measure for both the energy supplied by food and the energy used by the body. Fat in foods contains over twice the calories of an equal weight of carbohydrates or protein. Fat should contribute to 30 percent or less of your total calories. A diet high in saturated fat and cholesterol increases the risk of heart disease.

4. **Choose a diet with plenty of grain products, vegetables, and fruits.** Vegetables, fruits, and grain products are good sources of starch, fiber, vitamins, and minerals. These foods are usually low in fat content. Be certain to include a daily source of fiber and vitamins C, E, and A. Fiber moves food through your digestive system and helps you have a daily bowel movement. This reduces your risk of colon cancer. Vitamins C, E, and A might help lower your risk of heart disease and cancer.

5. **Choose a diet moderate in sugars.** Sugars add calories to foods, but they are limited in nutrients. Eating too many foods that have a high sugar content can contribute to weight gain and tooth decay.

6. **Choose a diet moderate in salt and sodium.** Sodium is a mineral that your body needs in small amounts. Table salt is a source of sodium. Your body needs only 1/4 teaspoon of salt daily. Most teens consume ten times more salt than they need. Too much salt and sodium might increase blood pressure. You can reduce the amount of salt and sodium in your diet by limiting the amounts of these foods: luncheon meats, salty snack foods, cheeses, and fast foods. Avoid adding salt to foods.

7. **Adults who drink alcoholic beverages should do so in moderation. Teens should not drink alcoholic beverages.** Alcohol can harm brain cells, the liver, and other body organs. Alcohol alters the use of some essential nutrients in the body. Alcoholic beverages are high in calories. They do not contain the vitamins and minerals needed for good health. For good health, avoid drinking alcohol now and later.

Diet and Heart Disease

Diets high in saturated fat and cholesterol increase the risk of heart disease. **Cholesterol** (kuh·LES·tuh·rawl) is a fat-like substance made by the body and found in many foods. A certain amount of cholesterol is needed for the protective coatings of the brain, skin, and nerve cells. Foods high in cholesterol are egg yolks, dairy products, and organ meats, such as liver.

Too much cholesterol in the blood is harmful to health. Cholesterol can stick to the inner walls of the blood vessels and form plaque. **Plaque** is hardened fatty deposits in blood vessels. This leads to atherosclerosis. **Atherosclerosis** (A·thuh·ROH·skluh·ROH·sis) is a disease in which fat deposits on artery walls. Blood pressure increases in an effort to supply blood to cells. Heart attack and stroke are more likely to occur.

Two important ways to reduce cholesterol in the blood are regular exercise and a balanced diet.

Exercise affects lipoproteins. **Lipoproteins** are substances that transport cholesterol in the bloodstream. **High density lipoproteins (HDLs)** are substances that carry cholesterol to the liver for breakdown and excretion. **Low density lipoproteins (LDLs)** are substances that carry cholesterol to body cells. People with greater levels of HDLs and lower numbers of LDLs are less likely to have diseases of the blood vessels. Regular vigorous exercise increases the level of HDLs.

A balanced diet containing antioxidants might lower the risk of heart disease. **Antioxidants** (an·tee·AHK·suh·duhnts) are substances that protect cells from being damaged by oxidation. Vitamins C and E and beta-carotene are anti-oxidants. Carrots, sweet potatoes, oranges, broccoli, whole grain bread, and green leafy vegetables are good sources of these vitamins.

Dishes That Contain Beans

Do you enjoy eating bean soup? Do you add beans to vegetable soup? Do you put beans with your rice? Beans help to lower blood choles-terol. And they are a good source of protein, too. Browse through a recipe book. Find a bean recipe to share with your family.

Six Ways to Reduce Cholesterol in Your Diet

Another way to reduce cholesterol in the blood is to reduce the amount of saturated fats and cholesterol in your diet.

1. Choose lean red meat, fish, chicken, turkey, and dry beans as protein sources.

2. Cut down on the number of eggs and organ meats, such as liver, that you eat.

3. Limit the amount of butter, cream, cheese, and whole milk in your diet.

4. Trim excess fat from meats.

5. Broil, bake, or boil rather than fry foods.

6. Read labels carefully to determine both amount and types of fat contained in foods.

Diet and Cancer

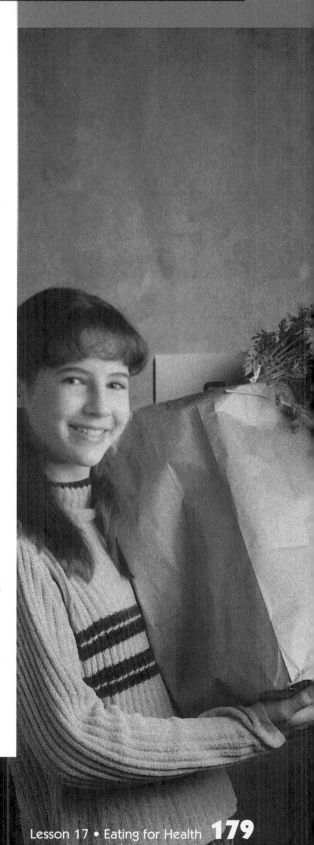

The National Research Council, a committee of the National Academy of Sciences, and the National Cancer Institute have worked together to develop a set of guidelines to reduce the risk of cancer through healthful diet. Following these guidelines is not a guarantee that you will not get cancer. However, you will decrease your chances of cancer.

The guidelines suggest that you eat plenty of fruits and vegetables. Fruits and vegetables play a protective role in reducing the risk of cancers of the lung, stomach, colon, bladder, pancreas, mouth, larynx, cervix, ovary, and breast. Foods rich in fiber play a protective role against colon cancer, which is the second leading cause of death from cancer in the United States. Consuming foods in the cabbage family might reduce your risk of developing colon and rectal cancers. Cauliflower, broccoli, and brussels sprouts are members of the cabbage family.

Antioxidants also might play a role in reducing the risk of cancer. A diet rich in vitamin A might reduce the risk of lung, gastrointestinal, and bladder cancers. Vitamins C and E are helpful in reducing cancer growth. These vitamins can be obtained from the foods you eat or from a standard multivitamin product.

The guidelines also suggest that you eat less of certain foods. Few salt-cured and smoked foods should be eaten. Cut down on bacon, ham, hot dogs, and luncheon meats.

Keep your diet low in fat, saturated fat, and cholesterol. Whenever possible, eat unsaturated fats instead of saturated fats. A diet high in saturated fats has been linked to breast, colon, and prostate cancers.

The guidelines warn against drinking alcoholic beverages. Drinking alcohol increases the risk of developing cancers of the mouth, esophagus, larynx, and liver. Your risk of developing these cancers increases if you drink alcohol and smoke cigarettes or marijuana.

Diet, Diabetes and Hypoglycemia

Diabetes (dy·uh·BEE·teez) is a disease in which the body produces little or no insulin or cannot use insulin. Diabetes occurs when the pancreas does not produce enough insulin. **Insulin** is a hormone that regulates the blood sugar level. Diabetes also results when insulin is produced but does not function correctly. People with diabetes need a diet rich in complex carbohydrates, high in fiber, and low in sodium and fat.

Hypoglycemia (hy·poh·gly·SEE·mee·uh) is a condition in which the pancreas produces too much insulin and the blood sugar level becomes low. People with hypoglycemia might become weak, dizzy, or irritable. People with hypoglycemia should eat small regular meals. The meals should be high in protein. They should avoid sweets because their bodies cannot regulate their blood sugar level.

Fried Is Frightful

Life Skill

I will follow the Dietary Guidelines.

Materials: Regular potato chips, low-fat potato chips, paper towels, paper, pen or pencil

Directions: Complete this activity to show how fat clings to arteries.

1. Place two paper towels in front of you.

2. Place a handful of regular potato chips on one paper towel.

3. Place a handful of low-fat potato chips on another paper towel.

4. Let the potato chips sit for a few minutes.

5. Remove or eat the potato chips from each paper towel. When the chips are gone, observe which paper towel has a film of oil on it. When you eat fried foods, the grease or oil sticks to your artery walls just as the oil stayed on the paper towel.

6. Write a summary of your demonstration. Explain why you should choose foods with low fat or no fat.

Activity

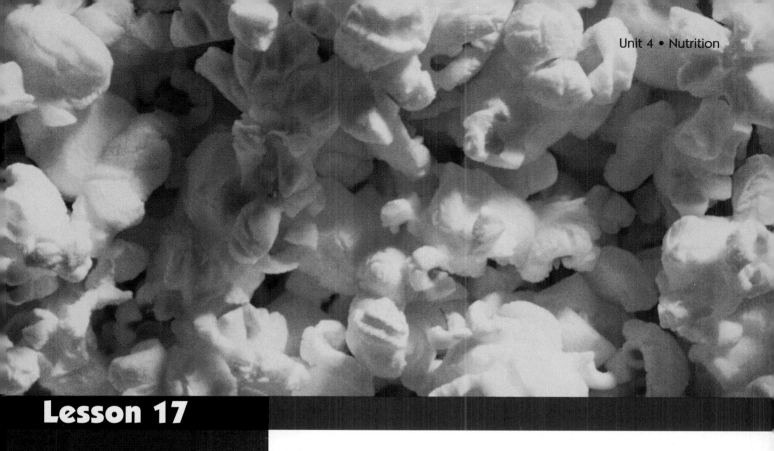

Lesson 17

Review

Vocabulary

Write a separate sentence using each of the vocabulary words listed on page 174.

Health Content

Write responses to the following:

1. Why do teens need to eat a variety of foods? **page 175**
2. Why do teens need to balance the food they eat with physical activity? **page 175**
3. Why do teens need to choose a diet low in fat, saturated fat, and cholesterol? **page 175**
4. Why do teens need to choose a diet with plenty of grain products, vegetables, and fruits? **page 176**
5. Why do teens need to choose a diet moderate in sugars? A diet moderate in salt and sodium? A diet that does not include alcohol? **page 176**
6. How are blood vessels affected by a diet high in cholesterol? **page 177**
7. How can regular exercise and a balanced diet reduce cholesterol in the blood? **page 177**
8. What are six ways to reduce the amount of saturated fats and cholesterol in the diet? **page 178**
9. What are dietary changes to reduce the risk of cancer? **page 179**
10. What are healthful dietary choices for people with diabetes? Hypoglycemia? **page 180**

The Cautious Consumer

Vocabulary

consumer

food label

Nutrition Facts

Serving Size

Servings Per Container

Amount Per Serving

daily value

Percent Daily Value

list of nutrients

vitamins and minerals required on a food label

daily values/calories footnote

ingredients listing

fast foods

junk foods

ethnic restaurant

foodborne illness

Salmonella

botulism

Life Skills

- **I will evaluate food labels.**
- **I will follow the Dietary Guidelines when I go out to eat.**
- **I will protect myself from foodborne illnesses.**

A **consumer** (kuhn·SOO·mer) is a person who chooses sources of health-related information and buys or uses health products and services. A cautious consumer pays attention to health-related information about foods. You are a cautious consumer when you: read food labels carefully; make healthful food selections when dining out; and consider food safety when making food selections.

The Lesson Objectives

- Interpret and evaluate the information on food labels.
- Identify healthful foods when dining out.
- List ways to prevent foodborne illnesses.

Food Labels

A **food label** is a nutrition panel of information that is required on all processed foods regulated by the Food and Drug Administration. A food label provides information that helps you make choices about the foods you eat. The information on a food label is based on a daily diet that provides 2,000 calories. A person who needs 2,000 calories each day can use this information exactly as it is. However, you might need to make some adjustments, depending on the number of calories you need each day.

Nutrition Facts is the title of the food label that is required on all processed foods regulated by the Food and Drug Administration. Use the following guide to check out food labels.

Nutrition Facts

Serving Size 1/2 cup (114g) ◄•••••••••••••••••••••• **Serving Size**
Servings Per Container 4

Amount Per Serving

Calories 90   Calories from Fat 30 ◄••••••• **Calories from Fat**

% Daily Value* ◄•••••••••••• **Percent Daily Value**

Total Fat 3g	**5%**
Saturated Fat 0g	**0%**
Cholesterol 0mg	**0%**
Sodium 300mg	**13%**
Total Carbohydrate 13g	**4%**
Dietary Fiber 3g	**12%**
Sugars 3g	
Protein 3g	

Vitamin A	80%	Vitamin C	60%
Calcium	4%	Iron	4%

◄•••••••••• **Vitamins and Minerals**

*Percent Daily Values are based on a 2,000 calorie diet. Your daily values may be higher or lower depending on your calorie needs.

◄•••••• **Daily Values/ Calories Footnote**

Total Fat	Less than	65g	80g
Sat Fat	Less than	20g	25g
Cholesterol	Less than	300mg	300mg
Sodium	Less than	2,400mg	2,400mg
Total Carbohydrate		300g	375g
Fiber		25g	30g

Calories per gram
Fat 9 • Carbohydrate 4 • Protein 4

Nutrition Facts

Serving Size

The **Serving Size** is the amount of a food that is considered a serving. Serving sizes are standardized to reflect the amount of foods people usually eat. The **Servings Per Container** is the number of servings that are in the container or package. Multiply the calories and nutrients by the number of servings you eat. This will help you determine your intake of calories and nutrients.

Percent Daily Value

The **daily value** is the amount of a nutrient that is needed each day for optimal health. The **Percent Daily Value** is the portion of the daily value of a nutrient provided by one serving of the food. The Percent Daily Value helps you get the nutrients needed for health. When the Percent Daily Value is 20 percent or higher, the food is a high source of the nutrient. When the Percent Daily Value is 10 percent or lower, the food is a low source of the nutrient.

Amount Per Serving

The **Amount Per Serving** states the number of calories in one serving and the number of Calories from Fat in one serving. Choose foods with a large difference between the total number of calories and the number of Calories from Fat.

List of Nutrients

The **list of nutrients** includes the Percent Daily Value for the nutrients that must be considered when planning a healthful diet. For good health, plan a diet with foods that have a low Percent Daily Value for total fat, saturated fat, cholesterol, sodium, and sugars. For total carbohydrates, dietary fiber, protein, vitamins, and minerals, the Percent Daily Value of the foods you eat should add up to 100 percent.

Vitamins and Minerals

The **vitamins and minerals required on a food label** are vitamins A and C and the minerals calcium and iron. Serious health problems can occur when the body does not have enough of these two vitamins and two minerals. Other vitamins and minerals might be included on the label, but they are not required.

Ingredients Listing

The **ingredients listing** is the list of ingredients in a food. The ingredients are listed by weight, beginning with the ingredient that is present in the greatest amount. The ingredients listing does not appear as part of the Nutrition Facts label, but appears somewhere else on the food container.

Daily Values/Calories Footnote

The **daily values/calories footnote** provides the amount of each nutrient needed each day based on a 2,000 and a 2,500 calorie diet. The following guidelines were used to determine the daily values for fat, saturated fat, carbohydrates, protein, and fiber.

- Fat intake should be less than 30 percent of total calories.

- Saturated fat intake should be less than 10 percent of total calories.

- Cholesterol intake should be less than 300 milligrams.

- Sodium intake should be less than one-quarter of a teaspoon of salt.

- Carbohydrate intake should be 60 percent of total calories.

- Fiber intake should be 11.5 grams for every 1,000 calories.

- Protein intake should be 10 percent of total calories.

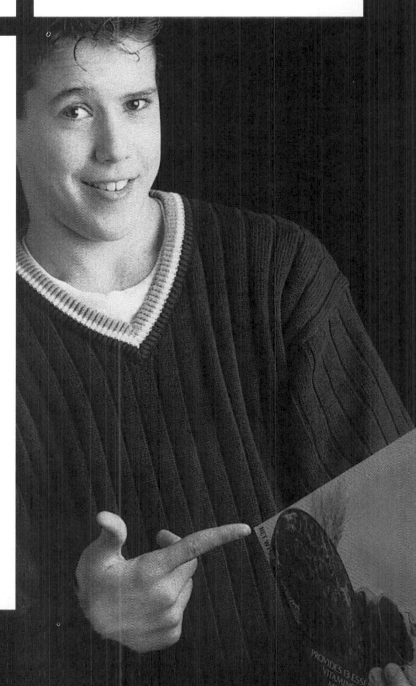

BUYER BEWARE

Suppose you are buying a box of cereal. Read the ingredients listing carefully. Perhaps oats is listed first in the ingredients listing. The ingredients that follow are the sugars sucrose, fructose, and glucose. The sum of these smaller amounts of sugars tells you the cereal contains a large amount of sugar. Even though oats are listed first, there might actually be more sugar than oats! If you combine the amounts of different sugars listed, it adds up.

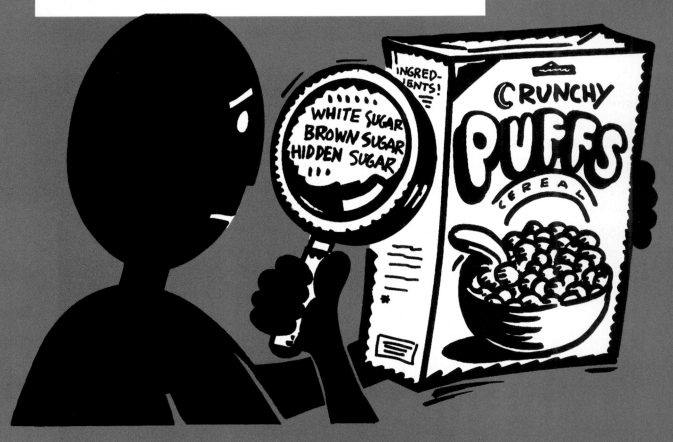

Food Selections When Dining Out

When you are dining out, you do not read food labels before you order. How can you be a cautious consumer when ordering fast foods or eating in a restaurant? Three suggestions for selecting foods when dining out are:

- **Select healthful foods from the Food Guide Pyramid.**
- **Follow the Dietary Guidelines.**
- **Follow guidelines for preventing heart disease and cancer.**

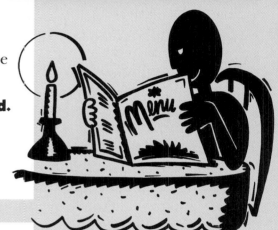

Fast Food Restaurants

Fast foods are popular with teens. **Fast foods** are foods that can be served quickly. They might be sold in walk-in or drive-through restaurants. Not all fast foods are junk foods. **Junk foods** are foods that are high in fat, sugar, or salt. Many junk foods are low in vitamins and minerals. Many teens choose junk foods when they eat at fast food restaurants. The typical fast food meal consists of a hamburger, fries, and a soft drink. This meal is high in calories, fat, and salt; it is low in vitamins and minerals.

You can make healthful food selections at fast food restaurants. A vegetable-topped pizza provides calcium (from the cheese) and other vitamins and minerals (from the vegetables). Many fast food restaurants now offer low-fat items, such as salads with fat-free or low-fat dressings, grilled chicken sandwiches, and low-fat or fat-free frozen yogurt.

Did you know...?

HOLD THE MAYO

Did you know that you can greatly reduce the amount of fat and the number of calories you consume when you hold the mayo? Suppose you put mustard on your sandwich each day rather than one teaspoon of mayonnaise. You would save 12,000 calories per year, or the equivalent of three and one-half pounds of body weight. You also can use low-fat or fat-free mayo.

Burger King

BK Broiler chicken sandwich–

379 calories, 18.0 fat grams

Egg/ham/cheese Croissanwich–

335 calories, 20.0 fat grams

Onion rings–

274 calories, 16.0 fat grams

Garden salad without dressing–

95 calories, 5.0 fat grams

Hamburger, single–

310 calories, 12.0 fat grams

Taco Bell

Nachos Bellgrande–

648 calories, 35.3 fat grams

Chicken fajita–

225 calories, 10.2 fat grams

Taco, regular–

183 calories, 10.8 fat grams

Light Chicken Soft Taco–

180 calories, 5 fat grams

Light Bean Burrito–

330 calories, 6 fat grams

Domino's Pizza

Cheese (16" pie)–

2 slices, 376 calories,

10.0 fat grams

Pepperoni (16" pie)–

2 slices, 460 calories,

17.5 fat grams

Deluxe (16" pie)–

2 slices, 498 calories,

20.4 fat grams

Fast Food Chart

McDonalds

Chicken McNuggets (4 oz.)–

290 calories, 16.3 fat grams

Filet-O-Fish sandwich–

440 calories, 26.1 fat grams

Quarter Pounder with cheese–

520 calories, 29.2 fat grams

Chocolate shake, low-fat–

320 calories, 2.2 fat grams

McChicken sandwich–

490 calories, 28.6 fat grams

Wendy's

Double cheeseburger–

796 calories, 48.1 fat grams

Potato, baked with bacon & cheese–

579 calories, 30.1 fat grams

Frosty–

398 calories, 16.0 fat grams

Chili–

228 calories, 7.5 fat grams

Chicken sandwich on multi-grain bun–

320 calories, 10 fat grams

KFC

Drumstick, Extra Tasty Crispy–

205 calories, 14.0 fat grams

Buttermilk biscuit–

235 calories, 11.7 fat grams

Mashed potatoes–

59 calories, 0.6 fat grams

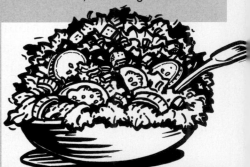

Data supplied by the companies to the Senate Select Committee on Nutrition and Human Needs.

Dining Out

You also can choose foods carefully when eating in a restaurant. Remember to follow the Dietary Guidelines. Many restaurant menus will indicate "heart healthy" or "light selections." Read the menu and ask how foods are prepared. Foods that are broiled, baked, or steamed are more healthful than fried foods. Ask about the ingredients used to prepare foods. Request healthful changes. For example, ask that your fish be grilled with lemon rather than butter. Ask to have salad dressing and sauces served on the side so that you can limit the amount you eat. The Restaurant Guide gives you some helpful hints for eating at ethnic restaurants. An **ethnic restaurant** is a restaurant that serves food eaten by people of a specific culture.

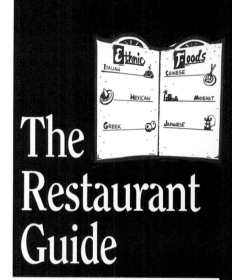

The Restaurant Guide

Italian

Select pasta, which is low in fat and loaded with carbohydrates.

Select dishes with lots of fresh vegetables, such as pasta primavera, that have a small amount of oil and are low in salt.

Choose linguine with white or red clam sauce.

Mexican

Choose shrimp or chicken burritos and enchiladas, instead of beef.

Select rice and bean dishes, which are high in fiber, low in fat, and are complete protein sources.

Ask for cheese and sour cream on the side.

Greek

Try pita bread, which is very low in fat.

Choose plaki—fish cooked with tomatoes, onions, and garlic, which is low in fat.

Limit your amount of olives and cheese, items that are high in fat and sodium.

Chinese

Choose healthful entrees that are steamed or lightly stir-fried in vegetable oil.

Avoid foods that are deep-fried.

Choose dishes with tofu or steamed rice.

Limit your use of soy sauce.

Middle Eastern

Choose dishes with couscous and bulgur wheat for healthful servings from the grain group.

Select shish kebabs with vegetables and lean meat for a nutritious choice.

Select melons, grapes, and other fresh fruits for dessert.

Japanese

Choose dishes with fresh vegetables that are lightly stir-fried in vegetable oil.

Select fish or poultry entrees instead of beef.

Food Safety

There are other ways to be a cautious consumer. Perhaps you have known someone who became ill after eating a certain food. This person had a foodborne illness. A **foodborne illness** is an illness caused by eating foods that have been contaminated by germs or by toxins produced by germs. Symptoms of foodborne illnesses include diarrhea, nausea, vomiting, and cramps.

Salmonella (sal·muh·NE·luh) is bacteria that contaminates foods. Symptoms of *Salmonella* include severe diarrhea, fever, vomiting, and cramps. *Salmonella* may result in death. **Botulism** (BAH·chuh·li·zuhm) is severe poisoning resulting from consuming foods with a preformed toxin. It results primarily from improperly canned foods. Botulism is rare but can be fatal. *Escherichia coli (E. coli)* are bacteria that usually are harmless. However, a certain type of *E. coli* can cause a foodborne illness.

Foodborne illnesses are generally treated by drinking water and other liquids, and bed rest. A doctor's care is needed. You can prevent foodborne illnesses.

- **Wash your hands before handling food.**
- **Wash countertops, utensils, and cutting boards after contact with food.**
- **Refrigerate food when necessary.**
- **Do not thaw frozen food at room temperature.**
- **Keep hot foods hot and cold foods cold.**
- **Thoroughly cook meat, poultry, and fish.**
- **Freeze or refrigerate leftovers promptly.**
- **Eat ground meat, poultry, and fish that are thoroughly cooked.**

Make Mine Well-Done

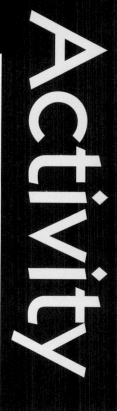

Life Skill — I will protect myself from foodborne illnesses.

Materials: Poster paper and markers

Directions: Read the information below. Then use your imagination to create a sign for food safety.

1. **Design a poster.** Your poster should warn people to eat only ground beef that is well done.

2. **Think of a slogan.** Write your slogan on your poster.

A certain type of *E. coli, E. coli* O157:H7, can contaminate ground beef. If contaminated ground beef is not cooked thoroughly before eating, *E. coli* O157:H7 can cause severe foodborne illness.

Lesson 18

Review

Vocabulary

Write a separate sentence using each of the vocabulary words listed on page 182.

Health Content

Write responses to the following:

1. What is the meaning of each heading on a food label? **pages 184–185**

2. What are three suggestions for selecting food when dining out? **page 187**

3. What are healthful foods that can be ordered at fast food restaurants? **page 188**

4. What are eight guidelines for preventing foodborne illnesses? **page 190**

5. Why should ground beef be cooked thoroughly before it is eaten? **page 191**

Weight-Conscious and Wise

Vocabulary

hunger

appetite

eating disorder

desirable weight

body composition

weight management

calorie

Life Skills

- **I will develop healthful eating habits.**
- **I will maintain a desirable weight and body composition.**

When you are weight-conscious and wise, you are aware of your eating patterns. You make an effort to be at a healthful weight. You exercise regularly to maintain a healthful percentage of body fat.

Hunger is the physiological need for food. **Appetite** is the desire for food that is determined by environmental and psychological factors. Weight management includes satisfying hunger as well as appetite.

The Lesson Objectives

- Give ways appetite can influence eating habits.
- List stressful situations for which teens might substitute harmful eating patterns for healthful ways of coping.
- Explain how to determine your desirable weight and body composition.
- Describe how to maintain your healthful weight.

Healthful Eating Habits

Have you heard the cliché, "Eat to live, don't live to eat?" When you "eat to live," you enjoy eating and are concerned about your health. Selecting foods from the Food Guide Pyramid and following the Dietary Guidelines help you "eat to live." You satisfy your need for food without letting your appetite get out of control.

Here are some ways your appetite might influence your eating habits.

- While watching television, you see a commercial for your favorite fast food restaurant. Suddenly you want to have a cheeseburger, fries, and a milkshake.

- You are at your friend's house and smell freshly baked chocolate chip cookies. Even though you are not hungry, you eat two cookies and drink a glass of milk.

- After a soccer game, you and your friends "pig out" on pizza to celebrate.

In each of these situations, eating habits were influenced by appetite rather than the need for food. It is not harmful to "pig out" occasionally. It is not harmful to eat when you are not hungry once in a while. You have healthful eating patterns if *most of the time* you make careful food selections and "eat to live."

Do Not "Pig Out!"

(too often)

Harmful Eating Habits

Now suppose you "live to eat." Your appetite controls your eating patterns. You are not eating to satisfy hunger, but to satisfy other needs. Many teens engage in harmful eating patterns to cope with their feelings and to deal with stressful situations. Let's look at some examples.

Maya is experiencing the body changes that accompany puberty.

She is uncomfortable with these changes and begins to feel that she is becoming fat. Rather than dealing with her feelings, she focuses on losing weight. Maya starves herself and develops an eating disorder. An **eating disorder** is a food-related dysfunction in which a person changes eating habits in a way that is harmful to the mind and body. An eating disorder is an extreme example of a harmful eating pattern. In Lesson 20, you will learn more about eating disorders.

Ashley is insecure around her friends.

She is never certain what she might do or say to feel more a part of the group. She likes to have something to nibble on in her hands. When she nibbles on food, she feels more secure. Nibbling can be a nervous habit to cover up for her feelings of insecurity.

Teisha has difficulty in school.

Whenever she tries to do homework, she becomes very frustrated. She immediately reaches for a snack. Snacking diverts her attention from her feelings of frustration.

Emilio is very angry about his family situation.

His parents have divorced. Emilio rarely sees his father, and his mother is now working very long hours. Emilio keeps his angry feelings to himself, but has begun to overeat. He has gained 15 pounds since his parents' divorce. Emilio stuffs himself rather than expressing his angry feelings.

Teens who have harmful eating patterns usually need help to learn new ways to cope with their feelings and to deal with stressful situations.

Desirable Weight and Body Composition

Desirable weight is the weight that is recommended for a person's age, height, sex, and body frame. See pages 196–197 to learn the range for your desirable weight. Compare your desirable weight with your actual weight.

Your body is made up of two types of tissues—fat tissue and lean tissue. **Body composition** is the percentage of fat tissue and lean tissue in the body. For good health, keep your percentage of body fat low. A healthful percentage of body fat for males your age is 14 to 17 percent. A healthful percentage of body fat for females your age is 21 to 24 percent. To keep your percentage of body fat low, you need regular physical activity.

Your Eating Habits

Have you thought about your eating habits? Are you aware of the situations that trigger your appetite? Do you turn to eating when you feel stressed or are unable to cope with feelings? Do you eat for healthful reasons? The first life skill listed for this lesson is **"I will develop healthful eating habits."** You need to practice this life skill before you can master the second life skill, **"I will maintain a desirable weight and body composition."** It is difficult to be at the best weight for you when you have harmful eating patterns.

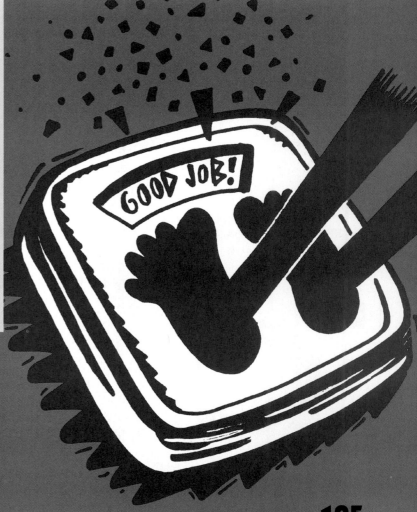

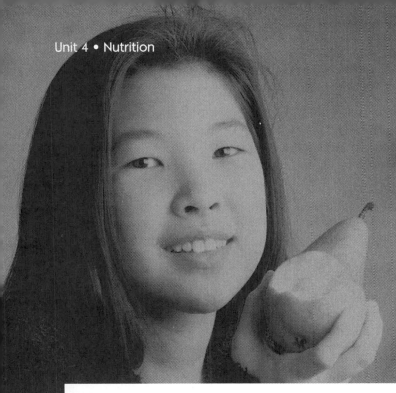

Range for Desirable Weight

Use a tape measure to measure your wrist and determine your body frame. If your wrist is:

- **less than 5 ½", you have a small frame;**
- **between 5 ½" and 6¼", you have a medium frame;**
- **over 6⅜", you have a large frame.**

Check the chart to determine the healthy weight range for your height and weight.

Female

Height (without shoes)	Weight (with light clothing, in pounds)		
	Small Frame	Medium Frame	Large Frame
4' 8"	85–91	89–100	97–112
4' 9"	87–94	91–103	99–115
4' 10"	89–97	94–106	102–118
4' 11"	92–100	97–109	105–121
5' 0"	95–103	100–112	108–124
5' 1"	98–106	103–115	111–127
5' 2"	101–109	106–119	114–131
5' 3"	104–112	109–123	118–135
5' 4"	107–116	113–128	122–139
5' 5"	111–120	117–132	126–143
5' 6"	115–124	121–136	130–147
5' 7"	119–128	125–140	134–151
5' 8"	123–133	129–144	138–156
5' 9"	127–137	133–148	142–161
5' 10"	131–141	137–152	146–166
5' 11"	135–145	141–156	150–171
6' 0"	139–149	145–160	154–176

Apply...

The Responsible Decision-Making Model™

You know that your weight is within your healthy weight range. Your physician has told you your weight is fine. Your friends say you would look better if you lost weight.

Answer the following questions on a separate sheet of paper. Write "Does not apply" if a question does not apply to this situation.

1. Is it healthful to try to lose weight when your weight is within your healthy weight range? Why or why not?

2. Is it safe to try to lose weight when your weight is within your healthy weight range? Why or why not?

3. Is it legal to try to lose weight when your weight is within your healthy weight range? Why or why not?

4. Will you show respect for yourself if you try to lose weight when your weight is within your healthy weight range? Why or why not?

5. Will your parents or guardians approve if you try to lose weight when your weight is within your healthy weight range? Why or why not?

6. Will you demonstrate good character if you try to lose weight when your weight is within your healthy weight range? Why or why not?

What is the responsible decision to make in this situation?

Male

Height (without shoes)	Weight (with light clothing, in pounds)		
	Small Frame	Medium Frame	Large Frame
5' 1"	100–108	106–117	114–129
5' 2"	103–111	109–121	117–132
5' 3"	106–114	112–124	120–136
5' 4"	109–117	115–127	123–140
5' 5"	112–121	118–131	126–144
5' 6"	116–125	122–135	130–149
5' 7"	120–129	126–140	135–154
5' 8"	124–133	130–144	139–158
5' 9"	128–138	134–148	143–162
5' 10"	132–142	138–153	147–167
5' 11"	136–146	142–158	152–172
6' 0"	140–150	146–163	156–177
6' 1"	144–155	150–168	161–182
6' 2"	148–159	155–173	166–187
6' 3"	152–163	160–178	170–192

Weight Management

Weight management is a diet and exercise plan that helps a person achieve and maintain his or her desirable weight and a healthful percentage of body fat. Look at the chart below. You will learn how long you need to do an activity to burn the calories contained in the foods on the chart.

	corn on the cob (1 ear) 83 calories	small French fries (1 serving) 220 calories	chocolate chip ice cream (1/2 cup) 260 calories
Do homework or watch TV for: (1.8 calories/minute)	46 minutes	122 minutes	144 minutes
Walk (3mph) for: (3.9 calories/minute)	21 minutes	56 minutes	67 minutes
Play football for: (4.8 calories/minute)	17 minutes	46 minutes	54 minutes
Rollerblade (9mph) for: (6.1 calories/minute)	14 minutes	36 minutes	43 minutes
Play tennis for: (7.2 calories/minute)	12 minutes	31 minutes	36 minutes
Run or jog (6mph) for: (10.6 calories/minute)	8 minutes	21 minutes	26 minutes

Weight management is a balancing act involving calories. A **calorie** is a unit of measure for both the energy supplied by food and the energy used by the body. You need to balance *calories in* (calories from the foods and beverages you eat and drink) with *calories out* (calories you use for physical activity and normal body functions).

To maintain weight, your *calories in* from foods and beverages and *calories out* from physical activity should be in balance. To gain weight, increase *calories in* by 250 calories each day. This will help you gain one-half to one pound a week. To lose weight, increase *calories out* by burning up 125 extra calories in activity and eating 125 fewer calories each day. This will help you lose about one-half to one pound a week.

cheeseburger 300 calories	macaroni and cheese (1 cup) 339 calories	tuna salad sandwich 399 calories
167 minutes	**188** minutes	**222** minutes
77 minutes	**87** minutes	**102** minutes
63 minutes	**71** minutes	**83** minutes
49 minutes	**56** minutes	**65** minutes
42 minutes	**47** minutes	**55** minutes
28 minutes	**32** minutes	**38** minutes

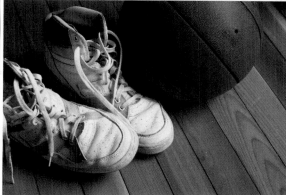

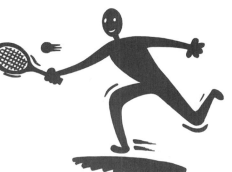

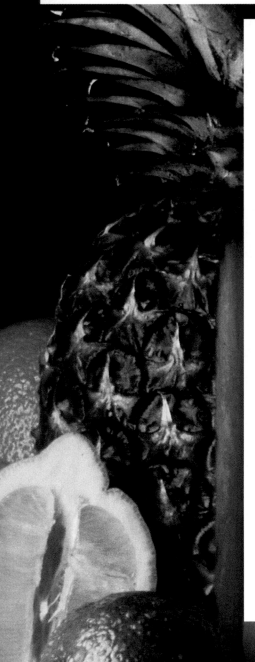

Steps for Gaining Weight

- **Eat extra servings of low-fat foods from the milk, yogurt, and cheese group.**
- **Eat extra servings from the bread, cereal, rice, and pasta group.**
- **Eat healthful snacks between meals.**
- **Exercise to increase muscle mass.**
- **Eat a healthful, balanced breakfast.**

Steps for Losing Weight

- **Eat a healthful, balanced breakfast.**
- **Participate in aerobic exercises to burn calories and reduce your body fat.**
- **Drink at least eight glasses of water a day.**
- **Drink a glass of water before eating meals and snacks.**
- **Chew your food thoroughly and eat slowly.**
- **Put smaller portions of foods on your plate and fill the rest of the plate with vegetables.**
- **Eat foods that are prepared in low-fat ways (broiled, skinless, baked).**
- **Do not add butter or oils to foods.**
- **Eat fewer than 150 calories from the fats, oils, and sweets group.**
- **Eat extra servings from the fruit group.**
- **Eat extra servings from the vegetable group.**
- **Eat meals and snacks while sitting down, instead of standing or walking around.**
- **Avoid eating while doing other activities such as watching television, doing homework, or talking on the telephone.**
- **Place eating utensils down between bites.**
- **Take a three-minute break halfway during each meal.**

Sample Menu for Weight Loss

Breakfast

Two pieces of whole-grain toast

All-fruit jam

One cup skim milk

One cholesterol-free egg substitute

Lunch

Turkey sandwich with mustard, lettuce, and tomato on whole wheat bread

One cup skim milk

Carrot sticks

Snack

Apple

Dinner

Salad with fat-free dressing

Grilled white-meat chicken

Broccoli

Plain baked potato

Sample Menu for Weight Gain

Breakfast

French toast with strawberries

Cereal with milk

One cup 2% milk

One cup orange juice

Lunch

Tuna fish salad sandwich with lettuce, mayonnaise, and tomato on whole wheat bread

One cup 2% milk

Apple

Snack

Carrot and celery sticks with ranch dressing

Wheat crackers with cheese

Dinner

Salad with low-fat dressing

Spaghetti with two meatballs

Roll with margarine

Lesson 19

Review

Vocabulary

Write a separate sentence using each of the vocabulary words listed on page 192.

Health Content

Write responses to the following:

1. What are ways appetite can influence eating habits? **page 193**

2. What are stressful situations for which teens might substitute harmful eating patterns for healthful ways of coping? **page 194**

3. How can you determine your desirable weight and body composition? **page 195**

4. How can you maintain your healthful weight? **page 199**

5. What are steps for gaining weight? For losing weight? **page 200**

Being Confident with Your Body Image

Vocabulary

body image

eating disorder

anorexia nervosa

malnutrition

bulimia

dehydration

obesity

metabolism

enabler

relapse

 Life Skill

• **I will develop skills to prevent eating disorders.**

Do you see someone special when you look in the mirror? Do you accept the appearance of your body? Are you proud of your body? Do you have a positive body image? Teens who feel good about themselves and have a positive body image are more likely to have healthful eating patterns.

The Lesson Objectives

• Discuss influences on your body image.

• Describe the causes, symptoms, and treatment for eating disorders.

• Identify factors that contribute to obesity.

• List health problems caused by obesity.

Body Image

Body image is the perception a person has of his or her body's appearance. You have a positive body image when you accept the appearance of your body. You have a negative body image when you do not accept the appearance of your body.

Many pressures and subtle influences can affect your body image. Television shows and magazine advertisements usually portray teens who are very attractive. Remember, these teens have been selected because they are models. It is very unrealistic to compare yourself to these teens. There is no "perfect teen" in real life. Some teens are tall, some are short, some are slender, some are muscular, and some are rounded.

Popular teen sports and activities might influence your feelings about your body. Too much emphasis is placed on weight in some sports. Wrestlers have to "make weight." Teens who wrestle might become obsessed with being at a specific weight to compete. They might develop a negative body image if they do not maintain a specific weight. Teens who participate in gymnastics, cheerleading, ice skating, and other activities also might be concerned about weight. Being preoccupied with being at a low weight is a cause of negative body image and low self-esteem.

Some teens develop a distorted body image. They do not see their body as it actually appears. Have you ever known someone that was a healthful weight who complained about being fat?

Other teens have difficulty accepting the body changes that accompany puberty. They feel uncomfortable and self-conscious when secondary sex characteristics develop. Some females will slouch when their breasts begin to develop. Some tall males slouch to be the same height as their classmates.

WARNING! If you:

- compare your appearance to that of a model;
- compare your appearance to that of a professional athlete;
- are obsessed with being thin or muscular;
- see yourself as fat when you have a healthful weight;
- do not accept the body changes that accompany puberty;

you might have a negative body image and need help.

Remember, to be a totally awesome teen, you must have a positive body image. You must have a healthful weight management plan and feel good about your body and appearance. Trusted adults can help you develop a positive body image.

Eating Disorders

Teens who have a negative body image are at risk for developing eating disorders. An **eating disorder** is a food-related dysfunction in which a person changes eating habits in a way that is harmful to the mind and body. Three common eating disorders are anorexia nervosa, bulimia, and obesity.

Anorexia Nervosa

Anorexia nervosa is an eating disorder characterized by self-starvation and a weight of 15 percent or more below normal. This eating disorder occurs in about 1 of 200 teenage females. Teenage males rarely develop this eating disorder. This might be due in some part to the fact that there is more pressure on females to be thin. Females with this disorder usually have difficulty accepting their changing bodies at puberty. They starve themselves as a way to deal with their emotions. They might vomit, use laxatives, take diuretics, or exercise to excess to achieve additional weight loss. These behaviors might damage the heart, kidneys, and other body organs. People with anorexia nervosa might suffer from malnutrition. **Malnutrition** is a condition in which the body does not get the nutrients required for good health. There have been cases where people have starved themselves to death.

Only a professional can correctly diagnose anorexia nervosa. Treatment for physical health problems is needed. A hospital stay often is necessary. The patient might need intravenous feedings of nutrients. Tests are required to assess damage to body organs. A healthful body weight must be achieved. Treatment for emotional problems also is needed.

Bulimia

Bulimia is an eating disorder in which a person has uncontrollable urges to eat excessively and then to rid the body of the food. A person will vomit, take laxatives and diuretics, use enemas, and exercise to excess to get rid of food eaten. Bulimia is often known as the "secret eating disorder." People with bulimia try to hide their behavior from others. They might "pig out" with friends and then excuse themselves, go to the restroom, and vomit.

Teens with bulimia need treatment for emotional problems. They often binge or "pig out" on food when they feel angry, lonely, depressed, or fearful. Then they feel guilty and try to rid their bodies of the excess calories. Counseling helps them learn healthful ways to cope with feelings.

Treatment for physical health also is needed. There can be serious damage to several body organs. Frequent vomiting causes stomach acids to injure the stomach lining, mouth, and throat. Stomach acids also damage the teeth and gums. Frequent use of laxatives and diuretics damages the kidneys. It can lead to dehydration. **Dehydration** is a condition in which the body does not have enough water. Teens with bulimia might suffer from malnutrition. They might lack the minerals needed for normal heart rhythm.

Obesity

Obesity is excessive body fat. A male is considered to be obese when he has a body fat percentage of 20 or more. A female is considered to be obese when she has a body fat percentage of 30 or more. Several factors contribute to obesity.

- **Genetics** There appears to be an inherited tendency toward obesity.

- **Slow body metabolism** **Metabolism** (muh·TA·buh·li·zuhm) is the rate at which food is converted to energy in the cells. The thyroid gland produces thyroxin which affects body metabolism. Too little thyroxin results in slow body metabolism. A physician can treat this condition.

- **Lack of physical activity** Body metabolism is slow without physical activity. Regular exercise speeds body metabolism and helps with obesity.

- **Eating too many calories and high-fat foods** Harmful eating habits contribute to obesity. Reducing the number of calories and high-fat foods helps with obesity.

- **Harmful eating patterns in which eating becomes a way of coping with feelings and problems**

Teens who are obese need to examine why they overeat. Treatment helps them recognize why they eat. They might reward themselves with food. They might "pig out" when they feel stress. They might overeat to cope with their sexuality during puberty. Attempts at weight loss rarely work without understanding these issues. Support groups can be very helpful.

Treatment for physical health might be needed. A physician will give a complete physical examination. The thyroid gland will be checked. An exercise plan and healthful weight loss diet will be designed. A physician will recommend the amount of weight that should be lost. The physician will also recommend how fast weight should be lost.

Obesity can cause serious health problems. Excessive body fat puts strain on body organs. The bones must support more weight than they should. The heart must beat more often to supply the excess fat cells with oxygen. Blood pressure increases to pump blood to body parts. Too much insulin from the pancreas is needed for the body to use the food. This can cause diabetes. Obesity has been linked to an increased risk for developing cancer.

Treatment for Eating Disorders

People with eating disorders usually are in a state of denial. They do not admit to themselves or others that they have a problem. They usually are unaware that the root of the problem is emotional, not physical. Of course, physical problems result.

Other people usually begin the process for getting help. For example, you might be aware of a friend who starves himself or herself or "pigs out" and vomits. You might contact the friend's parents or a school counselor and share your concerns. The school counselor will talk with your friend's parents. This begins the process for getting help for someone who needs it.

Treatment for anorexia nervosa and bulimia requires medical help and counseling. The person who helps with the counseling will ask many questions. People who have these conditions might have a relationship with an enabler. An **enabler** is a person who knowingly or unknowingly supports the harmful behavior of another person. The enabler might be a family member or friend. The enabler might deny what is happening. The enabler also might participate in the harmful behavior. Enablers need help changing their behavior.

Eating disorders are difficult to overcome. Many people with eating disorders must manage this behavior the rest of their lives. They want to avoid a relapse. A **relapse** is the return to addictive behavior after a period of having stopped it. They do not want to feel stressed or upset or anxious and repeat harmful eating patterns. There are support programs for teens with eating disorders. These programs emphasize the need for ongoing support and awareness.

Lesson 20

Review

Vocabulary

Write a separate sentence using each of the vocabulary words listed on page 202.

Health Content

Write responses to the following:

1. What factors influence your feelings about your body? **page 203**

2. What are warning signs that indicate a teen might have a negative body image? **page 203**

3. What are the causes, symptoms, and treatment for anorexia nervosa? Bulimia? **pages 204–205**

4. What are five factors that contribute to obesity? **page 206**

5. What are health problems caused by obesity? **page 206**

Unit 4 Review

Health Content

Review your answers for each Lesson Review in this unit. Then write answers to each of the following questions.

1. What is the difference between saturated fats and unsaturated fats? **Lesson 16 page 163**

2. What can happen to health if a person does not get enough calcium, iron, magnesium, phosphorus, potassium, and sodium? **Lesson 16 page 166**

3. What are nutrients you can get from eating foods from each of the five basic food groups? **Lesson 16 page 172**

4. What are reasons to choose a diet moderate in sugars? **Lesson 17 page 176**

5. How can you reduce the amount of saturated fats and cholesterol in the diet? **Lesson 17 page 178**

6. What are guidelines for selecting food when dining out? **Lesson 18 page 187**

7. How are your eating habits influenced by appetite? **Lesson 19 page 193**

8. How can you lose weight? **Lesson 19 page 200**

9. How is your body image influenced? **Lesson 20 page 203**

10. What are five reasons a person might become obese? **Lesson 20 page 206**

Vocabulary

Number a sheet of paper from 1–10. Select the correct vocabulary word. Write it next to the corresponding number. DO NOT WRITE IN THIS BOOK.

amino acids	fiber
appetite	insulin
bulimia	junk foods
consumer	lipoproteins
desirable weight	nutrient

1. _____ are foods that are high in fat, sugar, or salt. **Lesson 18**

2. A(n) _____ is a person who chooses sources of health-related information and buys or uses health products and services. **Lesson 18**

3. _____ is a hormone that regulates the blood sugar level. **Lesson 17**

4. _____ is the weight that is recommended for a person's age, height, sex, and body frame. **Lesson 19**

5. _____ is an eating disorder in which a person has uncontrollable urges to eat excessively and then to rid the body of the food. **Lesson 20**

6. _____ are the building blocks that make up proteins. **Lesson 16**

7. _____ is the desire for food that is determined by environmental and psychological factors. **Lesson 19**

8. A(n) _____ is a chemical substance in foods that builds, repairs, and maintains body tissues; regulates body processes; and provides energy. **Lesson 16**

9. _____ is the part of grains and plant foods that cannot be digested. **Lesson 16**

10. _____ are substances that transport cholesterol in the bloodstream. **Lesson 17**

The Responsible Decision-Making Model™

You are at a restaurant with friends. You wait a long time before the waiter brings your food. Your friends are sharing a pizza. You ordered a hamburger. The hamburger is pink inside. You really do not want to wait any longer to eat. Answer the following questions on a separate sheet of paper. Write "Does not apply" if a question does not apply to this situation.

1. Is it healthful to eat hamburger that is pink inside? Why or why not?

2. Is it safe to eat hamburger that is pink inside? Why or why not?

3. Is it legal to eat hamburger that is pink inside? Why or why not?

4. Will you show respect for yourself if you eat hamburger that is pink inside? Why or why not?

5. Will your parents or guardian approve if you eat hamburger that is pink inside? Why or why not?

6. Will you demonstrate good character if you eat hamburger that is pink inside? Why or why not?

What is the responsible decision to make in this situation?

Health Literacy

Effective Communication

Create a menu for a restaurant that specializes in heart healthy foods. Design a cover for the menu. Give the restaurant a clever name.

Self-Directed Learning

Look up the home page for the United States Department of Agriculture (USDA). Find the Broadcasters Letter symbol. The Broadcasters Letter is a weekly summary of USDA news. Write down three stories.

Critical Thinking

The Food Guide Pyramid replaces the older "Four Food Groups." Find an older book that presents the four food groups. Write a summary stating why the change was made to the Food Guide Pyramid.

Responsible Citizenship

Collect menus from some of your favorite restaurants. Analyze the menus for healthful food choices. Highlight the food choices. Bring the menu with you when you eat at these restaurants.

Multicultural Health

Talk with a friend from another culture. Find out what fast foods are eaten in his or her culture. Analyze whether the fast foods eaten in yours and your friend's culture meet the Dietary Guidelines.

Family Involvement

Prepare a grocery list of foods for one week for your family. Include foods from each of the six groups in the Food Guide Pyramid. Volunteer to shop with your parent or guardian to help get these foods.

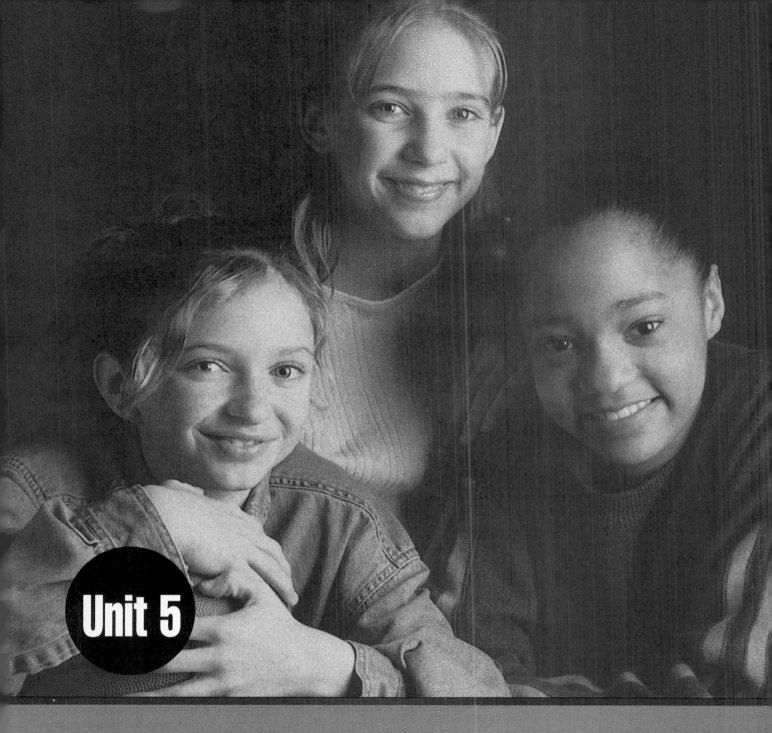

Unit 5

Personal Health and Physical Activity

Having a Neat and Clean Appearance

Vocabulary

grooming
anti-perspirant
deodorant
sebaceous glands
acne
dermatologist
dandruff
conditioner
lice
blister
callus
corn
ingrown toenail
lens
retina
optic nerve
pupil
cornea
iris
color blindness
astigmatism
hyperopia
farsightedness
myopia
nearsightedness
monovision
pinkeye
outer ear
sound waves
middle ear
eustachian tube
inner ear
decibel (dB)
noise pollution
audiometer

Life Skill • **I will be well-groomed.**

You never get a second chance to make a first impression. When you meet someone, that person forms an impression of you within ten seconds. **Grooming** is taking care of the body so that a person appears at his or her best. Grooming requires the regular cleaning of the body including the skin, hair, nails, and feet, as well as wearing clean clothes. Good grooming practices help keep you healthy by reducing the spread of germs from one part of the body to another. When you are neat and clean, your appearance is pleasing to others.

The Lesson Objectives

- Discuss ways to care for your skin, nails, and hair.
- Explain ways to care for your feet.
- Describe ways to care for your eyes and ears.

Taking Care of Your Skin and Nails

The skin is the largest organ of the body. In Lesson 11, you learned about the layers of the skin. Sweat glands lie beneath the dermis. Sweat glands allow perspiration to escape through the pores. Perspiration consists of water, salt, and waste products. When bacteria on the skin decompose, body odor results. You begin to have perspiration in your armpits during the teen years. Regular bathing and use of an anti-perspirant will help keep perspiration off the skin. An **anti-perspirant** is a product used to reduce the amount of perspiration. A **deodorant** is a product that reduces the amount of body odor and might reduce the amount of perspiration.

Besides sweat glands, there are other glands in the skin. **Sebaceous** (si·BAY·shuhs) **glands** are glands that secrete an oil to keep skin soft. During the teen years, hormones increase the amount of oil these glands produce. The extra oil may clog pores and cause acne. **Acne** is a skin disorder in which glands and hair follicles are inflamed. Pimples, whiteheads, and blackheads break out over the face, neck, shoulders, upper arms, and trunk. Acne is caused by the increased production of oil. It is not caused by diet. Eating chocolate, sweets, and fatty foods does not cause acne.

Acne is common in teens. Teens with severe acne might need treatment by a dermatologist. A **dermatologist** (duhr·muh·TAH·luh·jist) is a physician who specializes in the care of the skin. Acne is treated with topical medications, including antibiotics.

Acne that persists might be treated with oral medications. Teens with acne should avoid scrubbing areas affected by acne. Gently washing the skin and patting it dry helps prevent the spread of acne. Teens with acne should not squeeze or rub pimples, whiteheads, and blackheads. This harsh treatment might cause additional infections and scarring. Cosmetics should be used sparingly. Oily makeup can cause acne to become worse.

Another aspect of good grooming is having clean, trimmed fingernails. Keep your nails clean and avoid biting them. Nails that are dirty and broken are unattractive and unhealthy. Fingernails can collect dirt and bacteria. They should be cleaned and trimmed often. Trim nails straight across and not too close to the skin.

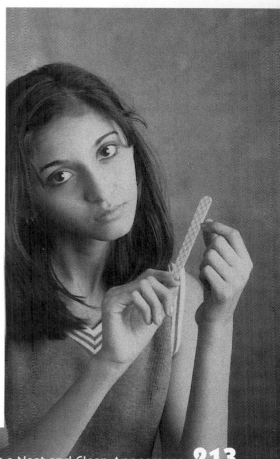

CHECKLIST

Ways to Care for Your Skin and Nails

- Bathe or shower each day.
- Take a bath or shower after exercising or being in hot weather.
- Use an anti-perspirant or deodorant under the arms to control body odor.
- Gently wash areas affected by acne with mild soap. Then pat dry.
- Never squeeze or rub pimples, white-heads, or blackheads.
- Use cosmetics, especially oily makeup, sparingly.
- Seek help from a dermatologist for severe acne.
- Protect your skin from the sun by wearing a sunscreen with a sun protection factor (SPF) of at least 15 and protective clothing (see Lesson 11).
- Seek proper medical care for skin rashes (see Lesson 11).
- Regularly check moles, warts, and freckles for changes in color, size, and shape (see Lesson 11).
- Keep fingernails clean and trimmed.

Your Skin

Your Nails

Taking Care of Your Hair

Hair care is an important part of grooming. Clean hair has a shiny appearance. Wash your hair at least twice a week to remove dirt and oil. If you are very active, perspire heavily, or have an oily scalp, you might need to shampoo daily. But do not overdo washing hair. Washing too often dries hair and makes it look dull.

Work suds through the hair once and rinse thoroughly. A second lathering is not necessary. It dries out your hair. Experiment with different shampoos to find the right one for you. There are special shampoos you can use if you have dandruff. **Dandruff** is flakes of dead skin cells on the scalp.

You might choose to use a conditioner after rinsing the shampoo from your hair. A **conditioner** is a product that coats the hair shaft making it feel smooth. Many conditioners and shampoos contain ingredients that remove tangles from hair. Follow directions for the amount of time to leave the conditioner on your hair.

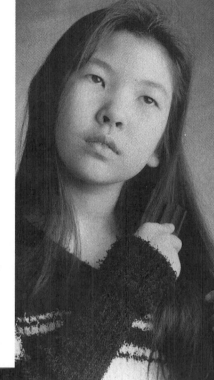

Comb your hair after rinsing it thoroughly. Brushing wet hair might cause it to break. If possible, allow your hair to dry naturally or use a blow dryer on a warm or cool setting. Curling irons and blow dryers on hot settings can over-dry your hair. They can cause your hair to become dry, brittle, and to have split ends.

Use hair products such as hairspray, mousse, and gel sparingly. If you use too much, these products can cause white flakes that look like dandruff. These products can also cause the hair to become dry, brittle, and to have split ends. A word of caution about aerosol hairsprays. Avoid inhaling aerosol hairsprays as they might contain ingredients that harm the air sacs in the lungs.

Take precautions to avoid being infected with head lice. **Lice** are insects that pierce the skin and secrete a substance that causes itching and swelling. Head lice attach themselves to hair on the head and other parts of the body. Head lice can be spread by sharing a brush, comb, or hat with a person who is infected. Do not share brushes, combs, or hats.

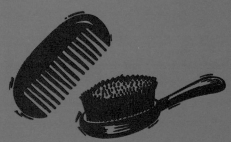

Hair-Raising Facts

1. Your hair grows faster than any other part of your body.

2. The part of your hair that you can see, the hair shaft, is made of dead cells.

3. Your natural hair color was passed to you from the genes of your biological parents.

4. Strands of your hair can be examined to determine your age, gender, and race.

5. Strands of your hair can be examined to determine if you are using certain drugs.

6. Your hair grows about one-half inch per month.

7. Your hair will not grow back thicker if you cut it.

8. Shampooing your hair twice at one time can dry out your hair.

9. Conditioners coat the hair shaft making it appear shiny, but they do not repair split ends.

10. The tiny white flakes on a person's blouse or shirt could be dandruff, or from a buildup of hairspray, gel, or mousse.

CHECKLIST

Ways to Care for Your Hair

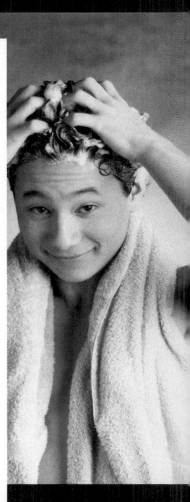

- Wash your hair at least twice a week.
- Wash your hair more often if you are very active, perspire heavily, or have an oily scalp.
- Select the shampoo that is best for your hair.
- Use a special shampoo if you have dandruff.
- Work suds through the hair once and rinse thoroughly.
- Follow directions carefully if you use a conditioner.
- Comb your hair instead of brushing it when it is wet.
- Allow your hair to dry naturally or use a blow dryer on a cool or warm setting.
- Do not overuse products such as hairspray, mousse, or gel.
- Avoid inhaling aerosol hairsprays because they might contain ingredients that damage the air sacs in the lungs.
- Do not share combs, brushes, or hats.

Taking Care of Your Feet

Your feet take you many places! Wear comfortable shoes that are the correct size. Wash feet daily. Wear clean socks. Keep toenails cut straight across. These habits help prevent blisters, calluses, corns, and ingrown toenails.

To avoid foot odor, wash and dry your feet often. Wear clean socks at all times. After wearing shoes, allow them to air out before wearing them again. Do not wear wet shoes.

A **blister** is a raised area containing liquid that is caused by an object rubbing against the skin. Often, the cause is shoes that fit poorly. If a blister develops, cover it with a bandage. If the blister breaks and oozes fluid, clean the area. Treat it with an antiseptic and cover it with a sterile bandage.

A **callus** is a thickened layer of skin due to excess rubbing. Calluses often appear on the feet. Determine what caused the rubbing and make changes to stop the rubbing. The callus will often heal without treatment.

A **corn** is a growth that results from excess rubbing of a shoe against the foot, or from toes being squeezed together. Special pads can be used to relieve the pain. If corns do not heal, check with a physician.

An **ingrown toenail** is a toenail that grows into the skin. Swelling and infection can result. A physician can treat this condition.

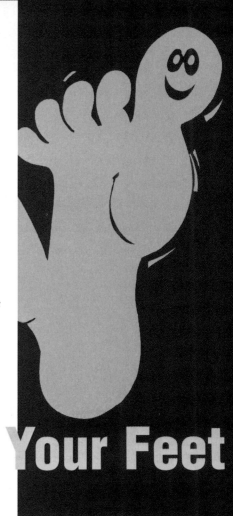

Your Feet

Ways to Care for Your Feet

- **Wear comfortable shoes that are the correct size.**
- **Wash your feet daily and dry them thoroughly.**
- **Wear clean socks.**
- **Allow shoes to dry thoroughly before wearing them again.**
- **Cut toenails straight across.**
- **Know how to prevent and treat blisters, calluses, corns, and ingrown toenails.**

Taking Care of Your Eyes

The appearance of your eyes is one of the best indications of your health. Your eyes have a healthy glow when you take care of yourself. When you are in good spirits, it almost appears as if your eyes are "smiling." When you have correct vision, your eyes help you learn. More than 80 percent of knowledge is gathered by what you see.

Your Eyes

The **lens** is the part of the eye that focuses light rays entering the pupil on the retina.

The **retina** is the inner lining of the eyeball where light rays are absorbed and changed to electrical messages. Images are focused on the retina.

The **iris** is the colored part of the eye that adjusts to the size of the pupil to regulate the amount of light that enters the eye.

The **cornea** is the clear tissue over the front of the eye that covers the iris and pupil.

The **pupil** is the black opening in the center of the iris that changes size to regulate the amount of light that enters the eye. In dim light, the pupil becomes larger to let more light enter. In bright light, the pupil becomes smaller to protect the eye from too much light.

The **optic nerve** is the nerve that carries the electrical messages from the retina to the brain. The interpretation of these messages by the brain results in what you see.

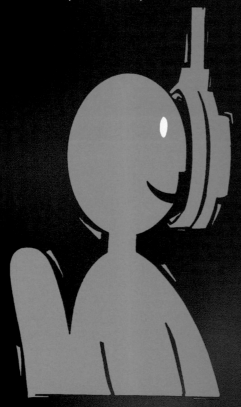

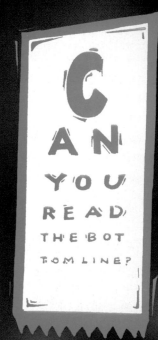

Vision Problems

During the teen years, you need an eye examination every 18 months to two years. An eye physician will review your health history and check for color blindness, lazy eye, and sharpness of vision. **Color blindness** is a condition in which a person sees colors differently than other people. It is usually caused by defects in light-sensitive pigments in the eye. Most vision problems are caused by defects in the shape of the eyeball. These defects keep images from focusing on the retina.

- **Astigmatism** (uh·STIG·muh·ti·zuhm) is a visual problem in which an irregular curvature of the lens or cornea causes blurred vision.

- **Hyperopia** (hy·puh·ROH·pee·uh), or **farsightedness**, is a visual problem in which close objects appear blurred while distant objects are seen clearly.

- **Myopia** (my·OH·pee·uh), or **nearsightedness**, is a visual problem in which distant objects appear blurred while close objects are seen clearly.

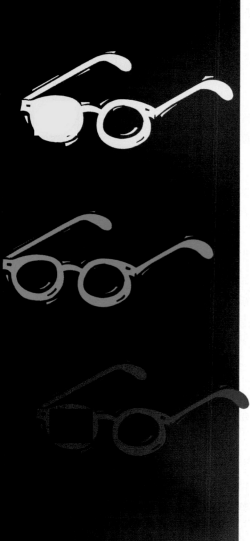

Eyeglasses and contact lenses can help correct vision problems. They help the lens of the eye focus the light on the retina so that vision is sharp. Eyeglasses often are made with plastic and nonbreakable glass to prevent injury if they are broken. An anti-reflective coating might be applied to prevent glare. Another coating might be applied to reduce exposure to ultraviolet radiation. If you wear eyeglasses, follow instructions for cleaning them to avoid scratching the lenses.

Contact lenses are worn directly on the cornea. Contact lenses help focus light on one place on the retina. For this reason, contact lenses can be used to correct astigmatism as well as nearsightedness and farsightedness. Because the shape of soft contact lenses adjusts to that of the cornea, they are very comfortable.

Both hard and soft contact lenses can be worn for monovision. **Monovision** is wearing one contact lens to see close objects and the other to see at a distance.

If you wear contact lenses, follow instructions for correct use. Different kinds of contacts are made to be worn for different lengths of time. For example, some people wear contact lenses designed to be worn for a day and then thrown away. Others are designed to be worn for several weeks and then thrown away. Still others wear the same contact lenses for a year. They must be removed and cleaned or disinfected at regular times. Special solutions are used to keep contacts clean and to prevent infection. Germs or dirt on contact lenses can cause infection of the cornea.

To protect your eyes, remove contact lenses if:

- **they are very uncomfortable;**
- **your eyes become red or tearful;**
- **vision becomes blurred;**
- **you have double vision;**
- **there are rings around the images that you see.**

CHECKLIST

Ways to Care for Your Eyes

- Have an eye examination every 18 months to two years.

- Wear eyeglasses and contact lenses if they have been prescribed to correct your vision. Follow instructions for cleaning and disinfecting contact lenses.

- Check with an eye physician if you experience blurred vision, see rings around images, or see double.

- Wear sunglasses and a visor to protect your eyes from ultraviolet radiation and glare.

- Wear safety glasses for sports in which there is a risk of eye injury and when using power tools.

- Avoid eyestrain by sitting at least six feet from the television.

- Place a lamp so that it shines on your school books when doing homework.

- Do not scratch or rub the eye if something gets in it. Rinse away the particle by splashing cool water in the eye.

- Apply an ice-cold compress and see an eye physician when there is a blow to the eye.

- Check with the school nurse if your eyes become red and itch. These might be signs of pinkeye or a viral infection. **Pinkeye** is an inflammation of the membranes covering the white of the eye and eyelid. It is caused by bacteria, and spreads easily from one person to another.

Your Eyes

Taking Care of Your Ears

Hearing is an important way that you gain information. Being able to hear certain sounds, such as an approaching car, can help you stay safe. Hearing also helps you communicate with others.

Your Ears

The **outer ear** is the part of the ear that collects sound waves. **Sound waves** are vibrations or movements of air.

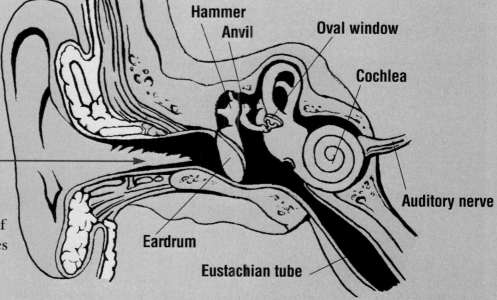

Hammer
Anvil
Oval window
Cochlea
Sound waves
Auditory nerve
Eardrum
Eustachian tube

The **middle ear** is the part of the ear in which sound waves push against the eardrum causing it to vibrate. When the eardrum vibrates, it moves three small bones. These three bones are the hammer, anvil, and stirrup. These bones carry the vibration to the oval window. The middle ear also contains the eustachian tube. The **eustachian** (yoo·STAY·shun) **tube** is a tube that helps keep the air pressure on both sides of the eardrum equal. It begins behind the eardrum and leads to the throat.

The **inner ear** is the part of the ear that sends messages to the brain and helps a person keep his or her balance. When the oval window vibrates, tiny hairs inside the cochlea feel the vibration. This causes electrical messages to travel along the auditory nerve to the brain. The brain interprets these messages. You hear these messages as specific sounds. The semicircular canals contain a special fluid and tiny hairs that are connected to nerve endings. As you move about, these tiny hairs send messages to the brain. In this way, the brain interprets your movements and helps you keep your balance.

Decibel Levels of Common Sounds

Rocket launch.........................180 dB

Jet engine at close range...........150 dB

Live rock concert.................118 dB

Power lawn mower............86 dB

City traffic........................81 dB

Normal conversation....58 dB

Whisper...............32 dB

Hearing Loss and Ear Problems

A **decibel (dB)** is a unit used to measure the loudness of sounds. The slightest sound that a person can hear has a loudness of 0 decibels (dB).

Sounds from 40 to 60 decibels are comfortable. Sounds above 70 decibels are annoying and can cause hearing loss. Serious hearing loss can occur if you are exposed to sounds of 120 decibels. Sounds measuring greater than 140 decibels might cause pain as well as hearing loss. You can suffer permanent hearing loss if you are exposed to sounds measuring more than 180 decibels.

Noise pollution is loud or constant noise that causes hearing loss, stress, fatigue, irritability, and tension. Each day you are exposed to noise pollution. In fact, you might already have some hearing loss. Over half of eighteen-year-olds have hearing loss. Much of this hearing loss could have been prevented by reducing exposure to loud noise.

Some other causes of hearing loss are being exposed to drugs or infections before birth, being born prematurely, having a birth defect, or having a viral infection. Middle ear infections, high fevers, and injuries are also causes of hearing loss.

Hearing examinations are needed to confirm hearing loss. An **audiometer** is a machine used to assess the range of sounds that a person can hear. If there is hearing loss, a hearing aid can be worn. Sometimes surgery is helpful in correcting hearing loss. But in most cases, prevention is the key.

Suppose you know someone who has a hearing loss. You can improve communication with this person. Look directly at the person as you speak. The person can listen and watch your lips form words. Suppose you sit by the person and talk. Ask the person if it makes a difference if you sit on his or her right or left side. Always speak slowly. Repeat what you have said if you are asked. Do not be impatient. Remember, communication requires the effort of all people involved.

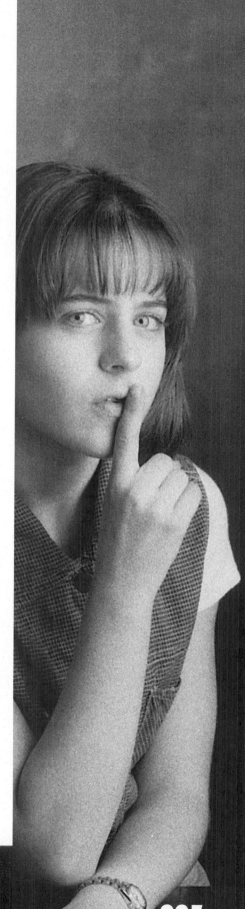

CHECKLIST

Ways to Care for Your Ears

- Clean the outer ear with a soft, clean washcloth to avoid wax buildup in the ear canal.
- Do not insert any objects (including cotton-tipped swabs) into the ear canal, because these objects might puncture the eardrum.
- Use the corner of a dry, clean towel to gently dry the ears after bathing or swimming.
- Wear earplugs when swimming to prevent water from entering the ear and causing ear infections.
- Consult a physician whenever an ear becomes infected or you have a bad cold or throat infection.
- Wear a hat, scarf, or earmuffs to prevent cold from irritating the middle ear.
- Keep the volume of radios, compact disc players, stereos, and the television at safe levels.
- Avoid listening to music at unsafe levels through headphones.
- Wear protective earplugs when operating loud machinery, using power tools, or attending rock concerts.

Your Ears

Apply...
The Responsible Decision-Making Model™

You and your friend are going to a rock concert. You are bringing protective ear plugs with you. Your friend says only geeks wear ear plugs.

Answer the following questions on a separate sheet of paper. Write "Does not apply" if a question does not apply to this situation.

1. Is it healthful not to wear ear plugs at the concert? Why or why not?

2. Is it safe not to wear ear plugs at the concert? Why or why not?

3. Is it legal not to wear ear plugs at the concert? Why or why not?

4. Will you show respect for yourself if you do not wear ear plugs at the concert? Why or why not?

5. Will your parents or guardian approve if you do not wear ear plugs at the concert? Why or why not?

6. Will you demonstrate good character if you do not wear ear plugs at the concert? Why or why not?

What is the responsible decision to make in this situation?

Lesson 21

Review

Vocabulary

Write a separate sentence using each of the vocabulary words listed on page 212.

Health Content

Write responses to the following:

1. How can you control body odor? Treat acne? **page 213**
2. What are eleven ways to care for your skin and nails? **page 214**
3. What are eleven ways to care for your hair? **page 217**
4. How do you care for a blister, callus, corn, and ingrown toenail? **page 218**
5. What are six ways to care for your feet? **page 218**
6. What are ways to correct astigmatism, hyperopia, and myopia? **page 221**
7. What are ten ways to care for your eyes? **page 222**
8. What are causes of hearing loss? **page 225**
9. What are changes in health that might be caused by noise pollution? **page 225**
10. What are nine ways to care for your ears? **page 226**

Having Medical and Dental Checkups

Vocabulary

personal health management

health history

physical examination

symptom

dental plaque

calculus

cavity

gingivitis

periodontal disease

orthodontist

malocclusion

braces

retainer

Life Skills
- **I will have regular examinations.**
- **I will follow a dental health plan.**

Personal health management is self-care that promotes optimal well-being. Personal health management includes: keeping your own personal health care records; choosing a lifestyle that promotes good health; having regular physical examinations; having regular dental checkups; and following a dental health plan. You, your parents or guardian, your physician, and your dentist work as a team to plan your health care.

The Lesson Objectives

- Discuss how your physician helps you be healthy.
- List symptoms for which prompt medical treatment is needed.
- Describe ways your dentist helps you keep your teeth healthy.
- Explain the purpose of wearing braces.
- Describe correct ways to brush and floss your teeth.
- Design a dental health plan.

How Your Physician Helps You

Your physician is an important part of your health care team. You and your parents or guardian need to select a physician. The physician will ask many questions when you meet for the first time. Prepare for this meeting by keeping a personal health care record. Write down important information such as your eating, exercise, and sleeping habits. Describe past health conditions and medical care. Your physician will use these facts for a health history. A **health history** is a record of a person's health habits, past health conditions, past medical care, allergies, and family's health.

Having a Physical Examination

Your physician will perform a physical examination. A **physical examination** is a series of tests that measure health status. Your height and weight will be recorded. The physician will listen to your heart and lungs and check your pulse and blood pressure. The physician might want you to have lab tests. Your urine and blood might be checked. After the physical examination, the physician will discuss the results with you and your parents or guardian. If the tests reveal a health problem, the physician will recommend treatment. Your physician will discuss your health habits with you.

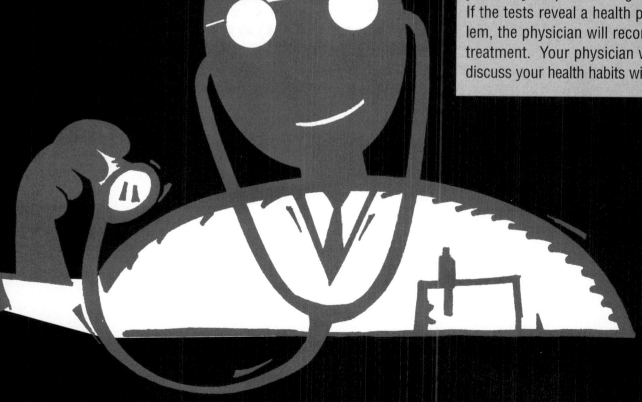

Checking Symptoms

There are other occasions when you need to see your physician. You might need to see a physician if abnormal or unusual symptoms appear. A **symptom** is a change in a body function or behavior from the usual pattern. A symptom might be an indication of a health problem. Some symptoms, such as constant headaches, interfere with a person's daily routine. A physician can tell ways to relieve the symptoms or treat the health problem causing the symptoms.

Visit your physician if you have any of the following symptoms:

- shortness of breath;
- loss of appetite for no obvious reason;
- blood in urine or bowel movement;
- blood coughed up;
- a constant cough;
- fever of 100°F (37.7°C) or higher for more than one day;
- swelling, stiffness, or aching in the joints;
- severe pain in any body part;
- frequent or painful urination;
- sudden weight gain or loss;
- dizziness;
- any warning signs of cancer;
- any warning signs of heart attack or stroke.

How Your Dentist Helps You

Your dentist and dental hygienist are also members of your health care team. They encourage you to have regular dental checkups and to follow a dental health plan. This plan should include taking a health history and having your teeth cleaned and examined every six months.

Dental plaque is an invisible, sticky film of bacteria on teeth, especially near the gum line. Brushing teeth helps remove plaque from the exposed surfaces of the teeth. Flossing helps remove dental plaque and bits of food stuck between the teeth. However, brushing and flossing might not remove plaque completely. Plaque might build up and harden. **Calculus** is hardened dental plaque. It can be removed during a dental treatment when the teeth are cleaned and polished.

You need to have your teeth cleaned and to have a dental checkup every six months. During a dental check-up, X-rays might be taken. X-rays show the insides of the teeth, gums, and the supporting bones.

The dentist might discover a cavity during your checkup. A **cavity** is a hole in a tooth. A filling is a material used to repair the cavity.

The dentist will also check your gums. **Gingivitis** (jihn·juh·VY·tis) is a condition in which the gums are red, swollen, and tender. They bleed easily. Gingivitis often is due to poor diet and lack of brushing and flossing. This condition worsens if it is not treated. **Periodontal disease** is a disease of the gums and other tissues that support the teeth. It often begins in teens with the buildup of plaque and calculus.

Wearing Braces

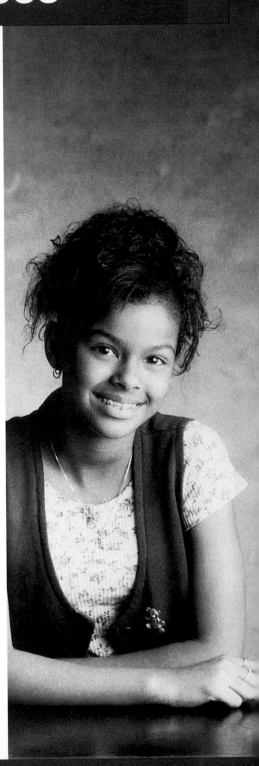

The dentist might recommend that you see an orthodontist. An **orthodontist** is a dentist who treats malocclusion. **Malocclusion** (ma·luh·KLEW·zhun) is the abnormal fitting together of teeth when the jaws are closed. It might be caused by heredity, jaw size, early loss of primary teeth, or injury. When teeth do not fit together properly, there is extra stress on the jaw. The teeth grind together too much. Plaque is more likely to collect and cause cavities.

Malocclusion can be corrected in a number of ways. Often it is treated by wearing braces. **Braces** are devices that are placed on the teeth and wired together to help straighten teeth. Children who get braces during childhood usually wear braces from 18 to 24 months. People who get braces as teens and adults usually need to wear them longer. After the braces are removed, a retainer is often worn. A **retainer** is a plastic device with wires that keep the teeth from moving back to their original places.

If you wear braces, it is important to brush your teeth and the braces carefully to prevent tooth decay. If you have a retainer, do not forget to wear it. Remember to keep your retainer clean.

If you wear braces, ask your orthodontist about your diet. Be careful what you choose. Hard candies might break off parts of your braces. Sticky foods such as caramels are hard to remove. Remember braces are expensive. You will not wear them forever. While you wear them, you must make wise choices.

Also, ask your orthodontist about mouthguards for sports. Your orthodontist can advise you on what to wear. Your orthodontist can discuss the proper fit.

Sometimes maloclussion is treated by reshaping teeth through dental restoration. In more serious cases, teeth might have to be removed. False teeth are teeth that might be used where teeth have been removed. False teeth also might be used if a person has lost a tooth after an injury.

Toothbrushing and Flossing

Toothbrushing is a way to clean teeth. Brush your teeth three times per day. Floss your teeth every day.

How to Floss

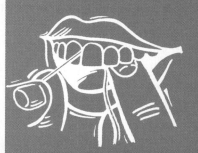

1. **Wrap dental floss around two fingers.**

How to Brush Your Teeth

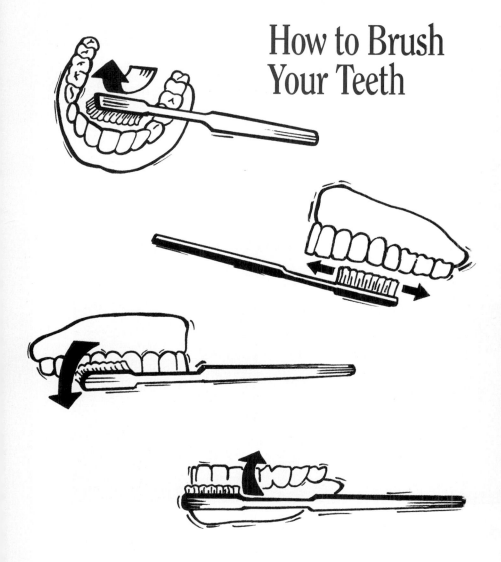

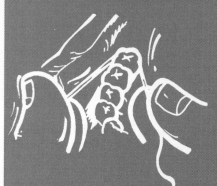

2. **Gently move floss between teeth to gum line.**

3. **Wrap floss around tooth and slide up and down.**

Follow a...

Health Behavior Contract

Copy the health behavior contract on a separate sheet of paper.

DO NOT WRITE IN THIS BOOK.

Name: _____ **Date:** _____

Life Skill: I will follow a dental health plan.

Effect On My Health: My teeth must last a lifetime. They help me chew foods and speak clearly. Healthy teeth give me a pleasant appearance. I must keep my gums healthy to support my teeth.

My Plan: I will write on my calendar actions I will take for the next week to have healthy teeth. I will brush and floss my teeth daily. I will choose foods and beverages that are sources of vitamin D, vitamin C, and calcium. I will limit sweet and sticky foods. I will protect my teeth from injury by wearing a safety belt when riding in a motor vehicle. I will wear a mouthguard for sports in which my teeth might be injured. At the end of each day, I will highlight the actions I have completed.

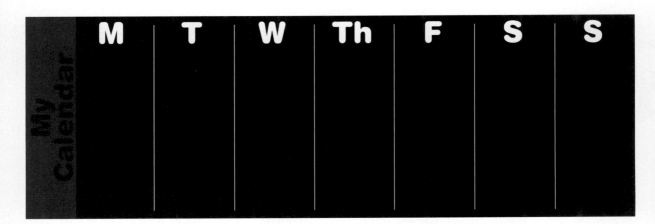

My Calendar	M	T	W	Th	F	S	S

How My Plan Worked: (Complete after one week.) At the end of the week, I will evaluate whether I followed my dental health plan. I will write in my journal actions on which I can improve. I will make a goal to follow my plan so that taking care of my teeth and gums becomes a habit for life.

Your Dental Health Plan

- Brush your teeth and tongue after each meal. Use a soft-bristle toothbrush to prevent injury to gums.

- Use a toothpaste that contains fluoride. Fluoride strengthens the teeth and helps prevent tooth decay.

- Floss your teeth each day.

- Have your teeth cleaned, polished, and checked every six months.

- Limit the amount of sweet and sticky foods that you eat.

- Eat foods that contain calcium, phosphorus, and vitamins C and D. These minerals and vitamins strengthen teeth and gums.

- Follow dental safety rules, such as wearing a safety belt in a car, to protect the mouth and teeth from injury in case of an accident.

- Wear a mouthguard for sports in which teeth might be injured.

- Avoid risk behaviors that might cause oral cancer and tooth decay. These risk behaviors include using smokeless tobacco and cigarettes, and drinking alcohol.

- Know the signs of oral cancer. Signs of oral cancer include a sore in the mouth that bleeds easily and does not heal, a red or white patch in the mouth, and difficulty in chewing and swallowing.

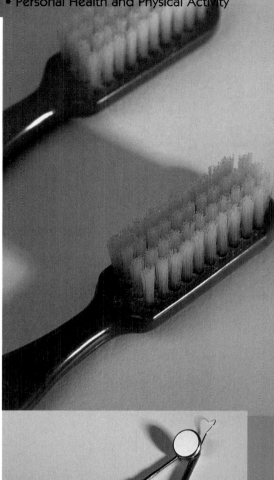

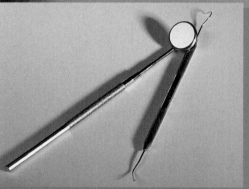

Lesson 22

Review

Vocabulary

Write a separate sentence using each of the vocabulary words listed on page 228.

Health Content

Write responses to the following:

1. What are ways physicians help keep you healthy? **page 229** Ways dentists help keep you healthy? **page 231**

2. What are thirteen symptoms for which prompt medical treatment is needed? **page 230**

3. Why are braces and a retainer worn? **page 232**

4. Describe the procedures for brushing and flossing teeth. **page 233**

5. What should you include in a dental health plan? **pages 234–235**

Being Energized with Physical Activity

Vocabulary

norepinephrine

beta-endorphins

stress

competition

body composition

essential body fat

adipose tissue

cardiac output

stroke volume

blood pressure

dynamic blood pressure

atherosclerosis

osteoporosis

osteoarthritis

anabolic steroid

sleep

insomnia

Life Skills

- **I will participate in regular physical activity.**
- **I will get adequate rest and sleep.**

Suppose you want to give yourself a gift. The gift would do the following: help you look terrific, enjoy others, live longer, and have fun. It is almost a sure bet you would like this gift. Actually, this is a gift you can give yourself right now. Participating in physical activity will provide you with all these things. SO GET OUT YOUR ATHLETIC SHOES AND GET ENERGIZED!

The Lesson Objectives

- List the Top Ten Reasons for Being Energized with Physical Activity.
- Explain how physical activity contributes to each of the Top Ten Reasons.

Top Ten

Top Ten

Top Ten

Top Ten

Top Ten

Top Ten

Top Ten

Top Ten

The Top Ten Reasons for Being Energized with Physical Activity

Physical activity...

1. gives you a feeling of well-being;
2. relieves your stress;
3. helps you develop social skills;
4. helps you learn how to compete;
5. helps you manage your weight;
6. strengthens your heart and lungs;
7. keeps your blood vessels healthy;
8. strengthens your bones;
9. tones your muscles;
10. helps you get a good night's sleep.

Physical Activity and Well-Being

Blood circulates through your body more vigorously when you participate in physical activity. As a result, you feel more refreshed and relaxed. The increased flow of blood carrying nutrients and oxygen to the brain helps you think more clearly. It is easier to concentrate and do your school work.

Physical activity can cause your body to produce higher levels of two substances. **Norepinephrine** (nor·eh·puh·NEH·frun) is a substance that helps transmit brain messages along certain nerves. **Beta-endorphins** (BAY·tuh·en·DOR·fihnz) are substances produced in the brain that help reduce pain and create a feeling of well-being. When high levels of these two substances are in the blood, they create a feeling of well-being.

To get your body to release norepinephrine and beta-endorphins into the bloodstream, you need to be physically active for at least 20 minutes or more. The effects of these substances will last for about 90 minutes after you have finished your workout. Participate in vigorous activities such as rollerblading, walking fast, running, biking, and swimming.

Being involved in regular physical activity has an added benefit for many females. Females usually begin their menstrual period somewhere between the ages of 8 and 14. Some females have menstrual cramps and pain. Physical activities that release the body's natural painkiller, the beta-endorphins, can help ease cramps and pain.

Some teens suffer from depression. Many physicians and mental health experts are now recommending physical activity to help treat depression.

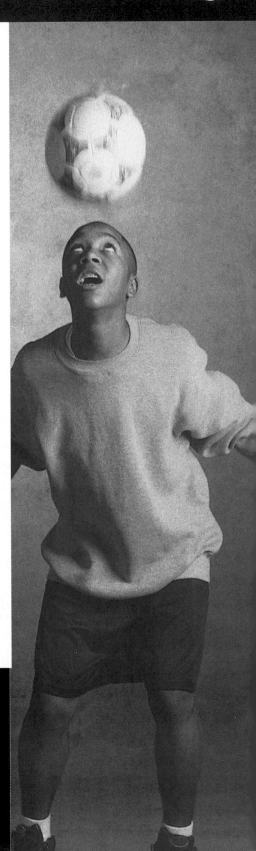

Physical Activity and Stress Management

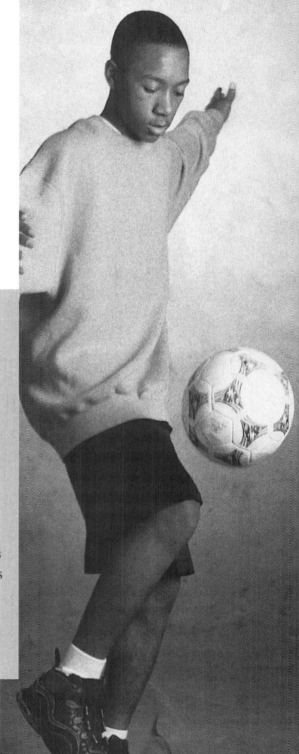

Stress is the response of the body to the demands of daily living. You learned about stress in Lesson 5. The body gets ready for action when you experience stress. Adrenaline is secreted into the bloodstream causing increased heart rate and blood pressure. Your muscles get ready for action.

These body changes are healthful when they help you meet the challenge of a stressor. After the challenge is met, your body returns to normal. But sometimes stress gets out of control. Your body needs help to return to its normal state. Vigorous physical activity relieves tension by providing an outlet for the energy that builds up with stress. It uses up the adrenaline. Your heart rate and blood pressure return to normal. Your muscles relax.

Here is some important advice. Do not wait for stress to get out of control. Be active and energized. Choose to be physically active to keep from becoming stressed-out.

Being energized with physical activity is a healthful way to cope with stress. You are less likely to participate in risk behaviors when you select healthful ways to manage stress. Do you know someone who feels stressed and drinks alcohol? Smokes cigarettes? Eats too much? Starts fights? These behaviors might be due to stress.

Physical activity keeps a person who is stressed busy. It is a good way to get away from the cause of stress. Sometimes when you are stressed you need a break. A hard workout releases beta-endorphins. Your outlook can change. You can be refreshed. The break allows you to come back, work on a problem, and solve it.

Physical Activity and Social Skills

Participating in physical activities gives you a chance to practice social skills. There are opportunities to meet and be with others. For example, you might join team sports such as volleyball, basketball, or baseball. You have the opportunity to talk and joke around. You gain a sense of belonging that is vital in the teen years. Remember, teens who feel "left out" are sometimes attracted to the wrong crowd. They are more likely to get into trouble.

Rollerblading, biking, dancing, and walking are activities that you can enjoy with others. You have the opportunity to be in the company of others in an enjoyable and relaxed situation.

Sharing physical activities is a good way for families to become closer. Physical activities can provide a time for family members to work together to reduce stress, build communication, and have fun.

Never underestimate the value of physical activity in strengthening relationships. As you mature and enter the workforce, you will notice something. Co-workers who participate in physical activities together get to know each other better. This often helps them work better with each other. You will notice that being able to discuss sports and being skilled in physical activities often can help people succeed at work.

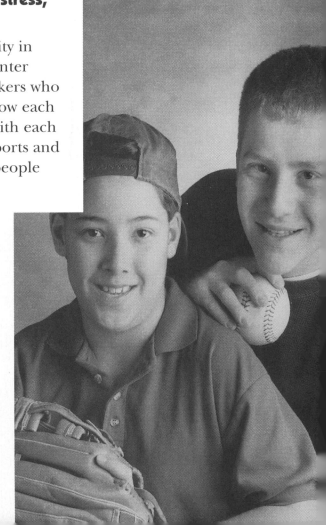

Physical Activity and Competition

Competition is the act of trying to win or gain something from another or others. Many aspects of life involve competition. You might already feel as if you are competing. Sometimes you compete with yourself. You try to outperform or be better at something than you have been in the past. For example, you want to better your score at bowling or improve your math scores from the last grading period. At other times, you compete with others. You compete for a grade, for a job, or for a position on an athletic team. Does this sound familiar?

You will compete with yourself and others throughout life. You will experience some successes or "wins." You also might experience some setbacks or "losses." Sports and games are physical activities that give you a chance to compete with yourself and others. Bowling, gymnastics, running, distance walking, and golf are sports in which you can compete with yourself to get a better score or time. You also can compete against others. Basketball, football, soccer, and tennis involve competing directly against others.

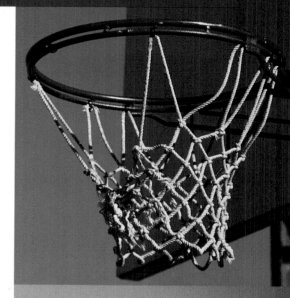

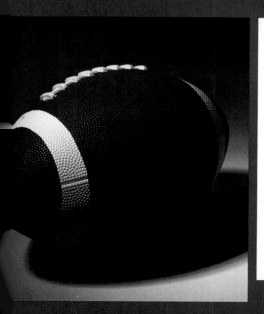

When you participate in sports and games, you learn skills needed to compete in other situations. You learn to:

- set performance goals and work to reach them;
- try your best at all times;
- win without bragging;
- handle defeat and make adjustments for a better performance;
- play by the rules.

Physical Activity and Weight Management

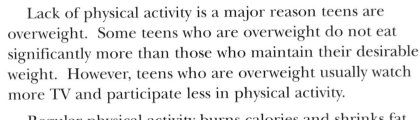

Lack of physical activity is a major reason teens are overweight. Some teens who are overweight do not eat significantly more than those who maintain their desirable weight. However, teens who are overweight usually watch more TV and participate less in physical activity.

Regular physical activity burns calories and shrinks fat cells. When you participate in regular physical activity, your appetite is decreased and you might not eat as much.

Regular exercise affects your body composition. **Body composition** is the percentage of fat tissue and lean tissue in the body. You learned that it is healthful to keep your percentage of body fat within a certain range. There are two kinds of body fat. **Essential body fat** is the fat that is located around such organs as the heart, lungs, liver, spleen, kidneys, and intestines. This type of fat protects these organs from injury and helps with body processes. **Adipose** (A·duh·pohs) **tissue** is the fat that accumulates around internal organs, within muscle, tissues, and under the skin. Having too much of this type of fat increases your risk of heart disease, diabetes, cancer, and arthritis. Having too much adipose tissue affects your appearance, too. Physical activity reduces the amount of adipose tissue.

Regular exercise also helps self-respect. Having self-respect is important in a plan for weight management. If you have self-respect, you take care of yourself. You are less likely to choose harmful ways to manage your weight. You also have something to do when you are stressed. Being stressed can cause teens to pig out and gain weight. Being stressed can cause teens to lose their appetite and drop weight.

The beta-endorphins released after a workout are helpful, too. When you feel good, your appetite is more likely to be normal. You do not eat too much or too little.

Physical Activity and the Heart and Lungs

Your muscle cells need more oxygen than usual during physical activity. Your cardiac output increases. **Cardiac output** is the amount of blood pumped by the heart each minute. Cardiac output is equal to your heart rate multiplied by your stroke volume. **Stroke volume** is the amount of blood the heart pumps with each beat.

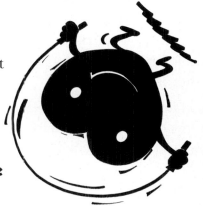

Your heart is a muscle that is composed of threadlike muscle fibers. Vigorous physical activity makes these fibers thicker and stronger. A strong heart muscle can pump more blood with each beat. When stroke volume is greater, the heart does not have to beat as often to supply cells with the same amount of oxygen. As a result, your resting heart rate is lower, allowing your heart to rest between beats.

Vigorous physical activity also lowers resting blood pressure. **Blood pressure** is the force of blood against the artery walls. High blood pressure exerts wear and tear on the arteries. It can harm tissues in the lining of the arteries. Vigorous physical activity keeps resting blood pressure in normal range. It lowers dynamic blood pressure. **Dynamic blood pressure** is the measure of the changes in blood pressure during the day. Sudden increases in blood pressure can harm blood vessels.

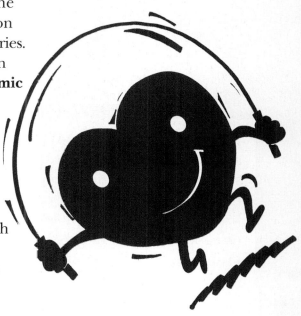

Regular physical activity strengthens the diaphragm muscle, which is just below the lungs. The diaphragm helps your lungs expand and contract when you inhale and exhale air. You are able to inhale more air with each breath when the diaphragm muscle is strong. More oxygen is available for your blood, and your heart works less. You also exhale more carbon dioxide.

Physical Activity and Blood Vessels

Physical activity helps prevent atherosclerosis. **Atherosclerosis** (A·thuh·ROH·skluh·ROH·sis) is a disease in which fat deposits on artery walls. The inside of the arteries narrow, causing reduced blood flow. The amount of cholesterol in the blood is linked to the development of atherosclerosis.

You learned about high density lipoproteins (HDLs) and low density lipoproteins (LDLs) in Lesson 17. Vigorous physical activity increases the number of HDLs and decreases the number of LDLs. The HDLs carry cholesterol to the liver for breakdown and excretion, thereby lowering the amount of cholesterol in the blood. Choose physical activities such as long-distance running, swimming, and biking to increase HDLs.

Physical Activity and Bones and Joints

Physical activities that are weight-bearing, such as running, walking, and rollerblading, strengthen bones and help prevent them from becoming thin and brittle. A lifetime habit of these activities helps prevent osteoporosis when you are older. **Osteoporosis** (ah·stee·oh·puh·ROH·sis) is a bone disease in which bone tissue becomes thin. As a result, the bone becomes extremely fragile and might fracture from even minor injuries.

Regular physical activity helps joints as well as bones. You are able to bend, twist, turn, and move in different directions when joints move easily. Stretching helps muscles lengthen. This allows your joints to move freely and easily through their full range of motion. You are less likely to become injured while doing everyday activities. A lifetime habit of stretching helps prevent osteoarthritis when you are older. **Osteoarthritis** (ah·stee·oh·ahr·THRY·tuhs) is a condition in which the movable parts of a joint break down. Stretching helps keep the joints movable throughout your life.

Physical Activity and Muscles

Physical activity strengthens muscles. Physical activity helps muscles work for longer periods of time. Muscles can then contract and relax repeatedly before tiring. Strong muscles are able to do more work.

Appropriate physical activity and a healthful diet are safe ways to make muscles stronger. Some teens mistakenly believe that anabolic steroids are safe to use to increase muscle growth and strength. An **anabolic steroid** (a·nuh·BAH·lik STIR·oyd) is a synthetic drug that is used to increase muscle size and strength. Anabolic steroids are injected or taken orally. There is evidence that use of anabolic steroids can harm physical and mental health. You will learn more about these substances in Lesson 29.

Physical Activity, Rest, and Sleep

Sleep is a restful state in which there is little or no conscious thought. Rest and sleep help your body rebuild and reenergize. While you sleep, your heart rate slows down about 10 to 15 beats per minute. Your blood pressure and breathing rate slow down. Your muscles are not as tense.

You might need between eight to ten hours of sleep each night. You might need more sleep if you are sick. Regular physical activity helps you have restful sleep. It helps reduce the likelihood of insomnia. **Insomnia** is a condition in which a person has difficulty sleeping.

Tips for Sound Sleeping

- Participate in regular physical activity, but no later than three hours before bedtime.

- Practice stress management skills when feeling stressed.

- Eat dinner before 6 p.m., and avoid snacking before bedtime.

- Avoid foods and beverages containing caffeine after 6 p.m.

- Unwind before bedtime by listening to relaxing music, reading, or taking a warm bath.

- Prepare a comfortable sleep environment by keeping your room dark and quiet.

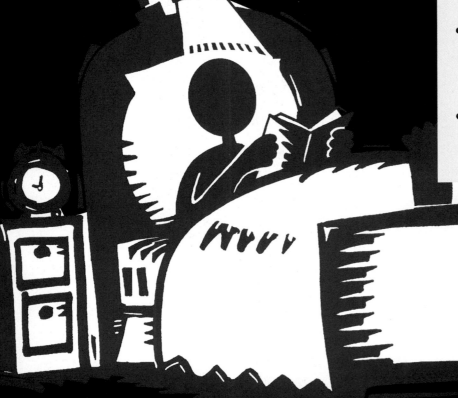

Hot Shots!

Life Skill I will participate in regular physical activity.

Materials: Notebook paper, scissors, pen or pencil for each of five groups; and one medium-sized ball, trash can or other container for the class

Directions: Play Hot Shots! to get some physical activity and to reinforce your knowledge of how physical activity benefits your health.

1. **Each group is assigned two headings by your teacher from this lesson.** One student in each group writes all the benefits of physical activity for that heading, one benefit per line. The other students help locate the benefits. Skip a line between benefits.

2. **Cut the benefits into strips and fold them.** Your teacher then collects them and mixes them up.

3. **Your class is then divided into two teams.** One by one, each student draws a strip and reads it. The student chooses how close to stand to the container. Then he or she tries to throw the ball into the container. The point scoring is: one point if one foot away, two points if two feet, and so on. The team with the most points wins.

Activity

Lesson 23

Review

Vocabulary

Write a separate sentence using each of the vocabulary words listed on page 236.

Health Content

Write responses to the following:

How does physical activity:

1. Affect the levels of norepinephrine and beta-endorphins? **page 238**

2. Help the body return to its normal state when a person feels stressed? **page 239**

3. Give you chances to practice social skills? **page 240**

4. Help you learn how to compete? **page 241**

5. Help with weight management? **page 242**

6. Help the heart and lungs? **page 243**

7. Change the amount of HDLs and LDLs? **page 244**

8. Help bones and joints? **page 244**

9. Help muscles? **page 245**

10. Help with rest and sleep? **page 246**

Designing a Physical Fitness Plan

Vocabulary

physical fitness
health-related fitness
muscular strength
muscular endurance
flexibility
cardiorespiratory endurance
healthful body composition
isotonic exercise
isometric exercise
isokinetic exercise
anaerobic exercise
aerobic exercise
target heart rate
maximum heart rate
lifetime sports and
physical activities
skill-related fitness
fitness skills
agility
balance
coordination
reaction time
speed
power
physical fitness plan

Life Skills

- **I will develop and maintain health-related fitness.**
- **I will develop and maintain skill-related fitness.**
- **I will follow a physical fitness plan.**

Participating in regular physical activity can help you gain physical fitness. What is health-related fitness? What types of exercises help you gain health-related fitness? Why is it important to participate in physical activities that you can participate in for a lifetime? What is skill-related fitness? What should your physical fitness plan include? These questions will be answered in this lesson.

The Lesson Objectives

- Describe the five areas of health-related fitness.
- Identify exercises used to measure physical fitness.
- Explain the benefits of exercises for health-related fitness.
- State examples of lifetime sports and physical activities.
- List skills you need for skill-related fitness.

The Five Areas of Health-Related Fitness

Physical fitness is the condition of the body that results from regular physical activity. **Health-related fitness** is the ability of the heart, lungs, muscles, and joints to perform well. Five areas of health-related fitness are shown on the chart. A person who has optimal health-related fitness has muscular strength, muscular endurance, flexibility, cardiorespiratory endurance, and a healthful percentage of body fat.

1. **Muscular strength**
2. **Muscular endurance**
3. **Flexibility**
4. **Cardiorespiratory endurance**
5. **Healthful body composition**

Health-Related Fitness

Areas of Health-Related Fitness	Examples of Exercise
Muscular strength: the ability to lift, pull, push, kick, and throw with force.	Lifting weights Doing pull-ups on a bar Doing push-ups Kicking a soccer ball Throwing a baseball
Muscular endurance: the ability to use muscles for an extended period of time.	Pedaling a bicycle for a mile Holding a weight above your head Rollerblading continuously for a long period of time
Flexibility: the ability to bend and move the joints through a full range of motion.	Touching your toes Doing a backbend
Cardiorespiratory endurance: the ability to do activities that require increased oxygen intake for extended periods of time.	Running a mile Swimming several laps
Healthful body composition: a high ratio of lean tissue to fat tissue.	Aerobic exercises

Physical Fitness Tests

Two tests have been developed to measure the physical fitness of young people. One test is part of the Prudential FITNESSGRAM program. The other test, the President's Challenge, was developed by the President's Council on Physical Fitness and Sports. Someone at your school might evaluate your fitness using either of these tests. If you have a high enough score for either test, you will earn an award.

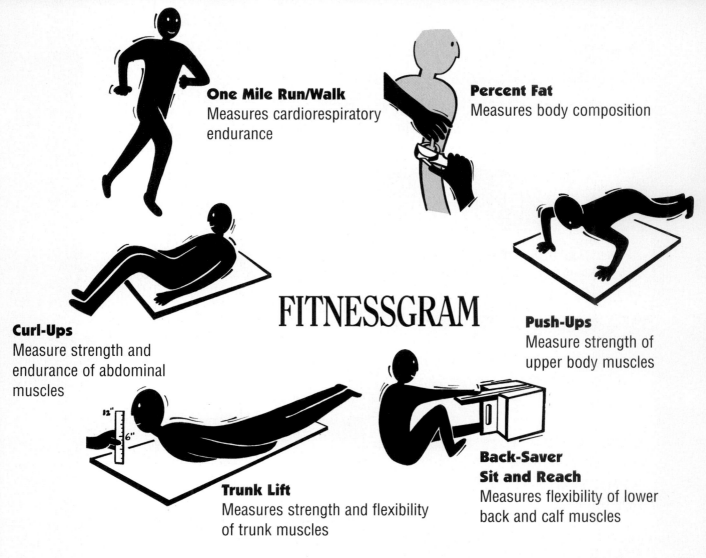

One Mile Run/Walk
Measures cardiorespiratory endurance

Percent Fat
Measures body composition

Curl-Ups
Measure strength and endurance of abdominal muscles

FITNESSGRAM

Push-Ups
Measure strength of upper body muscles

Trunk Lift
Measures strength and flexibility of trunk muscles

Back-Saver Sit and Reach
Measures flexibility of lower back and calf muscles

Reprinted with permission from The Cooper Institute for Aerobics Research, Dallas Texas.

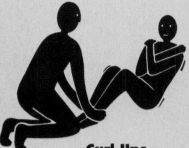

Curl-Ups
Measure strength and
endurance of abdominal
muscles

Pull-Ups
Measure strength and
endurance of upper
body muscles

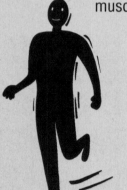

President's Challenge

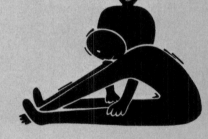

V-Sit Reach
Measures the flexibility of
lower back and calf muscles

Shuttle Run
Measures strength and
endurance of leg muscles

One Mile Walk/Run
Measures heart and
lung endurance

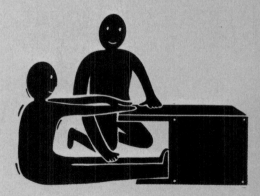

**Sit and Reach
(option to V-Sit Reach)**

Measures the flexibility of
lower back and calf muscles

Adapted from the President's Challenge, President's Council on Physical Fitness and Sports.

Types of Exercises to Develop Health-Related Fitness

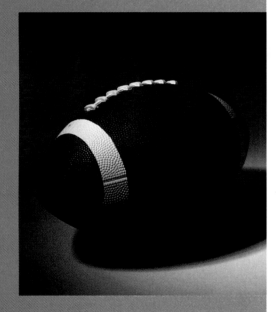

A variety of exercises help develop the five areas of health-related fitness. Each type of exercise provides specific and different results.

An **isotonic exercise** is an exercise in which there is a muscle contraction that causes movement. Curl-ups, push-ups, and lifting weights are examples. Isotonic exercises increase muscular strength, muscular endurance, and flexibility. They do not help cardiorespiratory endurance.

An **isometric exercise** is an exercise in which muscles are tightened for five to ten seconds without movement of body parts. Holding the abdominal muscles in tightly is an example. Isometric exercises make the muscles larger and stronger. They improve muscular strength. However, they do not help muscular endurance, flexibility, or cardio-respiratory endurance.

An **isokinetic exercise** is an exercise in which a weight is moved through an entire range of motion. Many schools and health clubs have exercise machines with weight plates and air pressure. These machines are used for this purpose. Instructors teach participants how to use the machines safely. Without proper instruction, it is easy to become injured. Isokinetic exercises promote muscular strength, muscular endurance, and flexibility. These exercises are of little benefit for cardiorespiratory endurance.

An **anaerobic** (an·uh·ROH·bik) **exercise** is an exercise in which the body's demand for oxygen is greater than the supply. You can continue the activity for only a short period of time before needing to stop and catch your breath. Swimming a quick lap and running sprints are examples. These exercises improve muscular strength, muscular endurance, and flexibility. They have limited value in improving cardiorespiratory endurance.

An **aerobic** (uh·ROH·bik) **exercise** is an exercise that requires a continuous use of oxygen over an extended period of time. Your demand for and use of oxygen are the same throughout the exercise. They are the most popular exercises for developing cardiorespiratory endurance. However, aerobic exercises must be done at your target heart rate. The **target heart rate** is a heart rate of 75 percent of maximum heart rate. **Maximum heart rate** is a heart rate of 220 beats per minute minus age. Besides helping you develop cardiorespiratory endurance, aerobic exercises decrease your percentage of body fat. Rollerblading, running, swimming, and bicycling distances are examples of aerobic exercises.

Remember to vary the types of exercises you choose. This is the only way to achieve health-related fitness. For example, suppose you enjoy in-line skating. Every day after school you in-line skate for an hour. You also skate for an hour each day of the weekend. This means you get seven hours of aerobic exercise each week.

In-line skating helps you develop cardiorespiratory endurance. You develop a lean and trim appearance. This is because skating helps you to have a high ratio of lean tissue to fat tissue. Skating also makes leg muscles strong. You develop muscular strength and endurance in your leg muscles.

But in-line skating is not enough to have total health-related fitness. You need to exercise other muscles groups in your body, such as your arms. You also need to develop flexibility. As you skate, you move some joints through a range of motion. But there are others you do not move. In-line skating is an excellent workout. But it is not enough. Include several types of exercises in your workout.

Lifetime Sports and Physical Activities

During the teen years, you are developing habits that you can continue for the rest of your life. **Lifetime sports and physical activities** are sports and physical activities in which a person can participate as a person grows older. Examine the chart to determine the fitness benefits of different lifetime sports.

The chart below shows fitness benefits

5 = highest in fitness benefits

1 = lowest in fitness benefits

	Cardiorespiratory endurance	Upper body strength	Lower body strength	Flexibility	Healthful body composition
Step aerobics	5	2	2	3	5
Basketball	3	2	2	1	3
Fast walking	4	1	2	1	4
Rollerblading	5	1	3	1	4
Soccer	5	1	4	1	4
Weight training	1	5	5	1	4
Swimming	5	4	4	1	3
Tennis	4	2	3	1	3

Skill-Related Fitness

Skill-related fitness is the ability to perform well in sports and physical activities. Fitness skills help you enjoy lifetime sports and physical activities. **Fitness skills** are skills that can be used in physical activities, sports, and games. There are six fitness skills that you can develop and practice.

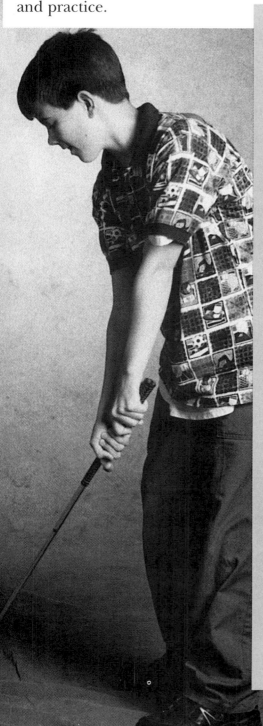

1. **Agility** is the ability to move quickly and easily. You use agility to change directions quickly, as when playing tennis or soccer.

2. **Balance** is the ability to keep from falling. You need balance for roller-blading, surfing, ice skating, and bicycling.

3. **Coordination** is the ability to use body parts and senses together for movement. You use your eyes and arms when you swing a racket at a ball.

4. **Reaction time** is the period of time it takes to move after a person hears, sees, feels, or touches a stimulus. The less time it takes you to move, the better your reaction time. A runner with a fast reaction time moves quickly when the starting signal is given.

5. **Speed** is the ability to move quickly. Moving quickly to kick a soccer ball requires speed.

6. **Power** is the ability to combine strength and speed. Throwing a baseball from the outfield to home plate requires power.

Follow a...

Health Behavior Contract

Copy the health behavior contract on a separate sheet of paper.

DO NOT WRITE IN THIS BOOK.

Name:_____ **Date:** _____

Life Skill: I will follow a physical fitness plan.

Effect On My Health: A **physical fitness plan** is a written schedule of physical activities to do to develop health-related fitness and skill-related fitness. A physical fitness plan will promote my cardiorespiratory endurance. I will reduce my percentage of body fat. I will increase my level of muscular strength, muscular endurance, and flexibility.

My Plan: I will list physical activities that I enjoy. Then I will evaluate each one using these five questions:

1. Is the facility I need available when I need it?
2. Can I afford to buy or rent the right equipment?
3. Can I afford to pay any fees required to participate in the activities?
4. Will I have enough time for the activities I choose?
5. Do I have the approval of my parents or guardian?

When I have narrowed my list to a few activities, I will decide how often and at what time of day to participate in these activities. I will write the times on my calendar. I will keep my calendar for one week.

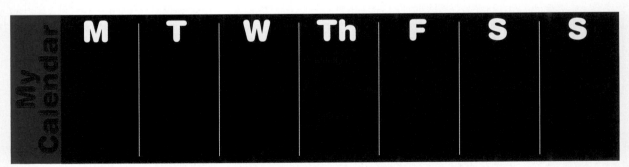

My Calendar | M | T | W | Th | F | S | S

Your Physical Fitness Plan

You can design a personal physical fitness plan using the health behavior contract on page 256. The physical activities you choose will depend on your health status, your body build, your current level of fitness, and your preferences. Remember to include physical activities that you can enjoy both now and when you are older. Also, remember that physical activities that promote cardiorespiratory endurance will reduce your percentage of body fat. Before you begin making your plan, determine your current level of physical fitness. Evaluate your body composition and your level of muscular strength, muscular endurance, flexibility, and cardiorespiratory

endurance. It is also desirable to get a medical checkup. Inform your physician you would like to begin a fitness program.

You will need to select equipment and clothing that are appropriate for the physical activities you choose. Your sessions will be more enjoyable when you are comfortable and your equipment is right for you. By following training principles and by knowing how to prevent and treat injuries, you will get the most benefit from your personal physical fitness plan. In addition, you should reevaluate your fitness level at regular intervals. To maintain physical fitness, you will need to establish new goals, and make and follow new plans.

Lesson 24

Review

Vocabulary

Write a separate sentence using each of the vocabulary words listed on page 248.

Health Content

Write responses to the following:

1. What are examples of exercises for each of the five areas of health-related fitness? **page 249**

2. What exercises are used to measure physical fitness in the FITNESSGRAM and the President's Challenge? **pages 250–251**

3. What are the benefits of isotonic exercises? **page 252**

4. What are the benefits of isometric exercises? **page 252**

5. What are the benefits of isokinetic exercises? **page 252**

6. What are the benefits of anaerobic exercises? **page 252**

7. What are the benefits of aerobic exercises? **page 253**

8. What are examples of lifetime sports and physical activities? **page 254**

9. What are six fitness skills? **page 255**

10. What should you include in a physical fitness plan? **pages 256–257**

Preventing and Treating Athletic Injuries

Vocabulary

training principles

warm-up

cool-down

specificity

overload

progression

frequency

physical profiling

biomechanics

RICE treatment

sports spectator

sports participant

Life Skills

- **I will prevent physical activity-related injuries and illnesses.**
- **I will be a responsible spectator and participant in sports.**

To be totally awesome is to follow through and do what is best for you. You have developed a personal physical fitness plan. You will get the most from your plan if you follow training principles and treat injuries promptly and correctly. Sports can be an enjoyable part of your physical fitness plan. You need to behave in a responsible manner when you are a spectator or participant in sports.

The Lesson Objectives

- Explain the meaning and purpose of training principles.
- Discuss ways to prevent injuries when participating in physical activity.
- Describe ways to be a responsible spectator and participant in sports.

Training Principles

Training principles are guidelines to follow to derive the maximum benefits from physical activity and to prevent injury. Six training principles will help you benefit from physical activity.

1. **The principle of warming up**
   A **warm-up** is three to five minutes of easy activity to prepare the muscles for more work. After warming up, stretch your muscles. Before bicycling fast, you might cycle a few minutes at a slower pace. During this time, the heart rate increases, the muscles stretch, and body temperature increases.

2. **The principle of cooling down**
   A **cool-down** is at least three to five minutes of reduced activity, such as after a workout. The heart rate slows and body temperature decreases during this time. After physical activities such as running or bicycling, blood is pooled in the legs. Cooling down helps the blood return to the heart.

3. **The principle of specificity**
   Specificity is choosing a physical activity for its desired benefit. If you want to develop cardiorespiratory endurance, you might choose speed walking rather than golf.

4. **The principle of overload**
   Overload is an additional activity that increases the body's capacity to do work. Suppose you do push-ups each day. You will need to increase the number you do to continue to increase muscular strength.

5. **The principle of progression**
   Progression is the gradual increase in intensity and duration of physical activity. Intensity is how hard you work during physical activity. Duration is the length of time of your workout. For example, you might walk on a treadmill. You can increase the incline at which you work to increase the intensity. Walking for a longer period of time will increase the duration.

6. **The principle of frequency**
   Frequency is the number of times a person participates in physical activity each week. Participating in physical activity once a week will not be enough. Participating in physical education classes might not be enough. You need to be involved in physical activities at least three to five times per week to be physically fit.

Preventing Injuries

Each year many teens are injured when participating in physical activities, including sports and games. You can avoid injuries by following some guidelines.

Know your body's limits. **Physical profiling** is a method of testing a person's physical limits to determine what types of physical activities are best. For example, running is not the best activity for someone with back problems. Rollerblading might not be the best activity for someone with weak ankles.

Work to develop skill-related fitness. **Biomechanics** is the study of how the body functions during movement. Many coaches videotape players to see if their movements are correct. An incorrect tennis grip might result in an elbow injury. Using exercise machines incorrectly is another cause of injury.

Follow safety rules. Safety rules for particular sports and games have been developed by experts. Experts know the dangers involved and how injuries might be prevented.

Get treatment for injuries. You might cause further harm if you continue to work out when you have an injury. Most injuries are musculoskeletal injuries. They might take several days or weeks to heal. The **RICE treatment** is a technique for treating musculoskeletal injuries. This treatment consists of rest, ice, compression, and elevation to promote faster healing. See your physician when an injury causes severe pain, joint problems, infection, or fever.

Wear appropriate clothing. Pay special attention to the clothing you wear when working out. Choose loose-fitting clothing to allow your skin to breathe. Shirts should be lightweight for proper ventilation. Wear shoes that fit correctly. Socks should be worn to cushion feet and to absorb perspiration. Wear light-colored clothing with reflective covering if you are outside at night.

Dress for the weather. If you are outside, wear clothing that is appropriate to the weather. Wear several thin layers of clothing in cold weather. Wearing thin layers allows the body to keep warm. The layers absorb the perspiration more easily than if thick layers are worn. Layers of clothing can be removed if you get too warm. If it is cold outside, wear gloves and a hat to protect fingers and ears.

Sports Show

Life Skill

I will prevent physical activity-related injuries and illnesses.

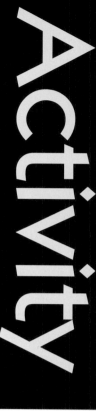
Activity

Materials: Paper, pen or pencil, books on sports, sports magazines, props as needed

Directions: In this activity, your group will prepare for a sports show. You will research and present information about training principles and prevention of injuries for your sport.

1. **Groups of four of five will sign up for a popular sport.** Your group will research and prepare a report that includes the following for your sport:

   - A list of activities for each training principle on page 259. For example, you might write that a warm-up activity for playing football is running in place.

   - A list of examples for each guideline on page 260. For example, you might research and record safety rules for playing soccer.

2. **Plan how your group will dress or carry props that represent your sport.** For example, if your sport is tennis, your group might wear white. One person might carry a tennis racket and another person might carry tennis balls.

3. **On the day of the Sports Show, each group will "model" by walking down a "runway" in the middle of the classroom.** One student will read the information that your group researched.

Being a Sports Spectator or Participant

Have you ever played team sports and been yelled at or booed by spectators? How did it make you feel? Embarrassed? Angry? Disrespected? When you are a sports spectator, treat the players the way you would want to be treated if you were playing. A **sports spectator** is a person who watches and supports sports without actively participating in them. People who are participating in sports usually are doing their best. They need support, not putdowns, from fans. When you are a sports spectator, do not boo or hiss at players, coaches, or referees. Show respect for the players and for the decisions of the referees. Respond with enthusiasm when your team makes a good play. Do not damage property or throw paper at the players or referees. Think how you feel when you are a sports participant.

A **sports participant** is a person who plays sports. When you are a sports participant, always put forth your best effort. Know the rules of the game. Respect and cooperate with your coach and teammates. Encourage your teammates. Maintain a healthful attitude toward winning and losing. If you not satisfied with your performance or you missed a play, do not mentally "beat yourself up." Everyone makes mistakes. Ask your coach for help and keep trying. Do not putdown or criticize a teammate who makes a mistake. Support your teammates the way you want them to support you. Keep sports in perspective. Chances are your academic skills are more important than your performance in sports for preparing to further your education and get a good job. Keep your grades a priority. Do not expect your coach or teachers to bend the rules on academic requirements for sports. If your grades slip and you are taken off the team, do not blame your teachers. YOU are responsible for your grades.

The RICE Treatment

The RICE treatment is a technique for treating injuries in which pain is lessened, swelling is limited, tissue damage is reduced, and faster healing is promoted.

Rest	Rest the injured part.
Ice	Apply cold, such as a cold compress, ice pack, or cold water.
Compression	Apply an elastic bandage to limit internal bleeding. Be careful not to apply the bandage too tightly. Check the body part for pain, numbness, change in color, or tingling. After 30 minutes, remove the bandage and the ice for 15 minutes. Then, reapply the ice and bandage for 30 minutes. Repeat the procedure for three hours.
Elevation	Elevate the injured part above the level of the heart. This helps drain blood and fluid from the injured area.

Lesson 25

Review

Vocabulary

Write a separate sentence using each of the vocabulary words listed on page 258.

Health Content

Write responses to the following:

1. What is the meaning and purpose of warming up? Cooling down? Specificity? Overload? Progression? Frequency? **page 259**

2. What are six guidelines to prevent injuries when participating in physical activity? **page 260**

3. What are ways you can be a responsible sports spectator? **page 262**

4. What are ways you can be a responsible sports participant? **page 262**

5. What are the steps in the RICE treatment? **page 263**

Unit 5 Review

Health Content

Review your answers for each Lesson Review in this unit. Then write answers to each of the following questions.

1. What should you do if you have a blister, callus, corn, or ingrown toenail? **Lesson 21 page 218**

2. How might noise pollution affect health? **Lesson 21 page 225**

3. For what symptoms should you visit your physician immediately? **Lesson 22 page 230**

4. What is the purpose of wearing braces and a retainer? **Lesson 22 page 232**

5. How can a person practice social skills when participating in physical activity? **Lesson 23 page 240**

6. What effect does physical activity have on muscles? **Lesson 23 page 245**

7. How do isometric exercises help you develop health-related fitness? **Lesson 24 page 252**

8. What fitness skills do you need to participate in lifetime sports and physical activity? **Lesson 24 page 255**

9. Why should you warm up before exercising? **Lesson 25 page 259**

10. How can you be a responsible sports spectator? **Lesson 25 page 262**

Vocabulary

Number a sheet of paper from 1–10. Select the correct vocabulary word. Write it next to the corresponding number. DO NOT WRITE IN THIS BOOK.

astigmatism	lice
muscular endurance	cardiac output
dental plaque	norepinephrine
gingivitis	specificity
isokinetic exercise	sports spectator

1. _____ is the amount of blood pumped by the heart each minute. **Lesson 23**

2. _____ is choosing a physical activity for its desired benefit. **Lesson 25**

3. _____ are insects that pierce the skin and secrete a substance that causes itching and swelling. **Lesson 21**

4. _____ is a visual problem in which an irregular curvature of the lens or cornea causes blurred vision. **Lesson 21**

5. _____ is a condition in which the gums are red, swollen, and tender. **Lesson 22**

6. _____ is a substance that helps transmit brain messages along certain nerves. **Lesson 23**

7. _____ is an invisible, sticky film of bacteria on teeth, especially near the gum line. **Lesson 22**

8. A(n) _____ is a person who watches and supports sports without actively participating in them. **Lesson 25**

9. _____ is an exercise in which a weight is moved through an entire range of motion. **Lesson 24**

10. _____ is the ability to use muscles for an extended period of time. **Lesson 24**

The Responsible Decision-Making Model™

A friend invites you to start running with him or her. You start to stretch before taking off. Your friend says, "Skip that. Only old people stretch before they run." Answer the following questions on a separate sheet of paper. Write "Does not apply" if a question does not apply to this situation.

1. Is it healthful not to stretch before running? Why or why not?

2. Is it safe not to stretch before running? Why or why not?

3. Is it legal not to stretch before running? Why or why not?

4. Will you show respect for yourself if you do not stretch before running? Why or why not?

5. Will your parents or guardian approve if you do not stretch before running? Why or why not?

6. Will you demonstrate good character if you do not stretch before running? Why or why not?

What is the responsible decision to make in this situation?

Health Literacy

Effective Communication

Refer to the chart in Lesson 21, Decibel Levels of Common Sounds. Design another way to show this information. For example, you might make a bar graph.

Self-Directed Learning

Choose a sport in which the players wear special clothing or equipment. Research the history of the sport. Find out whether the special clothing or equipment serves to protect health and in what ways.

Critical Thinking

Suppose you have a friend who is not physically active. (S)he does not enjoy sports. What are ways you can get your friend interested in health-related physical activities?

Responsible Citizenship

Look up the American Dental Association home page on the Internet. Find information on how to care for the teeth and gums. Make a print-out. Share it with your friends and family.

Multicultural Health

Choose a culture different from your own. Research the number one lifetime sport or physical activity in that culture in which people participate. Write a report that includes facts about the sport or activity.

Family Involvement

Make a list of grooming products your family uses. Visit a library or search the Internet to find sources of consumer information. Find out how the products your family uses are rated. Share your findings with your family.

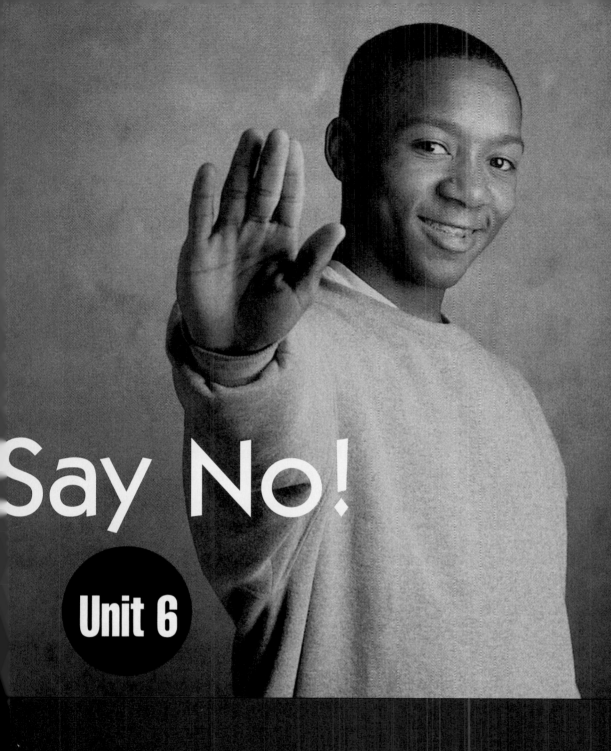

Say No!

Unit 6

Alcohol, Tobacco, and Other Drugs

The Responsible Use of Drugs

Vocabulary

drug
drug use
responsible drug use
drug misuse
drug abuse
suppository
receptor site
side effect
dose
solubility
medicine
prescription drug
prescription
pharmacist
brand-name drug
generic-name drug
over-the-counter (OTC) drug
tamper-resistant package
drug dependence
chemical dependence
chemical addiction
physical dependence
tolerance
withdrawal symptoms
psychological dependence

Life Skills

• **I will not misuse or abuse drugs.**
• **I will follow guidelines for the safe use of prescription and OTC drugs.**

A **drug** is a substance other than food that changes the way the body or mind works. **Drug use** is a term used to describe drug-taking behavior. **Responsible drug use** is the correct use of legal drugs to promote health and well-being. **Drug misuse** is the incorrect use of a prescription or over-the-counter drug. **Drug abuse** is the use of an illegal drug or the intentional misuse of a prescription or over-the-counter drug. Responsible drug use can promote your health and well-being. Drug misuse and abuse can ruin your health and your relationships.

The Lesson Objectives

• Explain ways drugs enter the body.
• Identify factors that determine the effects of drugs on the body.
• Describe differences between prescription drugs and over-the-counter, or OTC, drugs.
• List information found on the labels of prescription drugs and OTC drugs.
• State guidelines for the safe use of OTC drugs.
• Discuss types of drug dependence.

Ways Drugs Enter the Body

Drugs can enter your body in different ways: by mouth, by injection, by inhalation, and by absorption.

By Mouth

A drug taken orally is swallowed. A drug in the form of a pill, capsule, or liquid can be swallowed. After being swallowed, the drug travels to the stomach and small intestine. From the small intestine, the drug is absorbed into the bloodstream. The blood carries the drug throughout the body.

By Injection

When a drug is injected from a syringe or needle, it goes directly under the skin, into a muscle or blood vessel. A drug that is injected into a blood vessel can affect a person almost immediately.

By Inhalation

When a drug is inhaled through the nose or mouth, it travels to the lungs where it enters the bloodstream. Drugs that are inhaled also affect a person almost immediately.

By Absorption

When a drug is absorbed, it enters the bloodstream through the skin or mucous membranes. Ointments, creams, lotions, sprays, and patches can be applied to the skin or mucous membranes of the eyes, nose, mouth, anus or vagina. A **suppository** (suh·PAH·zuh·toh·ree) is a wax-coated form of a drug that is inserted into the anus or vagina. When the wax melts, the drug is released and absorbed into the bloodstream.

How Drugs Work Inside the Body

In many respects, your body cells are like a jigsaw puzzle. You cannot take just any piece of a puzzle and connect it to another piece. You cannot take just any drug and expect a certain action. Drugs have different effects on different body actions. A **receptor site** is the part of a cell where the chemical substance in a drug fits. Specific drugs work on specific receptor sites.

Sometimes drugs act on more than one receptor site. They might act on other receptor sites of other cells. For example, you might take a drug to treat an upset stomach. However, the drug might also act on other receptor sites and cause you to become dizzy. Being dizzy is an example of a side effect. A **side effect** is an unwanted body change that is not related to the main purpose of a drug. Tell a parent or guardian if you take a drug that causes side effects. You might need to stop taking the drug. Your parents or guardian might call your physician.

Suppose you get a drug from a pharmacy. Later, you will learn more about prescription drugs. The pharmacist might give you a printout about the drug. The printout will tell you what the drug is used to treat. It will tell you side effects that might occur. Read the printout carefully. Discuss the printout with your parents or guardian. Know what to expect.

You also might tell the pharmacist what other drugs you are taking. Of course you have already told your physician. But this serves as a double-check. Your pharmacist also can advise you if it is unwise to take two drugs together.

Remember, drugs change the way the mind and body work. Drugs can affect people in different ways. You must be cautious when taking a drug. Pay attention to side effects.

The effects drugs have on the body are determined by many factors.

The Way the Drug Enters the Body
The method of entry affects the speed with which the drug enters the bloodstream and affects a person.

Dose
The **dose** is the amount of a drug that is taken at one time. The greater the dose, the greater the effect of the drug and the more varied the effect might be.

Solubility
Solubility is the ability of a substance to be dissolved. Drugs can be water-soluble or fat-soluble. Drugs that are water-soluble dissolve well in water. Water-soluble drugs do not stay in the body for a long period of time. Fat-soluble drugs dissolve in fat tissue and can stay in the body for weeks or even months.

Weight, Age, and Health Status
A drug might have an increased effect on someone of a lower body weight, younger age, and poorer health status. A drug might have an increased effect in an older person.

Emotional State
How a person feels can determine the effects of a drug. If a person is depressed, using a drug that slows body actions can make the person even more depressed.

Use of Other Drugs
The reactions of more than one drug in the body at the same time can have unexpected effects. In one case, the effects of the drugs might be reduced. In another, the effects of the drugs might be increased. A physician should always be told what drugs you are taking to prevent harmful drug reactions.

Prescription Drugs

A **medicine** is a drug that is used to treat, prevent, or diagnose illness. Many medicines are prescription drugs. A **prescription drug** is a medicine that can be obtained only with a written order from a licensed health professional. A **prescription** (pri·SKRIP·shuhn) is a written order from a certain licensed health professional. Physicians and dentists are examples of licensed health professionals authorized to write prescriptions. Prescription drugs can be prepared and sold only by licensed pharmacists. A **pharmacist** is an allied health professional who dispenses medications prescribed by physicians. It is illegal to obtain a prescription drug without a prescription.

The following information is completed on the prescription by the physician: patient's name; type of medicine; number of pills, capsules, or tablets; dose; and directions for use. A pharmacist fills a prescription with either a brand-name or a generic-name drug. A **brand-name drug** is a registered name or trademark given to a drug by a pharmaceutical company. A **generic-name drug** is a drug that contains the same active ingredients as a brand-name drug. Generic-name drugs are usually less expensive than brand-name drugs.

Prescription Drug Label

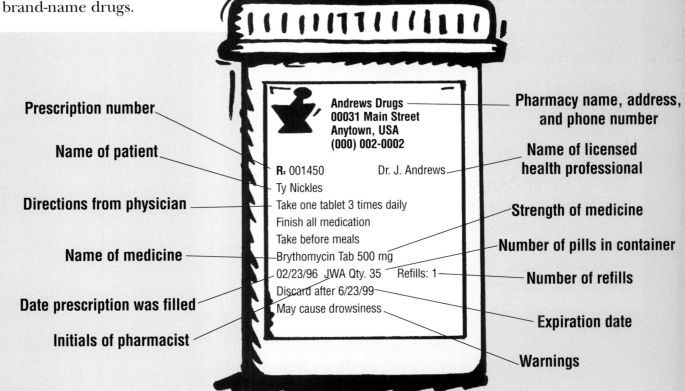

Prescription number

Name of patient

Directions from physician

Name of medicine

Date prescription was filled

Initials of pharmacist

Andrews Drugs
00031 Main Street
Anytown, USA
(000) 002-0002

R_x 001450   Dr. J. Andrews
Ty Nickles
Take one tablet 3 times daily
Finish all medication
Take before meals
Brythomycin Tab 500 mg
02/23/96 JWA Qty. 35   Refills: 1
Discard after 6/23/99
May cause drowsiness

Pharmacy name, address, and phone number

Name of licensed health professional

Strength of medicine

Number of pills in container

Number of refills

Expiration date

Warnings

Over-the-Counter Drugs

An **over-the-counter (OTC) drug** is a drug that can be purchased without a prescription. Many different OTC drugs can be bought in many kinds of stores. Generally, OTC drugs are taken to relieve signs and symptoms of an illness. These drugs often are not used to cure illnesses.

The Food and Drug Administration (FDA) requires that OTC drugs have labels with detailed information. They must be sold in tamper-resistant packages. A **tamper-resistant package** is a package with an unbroken seal that assures the buyer that the package has not been previously opened. Then the buyer knows that no one has tampered with the OTC drug in any way.

Guidelines for the Safe Use of OTC Drugs

- Take OTC drugs only with your parents' or guardian's permission.
- Read the label on an OTC drug before taking it.
- Take the dosage indicated rather than what you believe you should take.
- Use OTC drugs correctly. For example, drink water if the directions read, "Take with water."
- Discontinue use of the OTC drug and notify your physician if you experience side effects.
- Do not use OTC drugs that have been stored past the expiration date. The effectiveness of OTC drugs might change with time.
- Check with a physician or a pharmacist if you are going to use more than one OTC drug at the same time.
- Do not engage in activities in which there are safety concerns (riding a bicycle, playing a contact sport) if a medicine makes you drowsy.
- Do not purchase an OTC drug if its tamper-resistant seal is broken. Inform the store manager so the OTC drug can be removed from the shelf.

OTC Drug Label

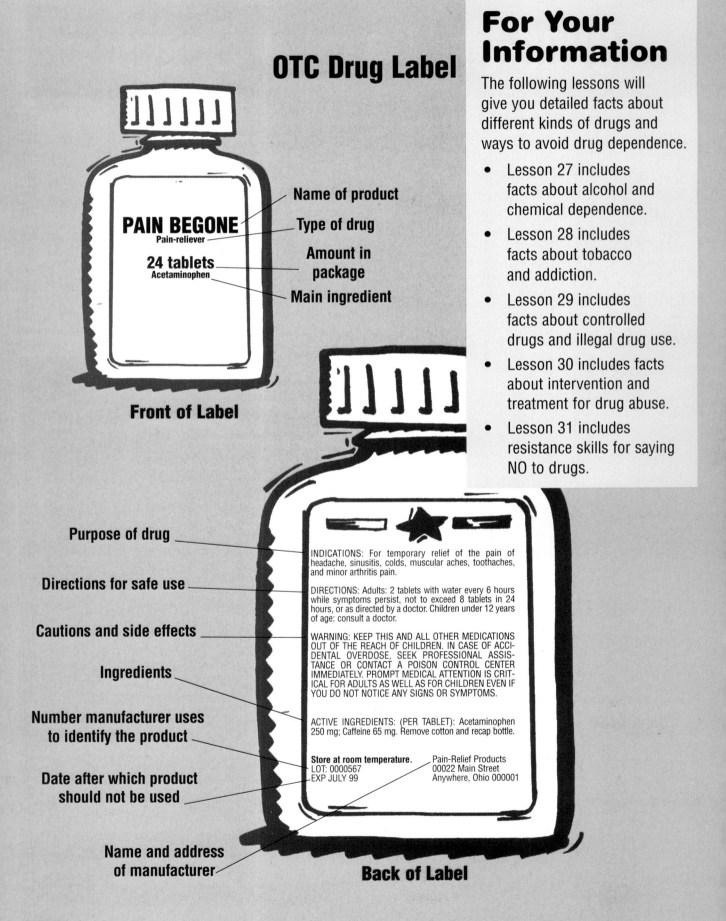

PAIN BEGONE
Pain-reliever

24 tablets
Acetaminophen

Name of product

Type of drug

Amount in package

Main ingredient

Front of Label

Purpose of drug

Directions for safe use

Cautions and side effects

Ingredients

Number manufacturer uses to identify the product

Date after which product should not be used

Name and address of manufacturer

INDICATIONS: For temporary relief of the pain of headache, sinusitis, colds, muscular aches, toothaches, and minor arthritis pain.

DIRECTIONS: Adults: 2 tablets with water every 6 hours while symptoms persist, not to exceed 8 tablets in 24 hours, or as directed by a doctor. Children under 12 years of age: consult a doctor.

WARNING: KEEP THIS AND ALL OTHER MEDICATIONS OUT OF THE REACH OF CHILDREN. IN CASE OF ACCIDENTAL OVERDOSE, SEEK PROFESSIONAL ASSISTANCE OR CONTACT A POISON CONTROL CENTER IMMEDIATELY. PROMPT MEDICAL ATTENTION IS CRITICAL FOR ADULTS AS WELL AS FOR CHILDREN EVEN IF YOU DO NOT NOTICE ANY SIGNS OR SYMPTOMS.

ACTIVE INGREDIENTS: (PER TABLET): Acetaminophen 250 mg; Caffeine 65 mg. Remove cotton and recap bottle.

Store at room temperature.
LOT: 0000567
EXP JULY 99

Pain-Relief Products
00022 Main Street
Anywhere, Ohio 000001

Back of Label

For Your Information

The following lessons will give you detailed facts about different kinds of drugs and ways to avoid drug dependence.

- Lesson 27 includes facts about alcohol and chemical dependence.

- Lesson 28 includes facts about tobacco and addiction.

- Lesson 29 includes facts about controlled drugs and illegal drug use.

- Lesson 30 includes facts about intervention and treatment for drug abuse.

- Lesson 31 includes resistance skills for saying NO to drugs.

Drug Dependence

Drug dependence can occur when directions for safe use of OTC and prescription drugs are ignored. Drug dependence can result from the use of alcohol, tobacco, or other drugs. **Drug dependence** is the continued use of a drug even though it harms the body, mind, and relationships. **Chemical dependence** and **chemical addiction** are other terms used for drug dependence.

Physical dependence is a condition in which a person develops tolerance and a drug becomes necessary, or the person has withdrawal symptoms. **Tolerance** is a condition in which the body becomes used to a drug and larger amounts are needed to produce the same effect. **Withdrawal symptoms** are unpleasant reactions that occur when a drug is no longer taken. **Psychological dependence** is a strong desire to continue using a drug for emotional reasons.

Lesson 26

Review

Vocabulary

Write a separate sentence using each of the vocabulary words listed on page 268.

Health Content

Write responses to the following:

1. What is the difference between responsible drug use, drug misuse, and drug abuse? **page 268**
2. What are four ways drugs enter the body? **page 269**
3. What are six factors that influence the effects drugs have on the body? **page 271**
4. What is the difference between brand-name and generic-name drugs? **page 272**
5. What kinds of information can be found on a prescription drug label? **page 272**
6. What are two differences between prescription and OTC drugs? **pages 272–273**
7. What is the purpose of tamper-resistant packaging? **page 273**
8. What are nine guidelines for the safe use of OTC drugs? **page 273**
9. What kinds of information can be found on an OTC drug label? **page 274**
10. What are two types of drug dependence? **page 275**

Choosing Not to Drink Alcohol

Vocabulary

alcohol

blood alcohol concentration (BAC)

oxidation

gastric ADH

immune system

pancreatitis

diabetes

cirrhosis

alcohol dementia

fetal alcohol syndrome (FAS)

problem drinking

problem drinker

alcoholism

blackout

enabler

codependence

Alcoholics Anonymous (AA)

Al-Anon

Alateen

Life Skill • **I will not drink alcohol.**

Suppose someone offers you a beverage. The person tells you it can interfere with your ability to reason. You might say and do things you will later regret. Your coordination might be affected. This might cause you to be injured. If you drink this beverage, you might be kicked off the sports team to which you belong. Would you choose to drink this beverage? The beverage you were offered was an alcoholic beverage. In this lesson, you will learn why saying NO is a responsible decision when you are offered an alcoholic beverage.

The Lesson Objectives

- Discuss the factors that affect blood alcohol concentration.
- Describe the effects of alcohol on the body and mind.
- Discuss alcoholism: progression of the disease, effects on family members, treatment, and recovery programs.
- Identify ten reasons teens make a responsible decision when they do not drink alcohol.

Alcohol Is a Powerful Drug

Alcohol is a drug in certain beverages that slows down the central nervous system and harms body organs. Beverages such as beer, wine, wine coolers, and whiskey contain alcohol. About 20 percent of the alcohol is quickly absorbed into the bloodstream through the walls of the stomach when a person drinks an alcoholic beverage. The rest is absorbed through the walls of the intestine.

Blood alcohol concentration (BAC) is the amount of alcohol in a person's blood. BAC is given as a percentage. The higher the BAC, the greater the effects of the alcohol. A person's BAC depends on several factors.

- **How much alcohol a person drinks** Beer, wine, wine coolers, and mixed drinks contain alcohol. The amount of alcohol in the beverage determines the effects of alcohol. The type of alcohol does not determine the effects.

- **How fast a person drinks** Alcohol is broken down by the liver and is excreted at a specific rate. Drinking alcohol quickly—slamming, chugging, or downing—is especially dangerous. There is little time for the liver to break down the alcohol and for the alcohol to be excreted. The BAC can reach life-threatening levels.

- **How much a person weighs** The greater a person's weight, the greater the volume of blood in the body. The same amount of alcohol produces a greater effect on someone who weighs less than someone who weighs more.

- **How a person feels** Alcohol is a depressant drug. Suppose a person is already depressed. Alcohol will increase the intensity of the depression.

- **How much a person has eaten** Alcohol passes more quickly into the bloodstream when the stomach is empty than when it is full.

- **When other drugs are in the bloodstream** The presence of a depressant drug in the bloodstream increases the effects of alcohol.

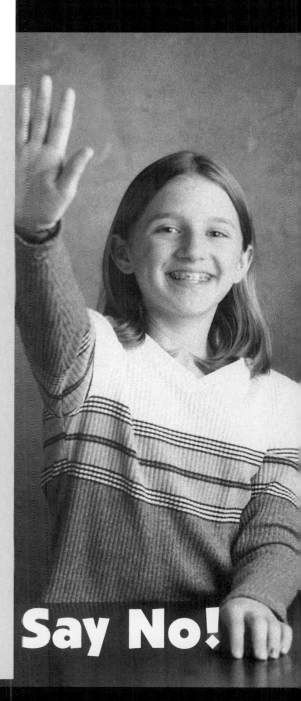

Say No!

Once alcohol enters the bloodstream, it goes to all body tissues before being excreted. Five percent of the absorbed alcohol is excreted through the lungs and urine. The remaining 95 percent must be oxidized by the liver. **Oxidation** (AHK·suh·DAY·shuhn) is the process by which alcohol is changed to carbon dioxide and water. The liver can oxidize about one-quarter to one-third ounce of pure alcohol an hour. This means it will take about two hours for the body to fully oxidize one ounce of alcohol.

Gastric ADH is an enzyme the liver needs in order to oxidize or break down alcohol for excretion. Females produce less gastric ADH than do males, even when other factors, such as weight and amount of alcohol consumed, are similar. This finding helps explain why females are affected by alcohol more quickly than are males. Females also develop liver disease more rapidly than do males.

The Amount of Alcohol in the Blood
Blood Alcohol Concentration (BAC)

Percent	Effects
0.02	A person feels very loose and relaxed. This might lead to a false sense of being comfortable in social situations.
0.06	Reaction time is slowed resulting in impaired coordination. Speech is slurred. Reasoning, judgment, and self-control are affected.
0.10	Reasoning, judgment, and self-control are seriously impaired. The ability to make responsible decisions is absent. In most states, a person is considered legally intoxicated.
0.12	There is further impairment of reasoning, judgment, and self-control. Vomiting can occur.
0.15	Behavior is seriously impaired. Staying awake is difficult.
0.30	A person is in a semi-stupor or deep sleep. Most people cannot stay awake to reach this BAC. A person who slams, chugs, or otherwise drinks alcoholic beverages quickly can reach this dangerous level of BAC.
0.50	Deep coma and death can occur.

Alcohol and the Body

Body Senses

You respond to dangerous situations in order to protect yourself when body senses are functioning well. The senses of sight, taste, touch, smell, and hearing are dulled as soon as alcohol in the bloodstream reaches the brain. You are more likely to have accidents when body senses are dulled.

Reaction Time and Coordination

Alcohol affects the part of the brain that helps coordinate body activities. Also, alcohol dulls the part of the brain responsible for reasoning and judgment. The result is that people who have been drinking might believe they can perform tasks when they cannot. Over 50 percent of all fatal accidents and more than 70 percent of all drowning deaths involve people who have been drinking.

Immune System

The **immune system** is the body system that contains cells and organs that fight disease. The number of infection-fighting cells is lowered when a person drinks alcohol. There is an increased risk of diseases. It is easier for abnormal cells to grow, thus increasing the risk of developing cancer.

Mouth, Pharynx, Larynx, and Esophagus

Drinking alcohol causes changes in the cells that line the mouth, pharynx, larynx, and esophagus. There is an increased risk of cancer of these organs.

Stomach

Drinking alcohol causes an increased flow of gastric juices in the stomach. With no food in the stomach, gastric juices may irritate the inner lining and cause ulcers. The risk of harm to the stomach is increased when alcohol and aspirin are used at the same time.

Warning:

Alcohol circulates in the bloodstream and affects all body organs. For a healthy and fit body, teens should not drink alcohol.

Pancreas

Drinking alcohol harms the pancreas. Excessive drinking can cause pancreatitis. **Pancreatitis** (pan·kree·uh·TY·tis) is the inflammation of the pancreas. This condition increases the risk of diabetes. **Diabetes** (dy·uh·BEE·teez) is a disease in which the body produces little or no insulin or cannot use insulin.

Liver

Alcohol causes more harm to the liver than it does to any other body organ. The liver filters alcohol from the bloodstream and chemically changes it to harmless products. Liver cells are eventually damaged with heavy drinking. This can lead to liver cancer and cirrhosis. **Cirrhosis** (suh·ROH·sis) is a disease in which the liver tissue is destroyed and replaced with scar tissue.

Heart and Blood Vessels

Alcohol causes blood vessels to dilate. Thus, in the short term, alcohol might lower blood pressure. Although someone who has been drinking feels warmer, body heat is being lost. Lowered body temperature can threaten health in cold weather. A person might be unaware of conditions that can cause frostbite. Drinking alcohol also increases the amount of sugar in the bloodstream. People who drink alcohol might develop atherosclerosis. Long-term use of alcohol can harm heart tissue. There is an increased risk of having an irregular heartbeat, high blood pressure, and stroke.

Brain and Nervous System

Drinking alcohol affects the cells in the brain. **Alcohol dementia** (di·MEN·shuh) is brain impairment with overall intellectual decline. When alcohol affects the nervous system, blackouts, seizures, and nerve destruction can occur.

Reproductive System

Alcohol can have immediate effects during puberty. Drinking alcohol can delay the first menstrual cycle and cause irregular periods in females. Drinking alcohol also can affect breast development. Females who drink as teens have an increased risk of breast cancer later in life. Males also are affected by drinking alcohol. Drinking alcohol can affect the size of the testes and the development of muscle mass. It can affect the age at which the voice deepens and the amount of body and facial hair.

The Developing Baby

Drinking alcohol during pregnancy can affect a developing baby. **Fetal alcohol syndrome (FAS)** is the presence of severe birth defects in babies born to mothers who drink alcohol during pregnancy. Among the defects are small eye slits, small head, and retarded physical and mental growth. FAS is the leading known cause of mental retardation.

Alcohol and the Mind

School Performance

Because alcohol is a depressant drug, it slows the activity of the brain cells. Drinking alcohol can affect learning. It is more difficult to think clearly and remember facts. Grades might suffer.

Decision-Making

The decisions you make should be healthful, safe, legal, respectful of self and others, follow parental guidelines, and show that you have moral values. When you drink alcohol, the part of your brain that helps you evaluate situations is dulled. Under the influence of alcohol, teens often make decisions they later regret.

Sexual Decision-Making

Teens experience sexual feelings. Sexual feelings increase and reasoning is dulled when teens drink alcohol. As a result, it is more difficult to say NO to becoming sexually active and stick to this decision. Teens who have been sexually active often report that they had been drinking at the time. The consequences of drinking and being sexually active are serious. More than half of teen females who became pregnant have reported they had been drinking when they had sex. Other teens who drink and become sexually active become infected with sexually transmitted diseases such as HIV.

Social Skills

Some teens feel awkward in social situations. They might drink alcohol to "take the edge off" and feel more comfortable. Using alcohol in this way interferes with the opportunity to learn how to be comfortable in awkward situations. Real self-confidence can be gained only by mastering social situations without using alcohol or other drugs as a crutch.

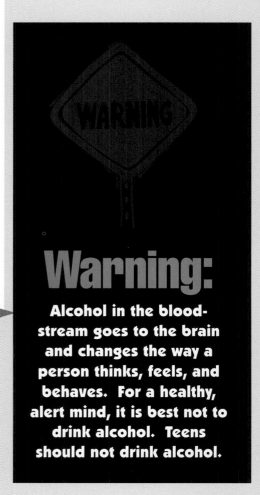

Warning:

Alcohol in the bloodstream goes to the brain and changes the way a person thinks, feels, and behaves. For a healthy, alert mind, it is best not to drink alcohol. Teens should not drink alcohol.

Violence

People who drink alcohol might become angry or aggressive. They might act on these feelings and harm others. Teens who drink or who spend time around others who do are at risk for being involved in fights, abuse, and murder. Teens who have been drinking alcohol also are more likely to engage in illegal behaviors such as shoplifting, damaging property, and selling drugs.

Depression and Suicide

The teen years are stressful. Some teens feel depressed at times. Because alcohol is a depressant, it can cause teens who are depressed already to feel even more depressed. Alcohol and other drugs are a factor in most suicide attempts. Teens who had been drinking or using other drugs were not thinking clearly when the suicide attempt was made. They were unable to see another way of handling problems. They did not seek the help that was needed.

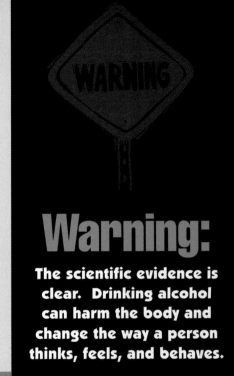

Warning:

The scientific evidence is clear. Drinking alcohol can harm the body and change the way a person thinks, feels, and behaves.

The Responsible Choice...

I will not drink alcohol.

Lesson 31 includes resistance skills you can use to resist pressure to drink alcohol.

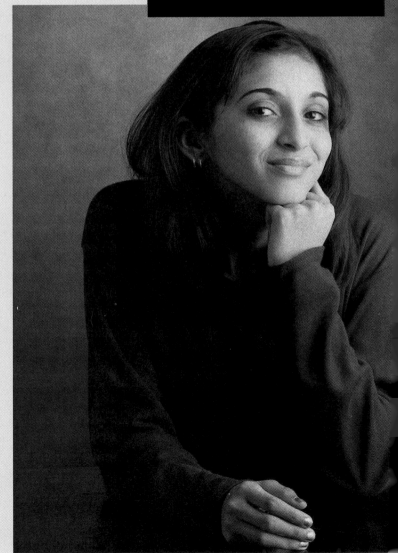

Problem Drinking and Alcoholism

Problem drinking is a pattern of drinking that produces difficulties in a person's life. A **problem drinker** is a person who causes problems for himself or herself or others when drinking. The difficulty can occur after only one drink. For example, it is illegal for you to drink alcohol. If you are pressured to drink and do so, you have done something illegal. You might experience serious consequences such as getting kicked off a sports team or being grounded by your parents or guardian.

There are other ways in which drinking causes difficulties in a teen's life. At your age, you are learning ways to relate with other teens. At times, you might feel awkward. This is normal and you get better with practice. A problem drinker might drink to avoid the uneasiness in social situations. This causes problems. The teen who is a problem drinker does not develop the skills he or she needs.

Other teens are aware of teens who drink. They know they should stay away from them. A problem drinker will have fewer social opportunities. The teens who want to hang out with a problem drinker accept wrong behavior. They might be problem drinkers as well. These are not the right kinds of relationships to have.

Teens who drink and choose wrong actions are problem drinkers. Suppose a teen drinks alcohol, does something, and regrets it later. This is a sign that the teen is a problem drinker. Perhaps the teen has an argument. Perhaps the teen gets into a fight. These are all signs that a teen is a problem drinker.

Tips for Recognizing Problem Drinking

- A problem drinker drinks alcohol even when it is illegal for him or her to do so.
- A problem drinker drinks alcohol to feel comfortable in social situations.
- A problem drinker gets into arguments and fights when drinking.
- A problem drinker does things (s)he later regrets when drinking.
- A problem drinker forgets what happened when (s)he was drinking.

When problem drinkers drink alcohol, they often lose control and act in ways that are not responsible. Problems drinkers need help. Problem drinking can lead to alcoholism.

Alcoholism is a disease in which there is physical and psychological dependence on alcohol. Many people are confused about alcoholism. They believe that a person with alcoholism is a person who drinks too much and too often. The fact is that people with alcoholism have different patterns of drinking. Some people drink too much and too often. But other people with alcoholism have different drinking patterns. A person can drink on weekends only and have alcoholism. A person can drink one drink or ten drinks at one time and have alcoholism. What determines whether or not a person has alcoholism is the dependence on alcohol.

People with alcoholism often have difficulty controlling their drinking. Blackouts might occur. A **blackout** is a period in which a person cannot remember what has happened. People with alcoholism usually deny that they have a drinking problem. Because alcoholism affects the thinking process, they do things they would not do if they had not been drinking. They might lie and choose actions that show little concern for others.

There are good reasons to know and understand facts about alcoholism. Alcoholism is a leading cause of disease and death. Alcoholism and other drug dependency is a leading cause of family dysfunction and relationship difficulties.

Family members and close friends are affected when a person has alcoholism. They often are enablers. An **enabler** is a person who knowingly or unknowingly supports the harmful behavior of another person. Enablers might develop codependence. **Codependence** is a mental disorder in which a person denies feelings and copes in harmful ways.

The treatment for alcoholism involves the family member with the disease as well as the other members of the family. It might involve counseling for close friends as well. Medical experts who treat alcoholism now agree that a person with the disease usually needs a 28-day treatment program at a special facility.

After completing a treatment program, a person with alcoholism needs support. The person is never cured of alcoholism. The disease lasts a lifetime. The person can never drink alcohol again.

The Effects of Alcoholism on Family Members*

Suspicion	Family members might feel suspicious and anticipate the next drinking occurrence.
Insecurity	Children of parents with alcoholism feel insecure.
Guilt	Family members often blame themselves. They might think that their shortcomings caused the drinking problem.
Fear	Family members are often afraid. They fear angry behavior. They worry that the family will break up.
Disappointment	Family members are disappointed because people with alcoholism are unreliable and relationships are broken.
Embarrassment	Family members might not want to bring friends home because the drinker's behavior embarrasses them.
Resentment	Family members are angry and resentful as the disease worsens.

*Close friends often feel the same effects that family members do.

Recovery programs are available for people with alcoholism, their family members, and close friends.

- **Alcoholics Anonymous (AA)** is a self-help treatment group in which people with alcoholism attend meetings and support each other to keep from drinking and to choose healthful behavior.

- **Al-Anon** is a support group for family members and friends of people with alcoholism and/or other addictions.

- **Alateen** is a support group for young people who have been affected by the behavior of someone with alcoholism and/or another addiction.

Alcohol and YOUR CHOICES: Points to Ponder

To ponder is to think. There are many points to ponder about alcohol. These points will help you make decisions regarding alcohol now and in the future.

POINTS TO PONDER

- **It is illegal for minors to drink or purchase alcoholic beverages.**

- **The number of ounces of alcohol that a person drinks, not the kind of alcoholic beverage, determines the BAC.** Beer, wine, wine coolers, and mixed drinks contain alcohol.

- **Drinking alcohol quickly—slamming, chugging, or downing—can raise the BAC to life-threatening levels before alcohol can be oxidized and excreted from the body.**

POINTS TO PONDER

- **Females have a tendency to produce less gastric ADH than do males, even when other factors such as weight and amount of alcohol consumed are similar.** Females will be affected by the depressant effects of alcohol more quickly than males. They develop liver disease more rapidly.

- **Sexual feelings are increased, and reasoning and judgment are dulled when teens drink.** As a result, it is more difficult to say NO to becoming sexually active. Teens who drink and become sexually active are at greater risk for becoming teen parents and being infected with STDs such as HIV.

- **Most acts of violence involve the use of alcohol or other drugs.** Teens who drink are more at risk for being involved in fights, abuse, and murder. They are more likely to engage in illegal behaviors such as shoplifting, damaging property, and selling illegal drugs.

- **A person who is depressed and drinks alcohol becomes even more depressed.** Alcohol is a depressant drug that is a factor in most teen suicide attempts.

- **The chances of developing alcoholism are much greater if someone to whom you are biologically related has this disease.**

- **A person with alcoholism has a disease and usually needs at least a 28-day treatment program at a special facility.**

- **Family members and close friends of a person with alcoholism should avoid being enablers and should join a recovery program if they show signs of codependence.** Protecting a person with alcoholism allows the person to continue the addiction. When family members or friends deny feelings or cope in harmful ways, they need to join a recovery program.

Drink to Your Health

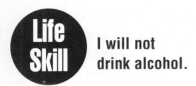

Life Skill
I will not drink alcohol.

Materials: Books with recipes of nonalcoholic beverages, pen or pencil, construction paper, markers

Directions: Create alcohol-free recipes of beverages and share the recipes with your family and friends.

1. **Look through recipe books for nonalcoholic drinks.**

2. **Choose a drink recipe that appeals to you.** You also can change the recipe or you can create your own recipe. Your recipe must feature one ingredient and how it keeps you healthy. For example, one ingredient might be a banana. You would write, "Bananas are the featured ingredient. They provide potassium and complex carbohydrates. They give you energy."

3. **Write this statement at the end of your recipe:** "This beverage contains no alcohol." Add a warning about the dangers of alcohol. Choose any one from this lesson.

4. **Copy your recipe onto construction paper.** Decorate the borders.

5. **Make another copy to take home.** You can make the beverage for your family.

6. **Display your decorated recipe.** Post the recipe on the bulletin board or have your teacher put all the recipes together to make a book.

Activity

Percentage of Alcohol in Different Beverages

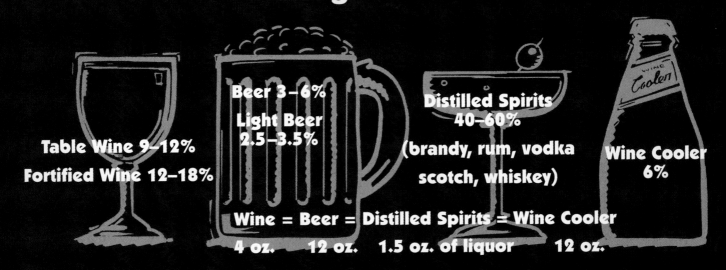

Table Wine 9–12%
Fortified Wine 12–18%

Beer 3–6%
Light Beer 2.5–3.5%

Distilled Spirits 40–60%
(brandy, rum, vodka scotch, whiskey)

Wine Cooler 6%

Wine = Beer = Distilled Spirits = Wine Cooler
4 oz.   12 oz.   1.5 oz. of liquor   12 oz.

Apply...

The Responsible Decision-Making Model™

Your friend invites you to his sister's wedding. There are two bowls of punch at the reception—one with alcohol and one without alcohol. Your friend hands you a glass of the alcoholic punch.

Answer the following questions on a separate sheet of paper. Write "Does not apply" if a question does not apply to this situation.

1. Is it healthful to drink the alcoholic punch? Why or why not?
2. Is it safe to drink the alcoholic punch? Why or why not?
3. Is it legal to drink the alcoholic punch? Why or why not?
4. Will you show respect for yourself and others if you drink the alcoholic punch? Why or why not?
5. Will your parents or guardian approve if you drink the alcoholic punch? Why or why not?
6. Will you demonstrate good character if you drink the alcoholic punch? Why or why not?

What is the responsible decision to make in this situation?

Lesson 27

Review

Vocabulary

Write a separate sentence using each of the vocabulary words listed on page 276.

Health Content

Write responses to the following:

1. What are six factors that affect blood alcohol concentration? **page 277**
2. Why is it life-threatening to slam, chug, or down alcoholic beverages? **page 277**
3. How is alcohol oxidized by the liver? **page 278**
4. Why do females experience the effects of alcohol sooner than males? **page 278**
5. What are ways alcohol affects the body? **pages 279–280**
6. Discuss fetal alcohol syndrome. **page 280**
7. What are effects of alcohol on the mind? **pages 281–282**
8. What are five characteristics of a problem drinker? **page 283**
9. Discuss alcoholism: progression of the disease, the effect on family members, treatment, and recovery programs. **pages 284–285**
10. What are ten reasons teens make a responsible decision when they do not drink alcohol? **pages 286–287**

A Tobacco-Free Lifestyle

Vocabulary

tobacco use

nicotine

carbon monoxide (CO)

stroke

tar

cilia

asthma

cancer

emphysema

chronic bronchitis

secondhand smoke

sidestream smoke

carcinogen

chewing tobacco

snuff

advertisement

assertive behavior

role model

tobacco cessation programs

media literacy

Life Skill

• **I will avoid tobacco use and secondhand smoke.**

Tobacco use is the use of any nicotine-containing tobacco products, such as cigarettes, cigars, and smokeless tobacco. Tobacco products contain an addictive drug. Smoking one cigarette or one cigar can result in addiction. Experimenting with chewing tobacco or snuff can result in addiction.

The Lesson Objectives

• Discuss the harmful effects of nicotine.

• List 15 reasons it is risky to smoke as a teen.

• Discuss ways smoking affects health, appearance, relationships, and spending habits.

• Discuss the risks of breathing secondhand smoke and ways to reduce your exposure to secondhand smoke.

• Discuss 13 reasons it is risky to use smokeless tobacco.

• Identify five reasons teens are tempted to use tobacco.

• Discuss seven resistance skills to resist pressure to use tobacco products.

• Describe ways to stop using tobacco.

Nicotine: A Highly Addictive Drug

Nicotine is a colorless, odorless drug in tobacco that stimulates the nervous system and is highly addictive. This drug dulls the taste buds, constricts the blood vessels, and increases heart rate and blood pressure. Nicotine produces tolerance; more and more nicotine is needed to produce the desired effect.

Physical dependence develops when the body becomes used to the effects nicotine produces. Nicotine stimulates the brain. The brain adapts to this level of stimulation. To remain stimulated, more nicotine is needed. Without it, withdrawal takes place. Withdrawal symptoms include nervousness, inability to sleep, and headaches. Many people who smoke or use smokeless tobacco say they do not enjoy it. However, the discomfort caused by withdrawal symptoms makes giving up the habit very difficult.

Psychological dependence develops when people feel the need to smoke or chew tobacco at certain times or for certain reasons. For example, a person might always smoke a cigarette after eating. Another person might chew tobacco when feeling stressed. These people are psychologically dependent on nicotine.

Psychological dependence is difficult to stop. People who are psychologically dependent might have to change their routine. For example, they might have to plan to do something right after eating. They might plan to do something such as take a walk. Then they can break the habit of having a cigarette after eating. They also might have to stay away from certain people. They might be used to lighting up with certain people.

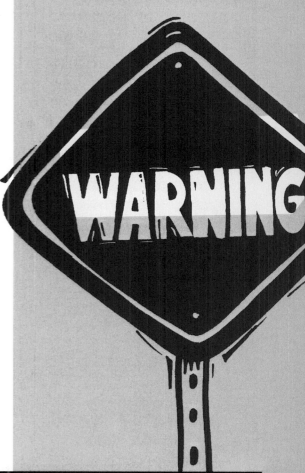

Many teens do not realize just how addictive nicotine can be. Some believe they can take a puff on a cigarette or chew tobacco and it will be no big deal. But the chances of getting hooked on nicotine make experimenting with tobacco risky.

"Come on, smoking one pack of cigarettes can't hurt you...."

"You're too young to get heart disease...."

"Cancer is for old people...."

If you believe these statements, guess again. Experimenting with smoking is risky RIGHT NOW. Smoking cigarettes will cost you—your health, your appearance, your relationships, and your money!

Warning:

Cigarette smoking has short-term physiological, cosmetic, social, and economic health consequences.

The Centers for Disease Control and Prevention

Centers for Disease Control and Prevention. Guidelines for school health programs to prevent tobacco use and addiction. MMWR 1994; 43 (No. RR-2): [inclusive page numbers].

Warning:

The probability of becoming addicted to nicotine after one exposure is higher than for other addictive substances...heroin, cocaine, and alcohol.

The Surgeon General's Report on Smoking and Health, 1994

Warning:

Cigarette smoking has direct health consequences.

The Centers for Disease Control and Prevention

Centers for Disease Control and Prevention. Guidelines for school health programs to prevent tobacco use and addiction. MMWR 1994; 43 (No. RR-2): [inclusive page numbers].

Smokers Speak Out Against Smoking

When asked, most tobacco users will tell you...DON'T START SMOKING. DON'T START USING SMOKELESS TOBACCO. It is very, very difficult to stop.

The majority of current smokers wish they had never started.

Gallup G. Jr., Newport F. Many Americans favor restrictions on smoking in public places. Gallup Poll Monthly 1990; 298: 19–27.

Most smokers who try to quit resume regular smoking within one year.

Pierce JP, Fiore MC, Novotny TE, Hatziandreu EJ, Davis RM. Trends in cigarette smoking in the United States: projections to the year 2000. JAMA 1989; 261(1); 61–5.

Three out of four teens who smoke have made at least one serious, yet unsuccessful, effort to quit.

CDC. Recent trends in adolescent smoking, smoking-uptake correlates, and expectations about the future. Advance data from vital and health statistics of the Centers for Disease Control and Prevention/National Center for Health Statistics; No. 221, Dec. 2, 1992.

Cigarette Smoking Is Risky Right Now

- You risk becoming addicted even if you smoke only one cigarette.

- Your level of physical fitness would be affected because smoking decreases stamina. You would become short of breath more easily.

- Your voice could become raspy and you would cough more often.

- You would get respiratory infections, such as the common cold and flu, more easily and you would recover from these infections more slowly.

- Your heart rate and blood pressure would increase, placing wear and tear on your heart.

- You would have more lipids (fat) circulating in your bloodstream and begin to develop fat deposits on the artery walls.

- Your condition would worsen if you have allergies or asthma.

- Your breath and clothes would smell like smoke.

- Your fingers and teeth might be stained yellow.

- Your peers might stay away from you because most teens do NOT smoke.

- Your parents or guardian would disapprove of your behavior.

- You could be breaking school rules if you smoke on school property or at school-sponsored functions.

- You would be more likely to make mistakes or have accidents because lighting and smoking a cigarette distracts your attention.

- You would be at increased risk for being in a fire caused by carelessness with your cigarette.

- You would be wasting money on a very expensive habit.

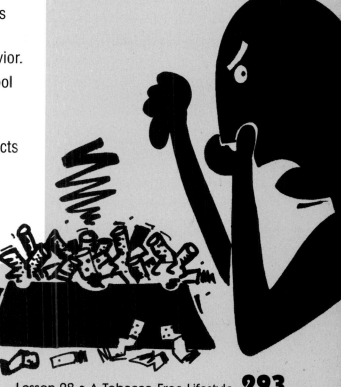

Cigarette Smoking Threatens Your Future

The behavior that you choose today influences your future health. If you begin smoking as a teen, it is very difficult to quit. When you smoke for several years, smoking begins to take its toll. Let's look at the price you pay on your health, your appearance, your relationships, and your money.

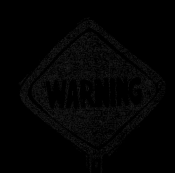

Warning:

Tobacco products contain other harmful substances in addition to nicotine.

The Centers for Disease Control and Prevention

Warning:

Cigarette smoking has direct health consequences.

The Centers for Disease Control and Prevention

Warning:

Cigarette smoking has long-term physiological, cosmetic, social and economic health consequences.

The Centers for Disease Control and Prevention

Centers for Disease Control and Prevention. Guidelines for school health programs to prevent tobacco use and addiction. MMWR 1994; 43 (No. RR-2): [inclusive page numbers].

Smoking and the Cardiovascular System

Smoking is a major cause of death from heart and blood vessel diseases. Nicotine in smoke raises the resting heart rate as many as 20 beats per minute. This places extra wear and tear on the heart.

Other substances in tobacco also have a harmful effect on the heart. One of these substances is carbon monoxide. **Carbon monoxide** (KAR·buhn muh·NAHK·syd) **(CO)** is an odorless, tasteless, colorless, poisonous gas. What happens when a person inhales smoke from a cigarette? The carbon monoxide tends to replace oxygen in the red blood cells. As a result, some red blood cells transport carbon monoxide in place of oxygen. However, body cells must still get enough oxygen to survive.

To deliver adequate oxygen to the cells, the heart must pump faster. This, too, causes strain on the heart. The combination of nicotine and carbon monoxide in cigarette smoke is responsible for the large number of smokers who develop heart disease.

Studies show that smoking also has harmful effects on blood vessels. Smoking speeds the development of fat deposits inside the arteries. Fat deposits reduce the space in the artery through which blood can flow. The risk of developing blood clots increases. A clot in the brain can result in a stroke. A **stroke** is a condition caused by a blocked or broken blood vessel in the brain. When someone has a stroke, body parts can be paralyzed. Death can result.

Smoking and the Respiratory System

Smoking prevents the lungs from working as effectively as they can. When a person smokes, tar lines the lungs and the air passages. **Tar** is a thick, sticky fluid that is produced when tobacco burns. There are over 200 harmful chemicals in tar. When tar is in the lungs, oxygen cannot pass easily to the blood. As a result, breathing becomes more difficult. Smokers become short of breath and usually find it difficult to participate in vigorous activities.

Tobacco smoke harms the cilia in the nose, throat, and bronchial tubes. **Cilia** (SIH·lee·uh) are hairlike structures in the respiratory tract that trap dust and other particles and remove them. Using a waving motion, they prevent harmful substances from entering the lungs. When a person smokes, the cilia become paralyzed. When the cilia stop functioning, harmful substances enter the air passages. A person must cough to get the air passages clean. This is known as smoker's cough. After a person has smoked for several years, the cilia may be destroyed.

Paralyzed cilia cannot work effectively to keep harmful substances from entering the lungs. These harmful substances increase the risk of respiratory infections, such as colds. Smokers have more respiratory infections than nonsmokers.

Smoking-Related Conditions and Diseases

Smoking affects the senses of taste and smell. It deadens the taste buds on the tongue. As a result, foods do not taste as they should. Smoking causes the sinuses in the nose to swell and become red. Therefore, the sense of smell is not as keen as it could be.

Smoking causes the air passages in the lungs to narrow. This makes breathing difficult. **Asthma** (AZ·muh) is a condition in which the bronchial tubes constrict, making breathing difficult. The combination of smoking and asthma can seriously affect a person's ability to breathe. Immediate medical treatment might be needed if an asthma attack results. During an attack, the person might not be able to get enough air into the lungs.

Smoking increases the risk of cancer. **Cancer** is a group of diseases in which there is uncontrolled multiplication of abnormal cells in the body. Smokers have high rates of cancer of the mouth, throat, lungs, and breast. Often, the tar causes healthy cells to change into cancer cells. Unlike some other types of cancer, lung cancer is rarely treated successfully. Smoking is the greatest cause of lung cancer. Lung cancer almost always causes death. If people did not smoke, the number of cases of lung cancer would be greatly reduced.

Smoking also causes emphysema. **Emphysema** (em·fuh·SEE·muh) is a disease in which air sacs in the lungs lose most of their ability to function. As a result, it is difficult for oxygen to be absorbed into the bloodstream from the lungs. Carbon dioxide builds up in the body because it cannot be expelled into the lungs from the bloodstream. A person must breathe more quickly to get enough oxygen into the bloodstream. Some people with emphysema must remain in bed. They are unable to walk across the room without becoming short of breath. The disease will not progress or will progress more slowly if a person stops smoking. However, any damage already caused cannot be reversed.

Smoking also causes chronic bronchitis. **Chronic bronchitis** (brahn·KY·tis) is a disease in which too much mucus lines the bronchial tubes. A person must cough frequently to help remove the mucus. The constant coughing irritates the cilia and bronchial tubes. Coughing cannot remove all the harmful matter from the air passage. Not removing this matter increases the risk of lung infections.

Smoking also causes asthma attacks. People who have asthma have difficulty breathing. Their air passages can become narrow. Nicotine affects the air passages. The harmful ingredients in smoke also affect the air passages. This increases the chance that a person who has asthma will have an attack. The person might wheeze.

Smoking and Your Appearance

When smokers smile, their yellow-stained teeth are noticeable. Cigarette smoking affects the mouth and gums. There is a greater chance of developing gum disease. In addition, there are still the obvious effects on appearance and grooming—smoker's breath and smelly clothes. People who smoke look older more quickly. Their skin wrinkles and they appear less fit than other people who are the same age.

Smoking and Relationships

Today, the majority of people do not approve of cigarette smoking. The risk to relationships can be costly. People who do not smoke often limit contact with those who do. Smoking can limit a person's social opportunities. Many people do not choose friends or dates who smoke. Many parents do not want people who smoke around their children. Many employers prefer not to hire people who smoke.

Smoking and Money

Cigarette smoking is costly. The price of a pack of cigarettes continues to increase. People who buy cigarettes are spending money that might be spent for a better purpose. Because people who smoke are at risk for many diseases and conditions, the medical costs are also high. And people who smoke are more likely to have expenses from fires and accidents caused by carelessness with cigarettes.

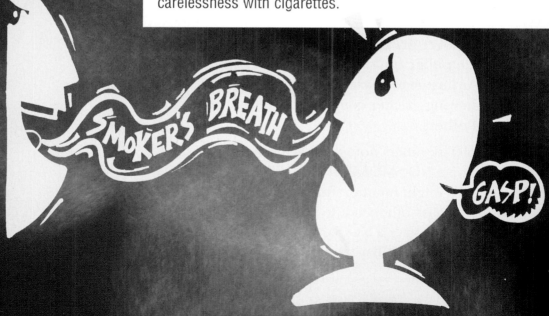

Stay Away from Secondhand Smoke

Have you ever been in a restaurant when someone sitting next to you was smoking a cigarette? Have you ever caught the odor of a cigar that someone was smoking clear across the room? **Secondhand smoke** is exhaled smoke and sidestream smoke. **Sidestream smoke** is the smoke that enters the air from a burning cigarette or cigar.

Just how dangerous is sidestream smoke? The Environmental Protection Agency recently classified environmental tobacco smoke as a Group A carcinogen. A **carcinogen** (kar·SIN·uh·juhn) is a substance that causes cancer. A Group A carcinogen is a known human carcinogen.

Secondhand smoke contains harmful substances. These substances can irritate the eyes, throat, and lungs, and can also cause headaches. People who have heart disease or respiratory problems, such as asthma, are especially affected.

Breathing secondhand smoke increases the risk of lung cancer and respiratory infections in nonsmokers. It also increases the risk of heart disease among nonsmokers. It also affects lung function. Babies and children of people who smoke have higher than normal rates of ear infections, bronchitis, and pneumonia.

Many steps are being taken to protect nonsmokers from secondhand smoke. Laws are being passed to prevent smoking inside public buildings, in schools, and in the workplace. Airlines have restricted smoking during flights. People are showing greater concern for their health and the health of others.

Many people ask others not to smoke in their homes. They might have a NO SMOKING sign. When they invite people over, they might mention that they do not allow smoking. Many people ask others not to smoke in their motor vehicle. They might have a NO SMOKING sign in their motor vehicle. You might have noticed one in a cab or bus.

FACT:

Maintaining a tobacco-free environment has health benefits.

The Centers for Disease Control and Prevention

Centers for Disease Control and Prevention. Guidelines for school health programs to prevent tobacco use and addiction. MMWR 1994; 43 (No. RR-2): [inclusive page numbers].

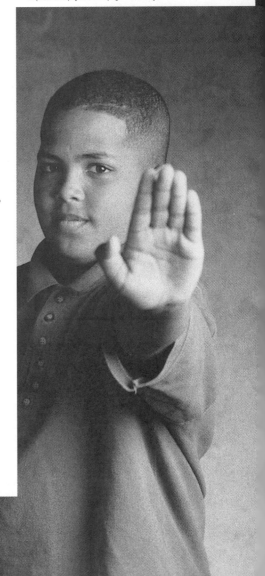

Use Honest Talk

Use honest talk to make your feelings known about secondhand smoke. Suppose someone lights up or starts to light up in your presence. Tell the person that you do not want to breathe cigarette smoke. Ask the person not to light up or to put the cigarette out. You might say, "I do not want to breathe secondhand smoke. I do not want you to smoke around me."

Give the reasons why you do not want to breathe secondhand smoke. You might say, "I want to protect myself from cancer. Smoking causes at least 30 percent of all cancers." Tell the person he or she is important to you. You might say, "I care about you and want to spend time with you." You also might add, "I know it is difficult to stop smoking. It is very addicting. I know you might be cranky while you are quitting. But I will support you during the hard times."

Think ahead about situations in which you know a person around you might smoke. For example, you might be hired by an adult who smokes to childsit. This adult might pick you up. You know that this adult might smoke in his or her car. You do not want to breathe secondhand smoke. Talk to your parents or guardian about what to do. You might want to tell the person when he or she calls that secondhand smoke bothers you. Be clear that you do not want to ride in a motor vehicle in which someone is smoking.

These situations can be difficult. But remember you must protect your health. You put yourself at risk every time you breathe secondhand smoke. There is no such thing as secondhand smoke that does not hurt you.

Sidestepping Secondhand Smoke

Steps you can take to reduce exposure to secondhand smoke include the following:

1. Avoid being in situations in which there will be secondhand smoke.
2. Sit in the nonsmoking section of restaurants.
3. Encourage your family to have a nonsmoking policy for your home.
4. Ask people who smoke not to smoke in your presence.

Smoking During Pregnancy

Studies show that eliminating smoking during pregnancy could prevent:

5 percent of infant deaths

20 percent of low birth weight babies

8 percent of premature deliveries

Females who stop smoking before becoming pregnant have babies with the same birth weight as females who never smoked.

Smokeless Tobacco Use Is Risky RIGHT NOW and LATER

Smokeless tobacco is manufactured and sold in two forms. **Chewing tobacco** is a tobacco product made from chopped tobacco leaves that is placed between the cheek and gums. **Snuff** is a tobacco product made from powdered tobacco leaves and stems that is placed between the cheek and gums. Both forms are harmful to a person's health.

Smokeless tobacco is not a safe alternative to smoking. Smokeless tobacco has the same harmful ingredients as tobacco in cigarettes. Nicotine in smokeless tobacco is absorbed into the bloodstream through the lining of the mouth. It produces tolerance and dependence. This makes the habit of using smokeless tobacco difficult to break.

Like cigarettes, smokeless tobacco increases the risk of cancer of the mouth. It irritates the lining of the mouth and throat, causing abnormal cells to grow. These abnormal cells can develop into cancer. Cancer cells can spread to other body parts and cause death.

Smokeless tobacco is placed between the cheek and gums. It often contains added sugar that causes tooth decay. Smokeless tobacco can contain sand that wears away the enamel on teeth. The teeth are less protected from decay. Smokeless tobacco also causes the gums to pull away from the teeth, exposing the roots. The teeth are then more sensitive and are more likely to fall out. Using smokeless tobacco causes yellow teeth and bad breath.

The evidence is clear. Using smokeless tobacco is neither cool nor smart.

Using Smokeless Tobacco Is Too Risky Right Now and Later

- You risk instant addiction even if you use smokeless tobacco just one time.

- Your heart rate and blood pressure would increase, placing wear and tear on your heart.

- Your breath would have an odor and your teeth would be stained.

- Your senses of taste and smell would be dulled. After some time, you would lose your sense of taste and smell.

- White spots (leukoplakia) would form on the inside of your mouth and on your gums. This is due to changes in the cells. After some time, these white spots could become cancerous.

- Your gums might bleed and soft tissue would be damaged. After some time, periodontal disease occurs and teeth might fall out.

- You might develop cavities from the sugar in the smokeless tobacco.

- You would develop sores in your stomach if you swallowed the smokeless tobacco.

- Others would find your behavior disgusting if you spit out the chewing tobacco or snuff.

- Many teens would stay away from you because most teens do not use smokeless tobacco.

- Your parents or guardian would disapprove of your behavior.

- You would be breaking school rules if you used smokeless tobacco on school property or at school-sponsored functions.

- You would be wasting money on a very expensive habit.

What Tobacco Advertisements DO NOT Tell You

Tobacco manufacturers are required to include warnings on their packages and in their advertisements. An **advertisement,** or ad, is a paid announcement about a product or service. These warnings are intended to educate you and others about the dangers of using tobacco products.

Tobacco manufacturers know that public opinion is very strong. It is no longer "in" to smoke or use smokeless tobacco. Tobacco manufacturers are spending more than six billion dollars a year to convince you and others that tobacco use is still "in."

When you look at an ad for a tobacco product, particularly for cigarettes, advertisers want to take your attention away from the warnings. To do this, they spend big bucks to develop ads which tell you that smokers have a certain image. Analyze ads for cigarettes, and you will recognize how they are designed to appeal to teens. People in these ads are models who are attractive, healthy looking, and well-dressed. They are having fun and are very appealing to members of the opposite sex. Do not be fooled.

What tobacco advertisements have not told you is that smoking cigarettes does not help you look healthy or attractive. Today, members of the opposite sex are likely to be turned off by your behavior, your breath, and your stained teeth. It is "in" to work out, be fit, eat low-fat foods, and take care of yourself. It is not "in" to smoke.

Warning:

Tobacco manufacturers use various strategies to direct advertisements toward young people, such as "image" advertising.

The Centers for Disease Control and Prevention

Centers for Disease Control and Prevention. Guidelines for school health programs to prevent tobacco use and addiction. MMWR 1994 43 (No. RR-2): [inclusive page numbers].

The tobacco industry and tobacco advertisers are well aware of the pressure on smokers to stop smoking. A new kind of ad is intended to help smokers combat this pressure. This ad tells you that smokers have the right to smoke. Again, do not be fooled. There is no "right" to smoke. The "right" to smoke would end where it harms another person. The majority of people do not want to breathe secondhand smoke. They want to be healthy.

Tobacco Teasers:
Reasons Teens Are Tempted

Teens might be tempted to use tobacco products for a variety of reasons.
Let's look at the truth about each of these tobacco teasers.

Tobacco Teasers	Truth
I want to be accepted by peers.	The majority of teens do not use tobacco products and do not approve of others doing so. You are likely to be criticized by your peers if you smoke.
I want to appear mature.	During the teen years, you are testing behaviors to see what will work for you as an adult. You want to appear adult-like and sharp. Today, sharp people do not smoke. They recognize that smoking adds nothing to their image. In fact, it hurts their image.
I want to cope with stress.	Reach for a cigarette to cope with stress? Use snuff or chew? No way. The nicotine in tobacco products actually triggers stress by causing adrenaline to be secreted. You get even more hyped up than you were. Use the stress management skills in Lesson 5 and stay away from nicotine.
I want to manage my weight.	Nothing is wrong with wanting to look your best. And being at your desirable weight has health advantages. But reaching for a cigarette to curb your appetite is short-sighted. It keeps you from forming healthful eating habits and leads to a harmful addiction.
I want to have a good image.	Health is "in" and tobacco is "out." Today, you have a good image when you work out, stay fit, eat low-fat foods, and take care of yourself. Your image is not good if your clothes smell bad and your teeth are yellow from tobacco.

The Majority of Teens Say NO

The majority of teens say NO to tobacco products. They say NO to cigarette smoking and they say NO to using smokeless tobacco. You can use assertive behavior and say NO, too. **Assertive behavior** is the honest expression of thoughts and feelings without experiencing anxiety or threatening others.

Put your resistance skills to work. (See Lesson 2.)

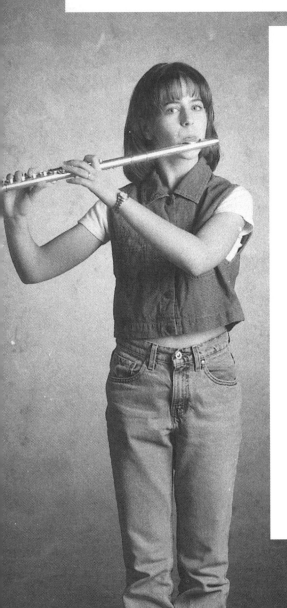

1. **Say NO in a firm and confident voice to tobacco use.**
   - Use assertive behavior.
   - Look directly at the person to whom you are speaking.

2. **Give reasons for saying NO to tobacco use.**
   - Explain that tobacco use is harmful, unsafe, addictive, and illegal for minors. Use of tobacco does not show respect for self or others. Tobacco use is against the guidelines of your family and school. Selling tobacco to minors is against the law.
   - Use one or more of the Reasons for Saying NO to Tobacco Use on page 340.

3. **Use nonverbal behavior to match verbal behavior.**
   - Do not hold a cigarette or pretend to inhale it.
   - Do not keep tobacco products for someone else in your locker or bookbag.

4. **Avoid being in situations in which there will be pressure to use tobacco products.**
   - Think ahead about whether or not activities will be tobacco-free.
   - Ask questions if you are not certain if there will be tobacco use.

5. **Avoid being with people who use tobacco.**
   - Choose friends who are tobacco-free.
   - Stay away from secondhand smoke.
6. **Resist pressure to engage in illegal behavior.**
   - Do not purchase tobacco products by lying about your age.
   - Do not purchase tobacco products from vending machines.
7. **Influence others to avoid tobacco use.**
   - Encourage others who smoke to quit.
   - Suggest smoking cessation programs.
   - Be a role model of a drug-free lifestyle.

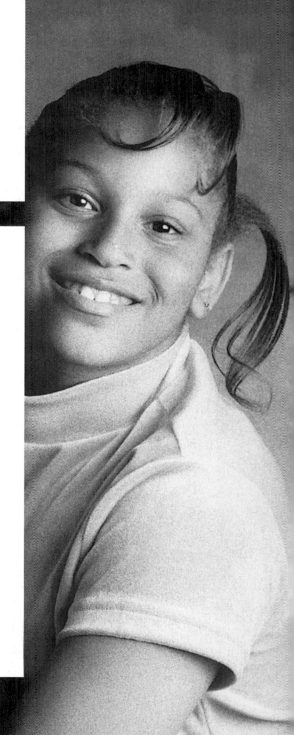

Rehearse what you might do if you are pressured to use tobacco.

"Just one puff cannot hurt you." "Just place a wad in your cheek, no one will see it." What else might peers say to you? Think ahead. Be ready. Rehearse what you will say. Practice with a friend or an adult.

Select healthful role models and be a role model for others.

A **role model** is a person who is an example or shows others how to behave. It is natural for teens to have heroes or adults whom they admire and respect. Some teens look up to their parents, their coach, their teacher, or a community leader. Other teens look up to a sports figure or television personality. Choose heroes and role models carefully. Their behavior should be responsible. Tobacco use is not responsible.

Be a hero to your peers and to younger children. Show others how to behave. Model what it is like to have a tobacco-free lifestyle.

Tobacco Cessation Programs

The best advice regarding tobacco use is DO NOT START. However, some teens have used tobacco products. Perhaps you smoke or chew...what should you do? STOP. Design a health behavior contract with the life skill "I will stop using smokeless tobacco" or "I will stop smoking." (See Lesson 1 on designing a health behavior contract.)

- Set a target date to quit.
- Make an appointment with the school nurse or a physician to help with your plan. Your physician might suggest a low-dose nicotine patch, prescription chewing gum with nicotine, or a smoking cessation program.
- Consider situations in which you usually have a cigarette or use smokeless tobacco. Change your routine to avoid these situations.
- Avoid people who use tobacco and places where tobacco will be used.
- Exercise vigorously to release beta-endorphins. Remember, these substances help you feel good. (See Lesson 23.)
- Form a support system. Tell people you are quitting and ask for their encouragement and support.

A tobacco cessation program can give you an extra boost to quit. **Tobacco cessation programs** are programs to help people stop smoking cigarettes and cigars or using smokeless tobacco. These programs are offered by:

- The local chapter of The American Cancer Society
- The local chapter of The American Lung Association
- The local chapter of The American Heart Association
- Your school
- The health department in your community
- Community providers, such as hospitals

FACT:

Laws, rules, and policies regulate the sale and use of tobacco.

All states have laws that prohibit the sale of cigarettes to minors.

The Healthy People Objectives for the Nation include a recommendation that all states have laws requiring that at least age 18 be the minimum age for purchase of tobacco products.

FACT:

Community organizations have information about tobacco use and can help people stop using tobacco.

Centers for Disease Control and Prevention. Guidelines for school health programs to prevent tobacco use and addiction. MMWR 1994; 43 (No. RR-2): [inclusive page numbers].

Voluntary Health Agency Cessation Programs

Many services and materials are available for people who wish to stop smoking:

- The American Lung Association offers the Freedom from Smoking Program that includes group stop-smoking programs, stop-smoking kits for females who are pregnant, and help-a-friend kits for nonsmokers to help smokers who are trying to quit.

- The American Cancer Society sponsors "The Great American Smokeout" each year on the Thursday before Thanksgiving. Smokers sign a pledge indicating they will not smoke on the day of the "Smokeout." The American Cancer Society also offers both group and self-help approaches for people who wish to stop smoking.

- The American Heart Association provides information on how to stop smoking, smoking and heart disease, and ways to avoid gaining weight when quitting smoking.

Health Benefits of Smoking Cessation

Quitting smoking has major and immediate health benefits for people of all ages.

People who quit smoking live longer than those who continue to smoke. People who quit smoking decrease their risk of:

Lung cancer

Cancers of the larynx, mouth, esophagus, pancreas, and bladder

Heart disease

Stroke

Respiratory infections

Ulcer

Tell It Like It Should Be

Life Skill

I will avoid tobacco use and second-hand smoke.

Materials: Magazines with ads of tobacco products, glue or tape, white paper, pen or pencil, scissors

Directions: **Media literacy** is the ability to recognize and evaluate the messages in media. Follow these steps to create an advertisement that discourages tobacco use.

1. Look through magazines for ads that promote a tobacco product.

2. Choose a statement from the list below that seems to go with the picture in the ad. For example, if the ad shows people talking, you might choose, "I will encourage others not to use tobacco."

3. Write the statement on a piece of paper that will fit over the text part of the ad. Tape or glue the paper over the text.

The Tobacco-Free Pledge

- I will take responsibility for my health.
- I will make a commitment to be tobacco-free.
- I will begin a smoking cessation program if I currently use tobacco products.
- I will use resistance skills if I am pressured to use tobacco.
- I will support decisions of others not to use tobacco.
- I will communicate knowledge and personal attitudes about tobacco use.
- I will encourage others not to use tobacco.
- I will support others who are trying to stop using tobacco.
- I will develop methods for coping with difficult personal situations other than by using tobacco.
- I will request a smoke-free environment.
- I will not be tempted by tobacco advertisements or other promotional materials.

Don't Get Caught Up in Cigar Smoke!

Have you seen ads that promote cigar smoking? This is just the latest trick to get you to start using tobacco. Don't fall for it! Teens might smoke cigars, thinking cigars are less harmful than cigarettes or smokeless tobacco. But one cigar has more nicotine and tobacco than one cigarette. Even if you do not inhale, you are still at risk for cancer of the mouth, tongue, larynx, and esophagus. Think it's cool to smoke cigars? There's nothing cool about bad breath, yellow teeth, and cancer!

Lesson 28

Review

Vocabulary

Write a separate sentence using each of the vocabulary words listed on page 290.

Health Content

Write responses to the following:

1. What are harmful effects of nicotine? **page 291**
2. What are 15 reasons it is risky to smoke as a teen? **page 293**
3. How does smoking affect the cardiovascular system and the respiratory system? **page 295**
4. Discuss smoking-related conditions and diseases: asthma, cancer, emphysema, chronic bronchitis. **page 296**
5. What are ways smoking affects appearance, relationships, and spending habits? **page 297**
6. What are the risks of breathing secondhand smoke and ways to reduce your exposure to it? **pages 298–299**
7. What are 13 reasons it is risky to use smokeless tobacco? **page 301**
8. What are five reasons teens are tempted to use tobacco? **page 303**
9. What are seven resistance skills to resist pressure to use tobacco products? **pages 304–305**
10. What are ways to stop using tobacco? **page 306**

Controlled Drugs and Illegal Drug Use

Vocabulary

controlled drug
illegal drug use
stimulants
tolerance
caffeinism
cocaine
crack
amphetamines
methamphetamines
look-alike drug
crank
ice
ADHD
sedative-hypnotic drugs
sedatives
hypnotic drugs
barbiturates
tranquilizers
psychological dependence
narcotics
morphine
codeine
heroin
marijuana, hashish
hallucinogens
LSD
flashback
PCP
mescaline
anabolic steroid
inhalants
huffing, sniffing, bagging
drug slipping

 Life Skill

• **I will not be involved in illegal drug use.**

A **controlled drug** is a drug whose possession, manufacture, distribution, and sale are controlled by law. Controlled drugs have powerful effects on the body and mind. A prescription is needed to obtain a controlled drug. A controlled drug must be dispensed by a pharmacist. Controlled drugs can be used legally only with a prescription. **Illegal drug use** is the wrong use, possession, manufacture, or sale of controlled drugs; and the use, possession, manufacture, or sale of illegal drugs.

The Lesson Objectives

- Discuss the effects and dangers of stimulant drugs; cocaine and crack; sedative-hypnotic drugs; narcotics; marijuana and hashish; and hallucinogens.
- Explain why it is dangerous to use anabolic steroids without a prescription and to abuse inhalants.

Stimulants

Stimulants are a group of drugs that increase the activities of the central nervous system. They increase the sense of alertness, and increase blood pressure and heart rate. Tolerance to stimulants occurs very quickly. **Tolerance** is a condition in which the body becomes used to a drug and larger amounts are needed to produce the same effect.

A person who has been using stimulants and stops will experience a marked reduction in energy. The person might become depressed and lose the ability to concentrate.

What Is Your CQ? (Caffeine Quotient)

Caffeine is a legal drug that is found in chocolate, coffee, tea, some soda pops, prescription drugs, and OTC drugs. Caffeine is not a controlled drug. However, because it is the most widely used stimulant, you will want to be aware of your CQ. Caffeine is a powerful stimulant, producing a "pick-me-up" effect. But this benefit is not without risk. Caffeine increases the likelihood of having irregular heartbeats. It irritates the stomach. Some people develop caffeinism. **Caffeinism** is a kind of poisoning due to heavy caffeine intake. Some signs include difficulty sleeping, mood changes, anxiety, muscle twitching, restlessness, headaches, depression, stomach pains, and a fast heartbeat.

For good health, keep that CQ low!

Check your CQ:

Coffee: 40–170 mg

Regular instant coffee: 30–130 mg

Decaffeinated coffee: 2–5 mg

High-caffeine cola: 42 mg

Chocolate: 6 mg

Tea: 25–100 mg

Cocaine and Crack

Cocaine (koh·KAYN) is a highly addictive stimulant drug obtained from the leaves of the coca bush. Cocaine can be absorbed through any mucous membrane, and is circulated to the heart, lungs, and other body organs. The effects are almost immediate. When inhaled, cocaine reaches the brain in three minutes; when injected, in 15 seconds; when smoked, in seven seconds. Dangers of cocaine use include:

- **increased heart rate, blood pressure, and respiration;**
- **anxiety and insomnia;**
- **fatigue;**
- **loss of interest in school work and other responsibilities;**
- **delusions, hallucinations, and paranoia;**
- **burns and sores on the nasal membranes;**
- **heart attack and stroke;**
- **increased aggressiveness;**
- **increased risk of hepatitis, HIV, and other infections from contaminated needles;**
- **increased involvement in crime in order to buy or sell cocaine;**
- **psychological and physical dependence;**
- **depression and suicide;**
- **overdose and death.**

Crack is a purified form of cocaine that produces a rapid and intense reaction. It is named for the sound it produces when smoked. The effects of crack are ten times greater than those of snorted (inhaled) cocaine.

Amphetamines and Methamphetamines

Amphetamines (am·FE·tuh·meenz) are chemically manufactured stimulant drugs that are highly addictive. They were used at one time as diet pills. They are no longer used for this purpose because of possible harmful effects.

Methamphetamines (meth·am·FE·tuh·meenz), or meth, are stimulant drugs within the amphetamine family. The use of meth produces effects similar to cocaine.

Is it an identical twin?... No, it is a look-alike drug.

A **look-alike drug** is a tablet or capsule manufactured to resemble amphetamines and mimic their effects. Look-alike drugs contain large amounts of legal nonprescription stimulants, such as caffeine. They are marketed as safe substitutes for illegal stimulants. Some states have declared look-alike drugs to be illegal.

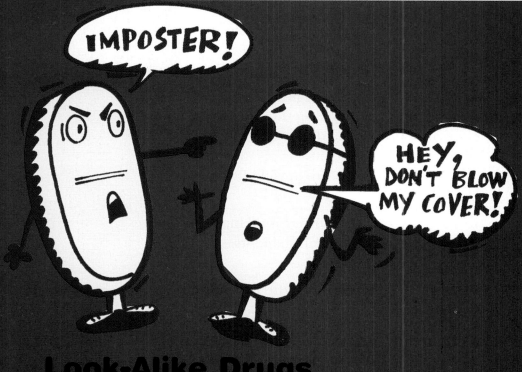

Look-Alike Drugs

New Generation Stimulants

The term "new generation stimulants" is being used for some of the illegal drugs. They are the latest stimulants people use. Crank and ice are two of the new generation stimulants. **Crank** is an illegal amphetamine-like stimulant. It is illegal to use crank. Crank has the same effects as crack and cocaine. But crank's effects last longer. A person who tries crank can be addicted right away. The person also can have serious health problems right away.

Ice is a smokeable form of pure meth. It is illegal to use ice. The effects of ice last longer than crack. A person who tries ice can be addicted right away. The person also can have serious health problems.

Use of Amphetamines for ADHD

Some teens have Attention Deficit Hyperactive Disorder (ADHD). **ADHD** is a developmental disorder characterized by inattention and hyperactivity. There are different ways to manage ADHD. Some teens who have ADHD take a drug to help manage it while other teens do not. The teen's parents or guardian and physician make a plan.

A physician might prescribe an amphetamine for a teen who has ADHD. The drug acts in such a way as to help the teen. It helps with the inattention. It tends to lessen the hyperactivity.

A physician knows the amount of the drug the teen needs. The teen follows directions for taking the drug. The teen must pay close attention to the dose. The teen must pay close attention to possible side effects. If there are side effects, the teen's parents or guardian will tell the physician right away.

A teen who requires a drug for this disorder is taking the drug as a medicine. The drug is used to gain benefits. The teen should not give any pills to someone else.

A physician will review use of the drug with the teen and his or her parents or guardian. They will check to see if the drug helps. They will record progress in learning.

Sedative-Hypnotic Drugs

Sedative-hypnotic drugs are a group of drugs that depress the activities of the central nervous system. **Sedatives** are drugs that have a calming effect on behavior. **Hypnotic drugs** are drugs that promote drowsiness and sleep.

Barbiturates (bar·BI·chuh·ruhts) are a type of sedative that was prescribed by physicians to help people sleep. Physicians rarely prescribe barbiturates today because they are dangerous. Some people get these drugs illegally. They buy them on the street.

There is no way to know how powerful they are. People who take them illegally might take them with another drug. Suppose a person takes a barbiturate and drinks alcohol. Suppose a person takes a barbiturate and another depressant drug. The combination of these drugs multiplies the depressant effects. The combination can be deadly. You might have read about a famous person who died this way. No doubt you were disappointed and/or angry this person chose such behavior.

Tranquilizers are sedatives that are prescribed by a physician to treat anxiety. If a physician prescribes this drug, it is used as a medicine. The drug is used for medical reasons. It provides health benefits to the person. A person who takes a tranquilizer must be very careful. The dose is very important. The person must pay attention to the warnings for safe use.

Sedative-hypnotic drugs slow reaction time. Using these drugs increases the likelihood of accidents. These drugs produce side effects, such as dizziness, nausea, and headaches. Their use can interfere with everyday activities, such as riding a bike, driving a car, and using equipment. These drugs can easily produce psychological dependence. **Psychological dependence** is a strong desire to continue using a drug for emotional reasons.

Sedative-hypnotics can lead to physical dependence when they are misused or abused. A person who stops taking these drugs might have serious withdrawal effects. The person might require treatment to get through the withdrawal.

All sedative-hypnotic drugs should be used only under a physician's care. They should not be used in combination with other depressants. Their use without a prescription is illegal and dangerous.

Narcotics

Narcotics are a group of drugs that slow down the central nervous system, cause drowsiness, and can be used as painkillers. Narcotics slow down body functions such as breathing and heart rate.

Some narcotics have medical uses when prescribed by a physician. **Morphine** is a narcotic that is used to control pain. When it is used, a patient has an altered perception of pain. **Codeine** (KOH·deen) is a narcotic painkiller produced from morphine. It is weaker than morphine. Codeine is found in some prescription cough syrups and pain relievers.

Heroin is an illegal narcotic drug derived from morphine. Heroin has no approved medical use. Users often share needles to inject heroin and risk infection with HIV and hepatitis B.

All narcotics are dangerous when misused or abused. They produce physical and psychological dependence. When narcotics are taken with a depressant such as alcohol, death can occur.

Cloud Nine

Life Skill I will not be involved in illegal drug use.

Materials: Cotton balls, construction paper, markers, yarn, hole-puncher, glue or tape

Directions: Follow these steps to create your own Cloud Nine and share your ideas with classmates.

1. **List nine ways you can get high without using drugs.** A high is a feeling of intense excitement or well-being. For example, you might write, "Throw a party for my friends" or, "Go to the movies with a person I really like."

2. **Make a cloud out of the cotton balls.** Attach nine pieces of yarn to the cloud.

3. **Copy each way to get high without drugs onto a separate piece of construction paper.** Punch holes in the papers and hang them from the cloud.

4. **Hang your clouds from your classroom ceiling.**

Activity

Marijuana

Marijuana is a drug containing THC that impairs short-term memory and changes mood. Marijuana is an illegal drug in some states. In other states, it is a controlled drug. Marijuana has limited medical use. Some physicians have been authorized to give marijuana to certain cancer patients. Marijuana helps these patients avoid nausea when undergoing chemotherapy.

Hashish is a drug that comes from the marijuana plant. Hashish is even stronger than marijuana. Over 150 different chemicals have been identified in marijuana and hashish.

Marijuana and hashish are dangerous for many reasons. Marijuana is harmful to mental health. When it is smoked, marijuana enters the bloodstream. Then it goes directly to the brain where it is stored. Smoking marijuana affects memory and interferes with concentration. Marijuana also affects judgment. It interferes with the ability to make responsible decisions.

When using marijuana, people often say and do things they later regret. They might take unnecessary risks that can harm health. For example, they might cross a street when a car is coming toward them.

Marijuana is harmful to physical health. Marijuana can damage lung tissue because it is inhaled deeply and held for a long period of time. It contains many of the same cancer-causing substances as tobacco. Marijuana harms the immune system. Its presence leaves a person at higher than normal risk for developing infections.

It is illegal to use marijuana. It is illegal to buy marijuana. It is illegal to sell marijuana or have it in your possession. Suppose a teen has marijuana in a locker or bookbag. This is a serious offense. Suppose a teen sells marijuana to another teen. This is a serious offense. Protect yourself. Stay away from teens who use, buy, sell, or possess marijuana.

Caution: THC Is Rising

In the past, marijuana usually had about 1 to 5 percent THC in it. Today, it can have as much as 8 to 15 percent THC in it.

Marijuana is fat-soluble. This means that THC can remain in the body for several weeks.

Hallucinogens

Hallucinogens (huh·LOO·suhn·uh·juhnz) are a group of drugs that interfere with the senses, causing people to see and hear things that are not real. Hallucinogens are also referred to as psychedelic drugs. The effects may last for hours or for days. Hallucinogens produce tolerance and psychological dependence.

LSD is a hallucinogen that is often sold illegally in powder, tablet, or capsule form. It can also be dissolved in sugar cubes or candy. LSD produces different effects. It can cause a person to feel confused or see things that do not exist. For example, a person might see colors or objects that do not exist. Different senses might blend with each other. A person might say (s)he sees sound or hears color. LSD produces a false sense of power. LSD use has resulted in many deaths. Some people who used LSD believed they could fly, so they jumped from buildings. Others felt they had the power to stop moving cars, so they jumped in front of them.

LSD is fat-soluble and stays in the body a long time. LSD produces flashbacks. A **flashback** is a sudden illusion that a person has long after having used certain drugs. For example, a person might see things that do not exist.

PCP, also known as angel dust, is a hallucinogen that can act as a stimulant or a depressant. PCP can cause body actions to speed up or slow down. It can cause slurred speech, vomiting, and loss of muscular control. It can also cause people to become aggressive and violent. PCP use also has resulted in many deaths.

Mescaline (MES·kuh·leen) is a hallucinogen made from the peyote cactus plant. It causes many of the same effects as LSD. Mescaline can affect the brain within 30 seconds after entering the body. Its effects can last for 12 hours.

What Is a Fat-Soluble Drug?

Take a dry sponge and feel its surface. Notice that it is not damp. Pretend the sponge is the body of a person who tries LSD. Pour water on the sponge. Now squeeze the water out of the sponge. Squeeze the sponge again and again. Feel the surface of the sponge. It will be damp. No matter how hard you squeeze, the sponge will be damp for a while. It needs time to dry. If a person uses marijuana, he or she has used a fat-soluble drug. It does not leave the body right after use. It stays in the body a long time.

Anabolic Steroids

An **anabolic steroid** (a·nuh·BAH·lik STIR·oyd) is a synthetic drug that is used to increase muscle size and strength. Anabolic steroids are injected or taken orally to stimulate increased muscle growth and strength. There is evidence that anabolic steroids are harmful. If taken during puberty, they might stunt growth. In males, they cause enlargement of breasts and damage to testicles. In females, they cause breast reduction, growth of body hair, and lowering of the voice. Their use by people of either sex might cause hardening of the arteries, high blood pressure, and liver damage.

Anabolic steroids affect behavior and mood. People who use them can have roid rage. This is very aggressive and violent behavior. People get into fights in which they or others are likely to be harmed. If they are playing sports, they are extra rough. They might not consider the safety of others.

Teens who use steroids and then quit might have withdrawal symptoms. The change in mood they got from the steroids changes. Their mood goes from being high to feeling very down. They often get bouts of serious depression. Teens who come off steroids are at risk for making a suicide attempt.

Suppose you know a teen who uses steroids. Talk to your parents or guardian. This teen needs help. This teen needs help as he or she withdraws from steroid use. The rapid mood swings that accompany withdrawal can be serious.

Muscled Off to Jail

Because of the physical and psychological dangers anabolic steroids pose to teens, laws have been passed prohibiting their use. Anyone who gives anabolic steroids to a minor can be sentenced to prison for ten years. Athletes who use steroids can be banned from athletic contests.

Inhalants

Inhalants are chemicals that are breathed in and produce immediate effects. Using inhalants to get a high is illegal. Inhalants are often household and industrial chemicals that are not intended to be inhaled. **Huffing,** or **sniffing,** is inhaling fumes from substances to get a high. **Bagging** is inhaling chemicals from a paper bag.

Some examples of inhalants are: glues and contact cement, gasoline, paint thinner, lighter fluid, spray-can propellant, paper correction fluid, liquid wax, shoe polish, fingernail polish remover, hair spray, furniture polish, and marker fluids. Because inhaled products contain different combinations of ingredients, the potential damage varies with the product.

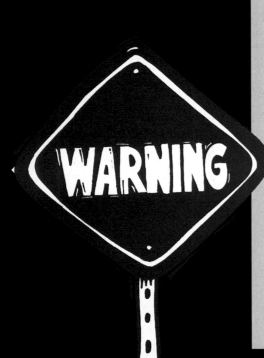

Huffing, sniffing, and bagging can cause:

- seizures and sudden death;
- altered states of consciousness;
- changes in behavior;
- kidney and liver failure;
- heart muscle damage;
- brain and nerve damage;
- leukemia;
- lead poisoning;
- ulcers around the mouth and nose;
- short-term memory loss and motor-skill impairment;
- brain damage.

Drug Slipping

Drug slipping is placing a drug into someone's food or beverage without that person's knowledge. These drugs usually do not have a taste or odor when mixed with food or beverages. The person eating the food or drinking the beverage cannot taste or smell the drug. Some drugs that are slipped into foods or beverages cause a teen to pass out. The teen might be raped when s(he) passes out. The teen usually has no memory of what happened. Drug slipping is illegal. A person who does this can be prosecuted.

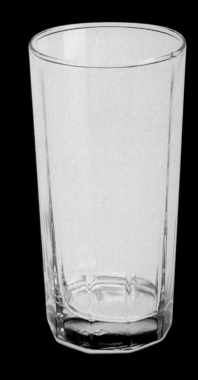

Lesson 29

Review

Vocabulary

Write a separate sentence using each of the vocabulary words listed on page 310.

Health Content

Write responses to the following:

1. What are the effects of stimulant drugs? **page 311**
2. What are the effects of cocaine and crack? **page 312**
3. What are the effects of amphetamines, methamphetamines, and new generation stimulants? **pages 313–314**
4. Why is it dangerous to use look-alike drugs? **page 313**
5. What are the effects of sedative-hypnotic drugs? **page 315**
6. What are the effects of narcotics? **page 316**
7. What are the effects of marijuana and hashish? **page 317**
8. What are the effects of hallucinogens? **page 318**
9. Why is it dangerous to use anabolic steroids without a prescription? **page 319**
10. What are eleven reasons it is dangerous to use inhalants to get high? **page 320**

Intervention and Treatment

Vocabulary

enabler

codependence

honest talk

formal intervention

inpatient care

outpatient care

relapse

student assistance program

parent support groups

 Life Skill • **I will be aware of resources for the treatment of drug misuse and abuse.**

Getting people who are drug-dependent to give up drugs is one of the most important tasks in the war on drugs. You can arm yourself with the knowledge and skills to help with this fight. Learn the signs of drug abuse. When someone you know abuses drugs, use honest talk to describe your thoughts and feelings. Keep informed of school and community resources for intervention and treatment.

The Lesson Objectives

- Explain how drug misuse and abuse progresses to drug dependence.
- List warning signs of drug abuse.
- Describe the behaviors of denial and of honest talk.
- Discuss different approaches to treatment and support programs for drug dependency.

Progression to Drug Dependency

When people misuse or abuse drugs, it can be difficult for them to stop. Drug misuse and abuse progress to drug dependence in the following way.

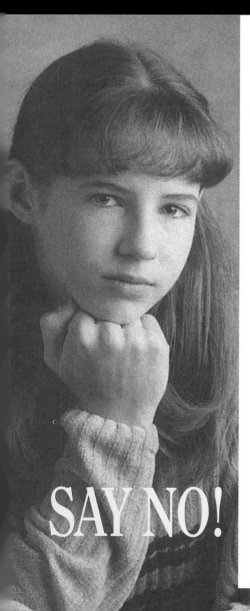

SAY NO!

"I will just try it."

A person is tempted to experiment with alcohol, tobacco, or another drug. The cycle starts.

"I like the feeling."

A person continues to use alcohol, tobacco, or another drug. (S)he might start spending less time with people who not use drugs and more time with those who do use drugs.

"I need some more of the drug to feel good."

A person develops tolerance.

"I do not have a problem with drugs."

A person stops recognizing his or her behavior and is in a state of denial. Denial is a condition in which a person refuses to recognize what (s)he is doing or feeling because it is extremely painful. The person will not admit to himself or herself or others that drug abuse is causing problems. Problems occur. The person might argue with others, not do school work, and break family rules. The person makes excuses for these behaviors.

"I just have to have it."

A person becomes drug-dependent.

Warning Signs of Drug Abuse

You can see how drug dependence begins with "I will just try it" and progresses to "I just have to have it." To stop this harmful progression, it is important to recognize some of the early warning signs of drug abuse.

Early warning signs of drug abuse include:

- talking about trying a drug;
- making plans to be in situations in which there will be drugs;
- giving up friends who do not use drugs;
- spending more time with people who use drugs;
- getting into trouble;
- showing no interest in activities;
- having a sloppy appearance;
- joining a gang;
- rebelling against authority;
- smelling like alcohol;
- having glassy eyes and a blank stare;
- stumbling;
- having slurred speech;
- hiding drugs;
- lying about drug use.

Denial Versus Honest Talk

Drug dependence is a disease. It harms people's bodies and minds. People who are drug dependent begin to think and act differently. Denial is one of the most common behavior changes. People who are drug-dependent will not admit the extent of their drug problem to themselves or others. They hide drugs and lie to others. They blame others for their behavior. They often become argumentative and violent. Their behavior is harmful.

Family members and close friends of those who are drug dependent respond in different ways. Some respond with harmful behavior and become enablers. An **enabler** is a person who knowingly or unknowingly supports the harmful behavior of another person. Enablers make excuses for a drug-dependent person. If someone else wants to confront the drug-dependent person, they get angry or avoid the topic. They want to keep things as they are rather than making changes.

People who are drug-dependent and those who are close to them often develop codependence. **Codependence** is a mental disorder in which a person denies feelings and copes in harmful ways. People with codependence lose touch with how they feel. They are numb to what is happening around them.

In many dysfunctional families, one or more family members are drug-dependent. Other family members respond with harmful behavior. They are enablers and codependent. Teens reared in these families are at risk for becoming drug-dependent. They are at risk for enabling the harmful behavior of others.

People who are healthy are not enablers. They are not codependent. They respond with honest talk. **Honest talk** is the straightforward sharing of a person's thoughts and feelings about a situation, a person, or a person's behavior. People who are healthy recognize when other people choose harmful behavior. They do not deny what they experience. They do not make excuses for what others do. They expect others to be accountable for their actions. They use honest talk and I-messages to express their feelings. Examples of I-messages are:

- **I cannot bring friends over, because I do not know if you have been drinking, and this makes me sad.**

- **I feel I cannot trust you when you lie about drug use, and this makes me stressed.**

People who are healthy know the importance of honest talk. When family members or friends choose harmful behavior, healthy people think this way: *Because I care about you, I do not find behavior that harms you or others acceptable. You must stop your harmful behavior and get help.*

Straightforward and Self-Assured

Stop for a moment to think about your relationships with others.

- **Do you expect people to be accountable for their actions?**
- **When people behave in harmful ways, do you tell them it bothers you?**
- **Are you comfortable with honest talk?**

If you answered NO to any of these questions, talk to a trusted adult. Remember, if you allow others to behave in harmful ways without putting your foot down, you are an enabler. You hurt yourself and others.

Formal Intervention and Treatment

Few people who are drug-dependent decide to seek treatment on their own. Remember, people who are drug-dependent usually deny that they have a problem. A person who uses honest talk knows that (s)he must confront the drug-dependent person in order for this person to get treatment. But confronting the drug-dependent person is tough to do. The help of a trained counselor is often needed. The counselor meets with family members and friends to plan a formal intervention. A **formal intervention** is an action by people, such as family members, who want a person to get treatment. During the formal intervention, they use honest talk to tell the drug-dependent person about his or her harmful behavior. They clearly say why treatment is necessary. A trained counselor often helps make a treatment plan.

There are different approaches to treatment. A drug-dependent person might require inpatient care. **Inpatient care** is treatment that is given to a person during a stay at a facility, such as a hospital. Inpatient care is often needed to help people who are drug-dependent with withdrawal symptoms. In many cases, people who are drug-dependent stay at a facility for 28 days. **Outpatient care** is treatment that does not require an overnight stay at a facility.

After completing a treatment program, people who are recovering need support. They are never completely cured. Without support, they might have a relapse. A **relapse** is the return to addictive behavior after a period of having stopped it. There are support programs for people who are drug-dependent, their family members, and their friends.

School and Community Resources

The types of school and community resources available for intervention and treatment of drug-related problems depend on where you live. Your parents or guardian can help you find resources in the school and community. Guidance counselors, school psychologists, school nurses, principals, teachers, and coaches are aware of resources.

Medical hospitals often provide special services for drug dependence. They offer medical treatment, counseling, and recovery programs. In many communities, there might be health care facilities that specialize in the treatment of drug dependence. There are many places within a community that provide recovery programs, such as Alcoholics Anonymous, Al-Anon, Alateen, and Narcotics Anonymous. Community agencies, such as the American Cancer Society, American Heart Association, and American Lung Association, offer help with tobacco cessation.

Your school might participate in intervention and treatment. There might be drug-free activities, resistance skills training, positive peer programs, and student assistance programs. A **student assistance program** is a school-based approach to the prevention and treatment of alcohol and other drugs. Student assistance programs use a referral process for getting appropriate and confidential help for students who need it. Schools might have special clubs that focus on positive actions students can take to stop risky behaviors. One such club is Students Against Drunk Driving. Schools might offer support programs. **Parent support groups** are groups formed by parents to help one another cope with problems.

How the Community Benefits

The community benefits when people who are drug dependent begin recovery programs. This is the first step in restoring health. It is a step in rebuilding relationships with family members and friends. It is a step toward asking for forgiveness for the pain caused to others. People who enter recovery take a step toward being productive again.

Honest Talk

Activity

Life Skill

I will be aware of resources for the treatment of drug misuse and abuse.

Materials: Paper, pen or pencil

Directions: The statements below represent responses of enablers. Write statements that represent honest talk. Then, make up your own situations and honest talk.

1. Think of three more situations and honest talk for each.

- "My brother really doesn't have a drug problem. He drinks only on weekends."

- "It's okay that my friend lost my jacket. I don't blame her for being zoned out on tranquilizers ever since her parents divorced."

- "My friend stood me up again. But I under-stand—he just broke up with his girlfriend and he needs to smoke joints to relax."

Lesson 30

Review

Vocabulary

Write a separate sentence using each of the vocabulary words listed on page 322.

Health Content

Write responses to the following:

1. How do drug misuse and abuse progress to drug dependence? **page 323**

2. What are 15 warning signs of drug abuse? **page 324**

3. How do you know a person is in denial? **page 325**

4. How can you recognize codependence? **page 325**

5. Why is it important to use honest talk with people who misuse or abuse drugs? **page 326**

6. What happens during a formal intervention? **page 327**

7. What happens during a relapse? **page 327**

8. Describe different approaches to treatment for drug dependency. **page 327**

9. What are some support programs for people who are drug-dependent, their family members and friends? **page 328**

10. What is the purpose of a student assistance program? **page 328**

Resistance Skills for Saying NO to Drugs

Vocabulary

drug-free lifestyle

risk factors

protective factors

peer pressure

resistance skills

victim of violence

drug trafficking

safe and drug-free school zone

injecting drug users

- **I will practice protective factors that help me stay away from drugs.**
- **I will use resistance skills if I am pressured to misuse or abuse drugs.**
- **I will choose a drug-free lifestyle to reduce my risk of violence and accidents.**
- **I will choose a drug-free lifestyle to reduce my risk of HIV, STDs, and unwanted pregnancy.**

A **drug-free lifestyle** is a lifestyle in which people do not use harmful and illegal drugs. When you choose a drug-free lifestyle, you have a sense of control over the direction of your life. You take responsibility for your behavior and decisions.

The Lesson Objectives

- Identify risk factors for harmful drug use in teens.
- Identify protective factors that help teens avoid harmful drug use.
- Outline resistance skills to resist harmful drug use.
- Explain why drug use increases the risk of crime, violence, accidents, infection with HIV and other STDs, and unwanted pregnancy.
- List reasons for saying NO to alcohol, tobacco, and other drug use.

Risk Factors

Some teens are more at risk for harmful drug use than are other teens. They have certain risk factors. **Risk factors** are ways that a person might behave and characteristics of the environment in which a person lives that threaten health, safety, and well-being. Some risk factors for harmful drug use are listed below. Some risk factors might describe your behavior or the environment in which you live. If so, you are at risk for using harmful drugs and need to work extra hard to resist the temptation. Risk factors refer only to the statistical probability that you might use harmful drugs. You have varying degrees of control over the risk factors. *You have control over whether or not you use harmful drugs.*

Risk Factors for Harmful Drug Use in Teens

- **Having difficult family relationships**
- **Having negative self-esteem**
- **Being unable to resist peer pressure**
- **Being unable to master developmental tasks**
- **Being economically disadvantaged**
- **Having one or more biological family members who are drug-dependent**
- **Lacking skills to cope with stressful situations**
- **Having difficulty achieving success in athletics**
- **Having a learning disability and/or doing poorly in school**
- **Having friends who misuse and abuse drugs**

Risk Factors a Person Cannot Control

Some teens have risk factors they cannot control. For example, some teens live in poverty. Some teens have one or more biological family members who are drug-dependent. These teens cannot use a risk factor as an excuse for drug use. Instead they must work extra hard. They must work to develop as many protective factors as possible. Protective factors are listed on the next page.

Protective Factors

Protective factors are ways that a person might behave and characteristics of the environment in which a person lives that promote health, safety, and well-being. Some protective factors for harmful drug use are listed below. Some protective factors might describe your behavior or the environment in which you live. If so, you already have some protection from being tempted to use drugs. Remember, the choice is always yours. *You have control over whether or not you use harmful drugs.*

Protective Factors That Help Teens Avoid Harmful Drug Use

- **Having close family relationships**
- **Having positive self-esteem**
- **Being able to say NO when pressured by peers to choose harmful behavior**
- **Having clearly defined goals and plans to reach them**
- **Living in a situation without economic difficulties**
- **Having family members who are not drug-dependent**
- **Having skills to cope with stressful situations**
- **Having a healthful attitude about competition and athletic performance**
- **Feeling a sense of accomplishment at school**
- **Having friends who do not misuse or abuse drugs**

Add a Protective Factor to Your Coat of Armor

Review the list of protective factors. Choose a protective factor to add to those you already have. For example, you might have difficulty saying NO when pressured by peers to choose harmful behavior. Rehearse. Practice using resistance skills with an adult. Then you have added a protective factor to your coat of armor.

Follow a...
Health Behavior Contract

Name:_____ **Date:** _____

Copy the health behavior contract on a separate sheet of paper.

DO NOT WRITE IN THIS BOOK.

Life Skill: I will practice protective factors that help me stay away from drugs.

Effect On My Health: If I practice protective factors that help me stay away from drugs, I can maintain a drug-free lifestyle. I will have a sense of control over the direction of my life. I will take responsibility for my behavior and my decisions. I will not risk committing or becoming a victim of crime or violence. I will reduce my risk of accidents, unwanted pregnancy, and infection with HIV and other STDs.

My Plan: One protective factor is having friends who do not misuse or abuse drugs. I will spend time with friends who do not misuse or abuse drugs. I will plan drug-free entertainment for each Friday and Saturday for one month. I will list activities on my weekend planner.

My calendar	Friday	Saturday
1st weekend		
2nd weekend		
3rd weekend		
4th weekend		

How My Plan Worked: (Complete after one month.) _____
_____
_____

Using Resistance Skills When Pressured to Use Drugs

Peer pressure is influence that people of similar age or status place on others to encourage them to make certain decisions or to behave in certain ways. Peers might pressure you to use harmful drugs. You must always say NO when you are pressured. **Resistance skills** are skills that are used when you want to say NO to an action or to leave a situation.

1. **Use assertive behavior.**

   • Stand tall.

   • Look directly at the person to whom you are speaking.

   • Say NO in a firm and confident voice.

   • Be confident because you are being responsible.

   • Be proud because you are obeying laws and respecting authority.

2. **Give reasons for saying NO.**

   • Explain that drug use is harmful, unsafe, and illegal. Using drugs shows no respect for self or others. Drug use is against the law and against family guidelines. Drug use interferes with good character.

   • Use one or more of the Reasons for Saying NO to Alcohol and Other Drugs on pages 338–339.

3. **Use nonverbal behavior to match verbal behavior.**

   • Do not send mixed messages to others. Remember that what you do must match what you say.

   • Do not pretend to use a drug; for example, do not pretend to sip a beer.

   • Do not hold or pass a cigarette or marijuana joint.

   • Do not touch a syringe or injection equipment that is for injecting drug use.

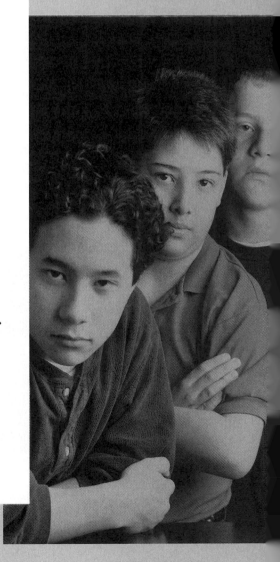

- Do not agree to buy a drug for someone else.
- Do not keep drugs for someone else in your possession, for example, hiding a stash in your locker, bedroom, or bookbag.
- Do not ride in a car with older teens who are attempting to buy alcohol at a drive-through store.
- Do not do anything that indicates that you approve of harmful drug use.

4. **Avoid being in situations in which there will be pressure to use harmful drugs.**
   - Think ahead about what peers will be doing when they invite you to join them.
   - Ask questions if you are not certain if there will be drug use.
   - Attend only drug-free activities.

5. **Avoid being with people who use harmful drugs.**
   - Choose friends who are drug-free.
   - Stay away from gang members.
   - Stay away from people who use or sell drugs.

6. **Resist pressure to engage in illegal behavior.**
   - Learn the laws that apply to drug use in your community and state.
   - Do not break laws.
   - Stay away from people who break laws.
   - Stay away from areas where there might be drug trafficking.

7. **Influence others to choose responsible behavior.**
   - Suggest drug-free activities.
   - Encourage those who pressure you to use drugs to change their behavior.
   - Be aware of places where teens who use drugs can get help.

Staying Drug-Free to Protect Against Violence and Accidents

People who use drugs might behave in aggressive and violent ways. They are less likely to respect the rights of others. When people use drugs, they drop their guard and do not protect themselves. They are more likely to become victims of violence. A **victim of violence** is a person who is harmed or killed by violence. People who are involved in drug trafficking are at extremely high risk of violence. **Drug trafficking** is the illegal purchase or sale of drugs.

People who use drugs have an increased risk of accidents. They do not think clearly. They take unnecessary risks. They have impaired reaction time and coordination.

SAFE AND DRUG-FREE SCHOOL ZONES

A safe and drug-free school zone is a defined area around a school for the purpose of sheltering young people from weapons and the sale of drugs. Increased penalties for using and selling drugs and having weapons have been set for these zones. School officials and law enforcement officers pay particular attention to safe and drug-free zones. They want to stop drug trafficking and crime. They want to reduce the risk of violence. They need your help and support. Encourage your friends to support safe and drug-free zones at your school.

Drugs and Violence: The Dangerous Connection

Protect yourself and others. Do not use drugs, and stay away from people who do. Harmful drug use increases the risk of violent behavior.

- **Fighting and assaults**
- **School expulsion**
- **Sexual assault and acquaintance rape**
- **Theft**
- **Domestic violence**
- **Suicide**
- **Homicide**

Staying Drug-Free to Protect Against HIV, STDs, and Unwanted Pregnancy

Using drugs increases the risk of getting HIV or another STD. HIV and other STDs are transmitted during intimate sexual contact. Teens who use drugs might not stick to their decision to practice abstinence. They do not think as clearly and make poor decisions. Most teens who have been sexually active were under the influence of alcohol or other drugs at the time.

Using drugs increases the risk of unwanted pregnancy. Teens who are using drugs do not consider possible consequences of their actions. One sexual contact can result in an unwanted pregnancy. Teens who use drugs are four times more likely to have an unwanted pregnancy than teens who do not use drugs.

SHARING NEEDLES IS RISKY BUSINESS

Injecting drug users are people who inject illegal drugs into their blood vessels with syringes and needles. People who inject drugs often share the needles they use to inject the drugs. A person infected with HIV who uses a needle to inject drugs can leave a small amount of his or her blood containing HIV on or in the needle. A second person who uses the same needle can become infected with HIV when the infected blood from the needle gets into his or her blood.

Reasons for Saying NO to Alcohol and Other Drugs

1. I do not want to dull my body senses.
2. I want to have a fast reaction time so I will not be injured in an accident.
3. I want to keep the number of infection-fighting cells in my immune system at a healthful level.
4. I want to protect myself from drug-related cancer.
5. I do not want to irritate the inner lining of my stomach and develop ulcers.
6. I do not want to develop cirrhosis of the liver.
7. I do not want to develop pancreatitis or diabetes.
8. I want to keep my heart and blood vessels healthy.
9. I want to prevent dementia, blackouts, seizures, hallucinations, and nerve destruction.
10. I want to have regular menstrual periods (females).
11. I want to reduce my risk of breast cancer (females).
12. I want my secondary sex characteristics to develop in a normal way.
13. I want to get good grades in school.
14. I want to make responsible decisions.
15. I want to stay in control of decision-making so that I can stick to my decision to abstain from sexual intercourse.
16. I want to stay in control of decision-making so that I abstain from sexual intercourse and do not become a teen parent.
17. I want to stay in control of decision-making so that I abstain from sexual intercourse and do not become infected with HIV or other STDs.

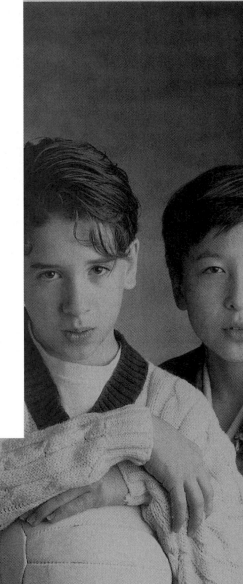

18. I want to be in social situations and gain social skills without the use of mood-altering drugs.

19. I do not want to become aggressive or violent and harm myself or others.

20. I do not want to become a victim because I am out of control or with other people who are out of control.

21. I do not want to become very depressed and think about suicide.

22. I want to obey laws.

23. I want to participate in school activities and not be thrown off school teams for drug use.

24. I want to be a role model of responsible behavior for younger brothers and sisters.

25. I want to be a responsible citizen.

26. I want to avoid needless medical bills for drug-related health problems.

27. I do not want to risk overdose, coma, and death.

28. I want to be physically fit.

29. I do not want to break school rules.

30. I do not want to waste money.

31. I want others to respect me.

32. I want to have healthful family relationships.

33. I want to cope with stress in healthful ways.

34. I want to be accepted by peers who are drug-free.

35. I want to do my part to help fight the war on drugs.

36. I do not want to be a juvenile offender.

37. I do not want to have a police record.

38. I want to be mentally alert to prepare for my future.

39. I want to compete fairly in athletic competition.

Reasons for Saying NO to Tobacco Use

1. I do not want to become addicted to nicotine.

2. I want to be physically fit.

3. I want to have a clear, pleasant voice.

4. I want to prevent respiratory infections, such as the cold and flu.

5. I want to keep my heart and blood vessels healthy.

6. I do not want to worsen allergies or asthma.

7. I want my clothes and breath to smell fresh and clean.

8. I do not want my teeth to be yellow and I want to have a nice smile.

9. I want to be accepted by peers who do not smoke.

10. I want my parents or guardian to approve of my behavior.

11. I do not want to break school rules or be prevented from attending school-sponsored functions.

12. I do not want to make mistakes or have accidents because I am lighting a cigarette.

13. I do not want to cause a fire.

14. I do not want to waste money on an expensive habit.

15. I do not want harmful gases, such as carbon monoxide, in my body.

16. I do not want to be short of breath.

17. I do not want to have smoker's cough.

18. I do not want to coat my lungs with tar.

19. I do not want to paralyze my cilia and prevent them from keeping harmful substances out of my lungs.

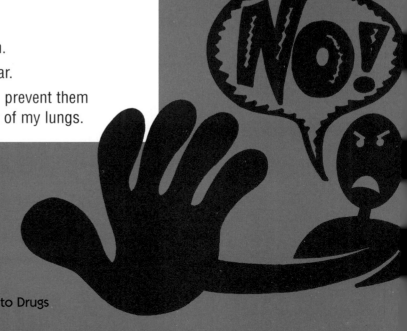

20. I want to taste and smell my food.

21. I do not want to develop emphysema or chronic bronchitis.

22. I do not want to develop gum disease or lose my teeth.

23. I do not want to develop the many kinds of cancers associated with tobacco use.

24. I do not want to age quickly and have wrinkled skin.

25. I do not want to produce secondhand smoke that harms others.

26. I do not want to waste money.

27. I do not want to offend others.

28. I do not want to develop cavities.

29. I do not want to disgust others by chewing and spitting.

30. I want to have a healthful, appealing appearance.

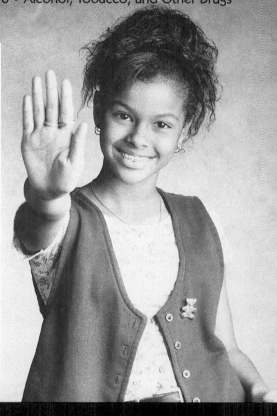

Lesson 31

Review

Vocabulary

Write a separate sentence using each of the vocabulary words listed on page 330.

Health Content

Write responses to the following:

1. How would you describe a drug-free lifestyle? **page 330**

2. What are ten risk factors for harmful drug use in teens? **page 331**

3. What are ten protective factors that help teens avoid harmful drug use? **page 332**

4. What are seven resistance skills you can use to resist harmful drug use? **pages 334–335**

5. Why does drug use increase the risk of crime, violence, and accidents? **page 336**

6. What are seven violent behaviors that are more likely to occur when people use drugs? **page 336**

7. Describe a safe and drug-free school zone. **page 336**

8. Why does drug use increase the risk of HIV, other STDs, and unwanted pregnancy? **page 337**

9. What are reasons to say NO to alcohol and other drug use? **pages 338–339**

10. What are reasons to say NO to tobacco use? **pages 340–341**

Unit 6 Review

Health Content

Review your answers for each Lesson Review in this unit. Then write answers to each of the following questions.

1. What influences the effects drugs have on the body? **Lesson 26 page 268**

2. What can you learn from the label on a container for an OTC drug? **Lesson 26 page 274**

3. What determines the amount of alcohol in a person's blood? **Lesson 27 page 277**

4. What are the effects of alcoholism on family members? **Lesson 27 page 284**

5. How are your heart and blood vessels affected by smoking? **Lesson 28 pages 294–295**

6. How can you resist pressure to use tobacco products? **Lesson 28 pages 304–305**

7. How do stimulants affect the body? **Lesson 29 page 311**

8. How do hallucinogens affect the body? **Lesson 29 page 318**

9. How do people who have drug dependence behave when they are in denial? **Lesson 30 page 325**

10. Why do you increase your risk of violence and accidents when you use drugs? **Lesson 31 page 336**

Vocabulary

Number a sheet of paper from 1–10. Select the correct vocabulary word. Write it next to the corresponding number. DO NOT WRITE IN THIS BOOK.

alcoholism	injecting drug user
crack	media literacy
dose	oxidation
drug dependence	relapse
inhalants	tar

1. _____ is a purified form of cocaine that produces a rapid and intense reaction. **Lesson 29**

2. _____ is the process by which alcohol is changed to carbon dioxide and water. **Lesson 27**

3. A(n) _____ is a person who injects illegal drugs into the body with syringes and needles. **Lesson 31**

4. _____ is the amount of a drug that is taken at one time. **Lesson 26**

5. _____ is the continued use of a drug even though it harms the body, mind, and relationships. **Lesson 26**

6. _____ is the ability to recognize and evaluate the messages in media. **Lesson 28**

7. _____ are chemicals that, when breathed in, produce immediate effects. **Lesson 29**

8. _____ is a disease in which there is physical and psychological dependence on alcohol. **Lesson 27**

9. _____ is a thick, sticky fluid that is formed when tobacco is burned. **Lesson 28**

10. A(n) _____ is the return to addictive behavior after a period of having stopped it. **Lesson 30**

The Responsible Decision-Making Model™

You go to a party at a friend's house. You see a teen slip something into another teen's drink when (s)he isn't looking. Should you keep quiet? Answer the following questions on a separate sheet of paper. Write "Does not apply" if a question does not apply to this situation.

1. Is it healthful to keep quiet about the drug slipping? Why or why not?

2. Is it safe to keep quiet about the drug slipping? Why or why not?

3. Is it legal to keep quiet about the drug slipping? Why or why not?

4. Will you show respect for yourself and others if you keep quiet about the drug slipping? Why or why not?

5. Will your parents or guardian approve if you keep quiet about the drug slipping? Why or why not?

6. Will you demonstrate good character if you keep quiet about the drug slipping? Why or why not?

What is the responsible decision to make in this situation?

Health Literacy

Effective Communication

The Centers for Disease Control and Prevention has identified these two categories of risk behaviors for teens: tobacco use; and alcohol and other drug use. Design a logo for each category that warns of the risks.

Self-Directed Learning

Research a famous person who abused alcohol or other harmful drugs. What factors led to the drug dependence? What was the outcome—did the person recover?

Critical Thinking

Cigars were popular several decades ago. For a time, only older people smoked cigars. Why do you think tobacco manufacturers are targeting teens today?

Responsible Citizenship

Containers of alcohol are required to carry warning labels. What would you include on a warning label? Design several labels and share them with your class.

Multicultural Health

Research drug laws for possession and use of illegal drugs in another country. Compare them to the laws in your country.

Family Involvement

Discuss with your family ways you have learned to manage stress. Ask your parent or guardian to share how they deal with stress.

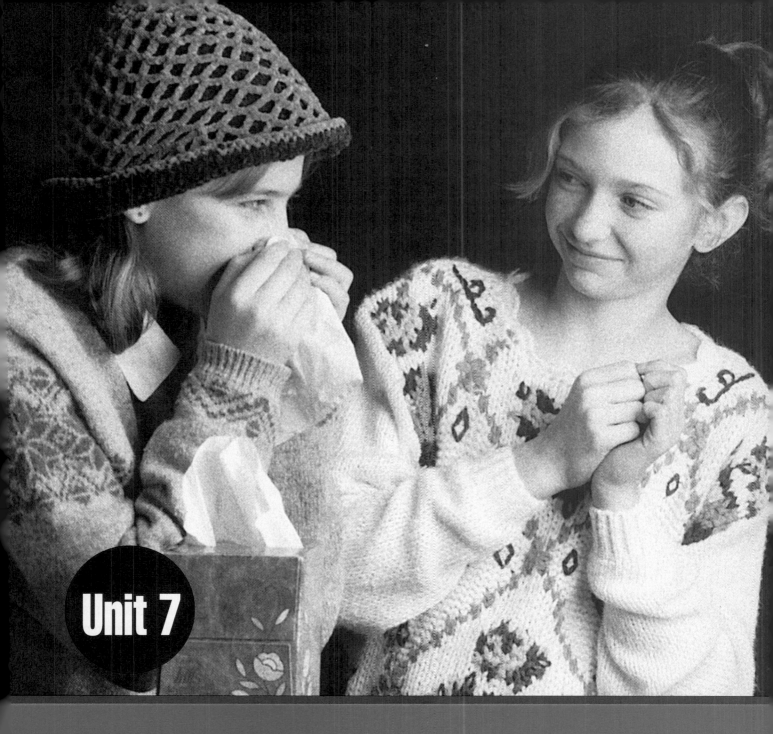

Unit 7

Communicable and Chronic Diseases

Common Communicable Diseases

Vocabulary

disease
communicable disease
pathogen
noncommunicable disease
viruses
bacteria
rickettsia
fungi
protozoa
direct contact
indirect contact
mucous membranes
mucus
fever
immune system
T cells
phagocytes
B cells
antibody
immunity
active immunity
vaccine
passive immunity
tetanus
lockjaw
symptom
diagnosis
antibiotic

Life Skills

- **I will choose behaviors to prevent the spread of pathogens.**
- **I will choose behaviors to reduce my risk of infection with communicable diseases.**

A **disease** is an illness. A **communicable** (kuh·MYOO·ni·kuh·buhl) **disease** is an illness caused by a pathogen. A **pathogen** is a disease-causing organism. The common cold is caused by pathogens, therefore, it is a communicable disease. A **noncommunicable disease** is an illness that is caused by something other than a pathogen. Heart disease is an example of a noncommunicable disease. It might result from hereditary factors, improper diet, smoking, or other factors. This lesson will focus on communicable diseases.

The Lesson Objectives

- List different kinds of pathogens and how pathogens can be spread.
- Discuss eight ways that the body defends itself against disease.
- Identify the causes, symptoms, diagnosis, treatment, and prevention for some communicable diseases.
- State 19 behaviors that reduce your risk of being infected with pathogens.

Disease-Causing Pathogens

There are five different kinds of pathogens.

Viruses

Viruses (VY·rus·es) are the smallest pathogens. They are programmed to infect only certain body cells. When a virus enters a cell, it directs the cell to make more viruses. Some viral diseases are the common cold, measles, chicken-pox, influenza, and herpes.

Bacteria

Bacteria (bak·TIR·ee·uh) are single-celled microorganisms. There are more than a thousand kinds of bacteria, but only about 100 are known to cause disease. Some diseases caused by bacteria are strep throat, tuberculosis, syphilis, gonorrhea, and Lyme disease.

Rickettsia

Rickettsia (ri·KET·see·uh) are pathogens that grow inside living cells and resemble bacteria. They are much smaller than bacteria. Two diseases they cause are Rocky Mountain spotted fever and typhus.

Fungi

Fungi (FUHN·jy) are single-celled or multicellular plantlike organisms, such as yeast and molds. Fungi can cause diseases of the skin, mucous membranes, and lungs. Some diseases caused by fungi are athlete's foot, ringworm, jock itch, nail infections, and candidiasis.

Protozoa

Protozoa (proh·tuh·ZOH·uh) are tiny, single-celled parasites. Some diseases caused by protozoa are malaria, African sleeping sickness, and dysentery. Giardia (jee·AHR·dy·uh) is a protozoan that might infect people who drink impure water in the United States.

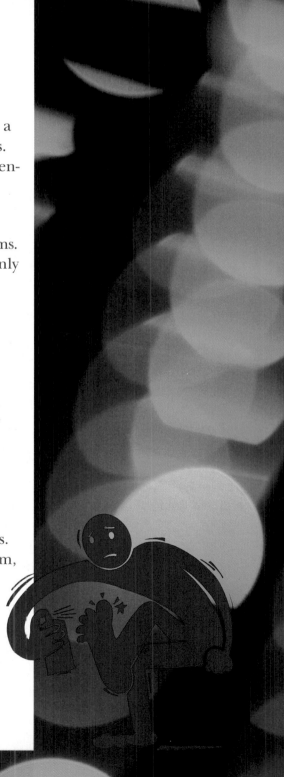

How Pathogens Are Spread

Pathogens can be spread in several ways.

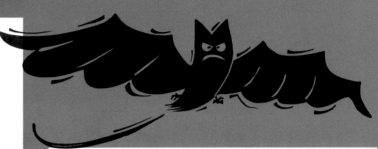

Direct contact with an infected person

Direct contact is the transfer of pathogens from an infected person to another person. Ways pathogens can be spread by direct contact with an infected person include:

- kissing;
- having sexual intercourse;
- receiving a transfusion of the person's blood;
- touching ulcers or sores;
- handling the person's body fluids, such as the blood or urine.

Contact with pathogens in the air

When an infected person coughs or sneezes, pathogens are released into the air. These pathogens can be inhaled by another person, who then becomes infected.

Contact with contaminated objects

Indirect contact is contact with an object that has been used by an infected person. A person can become infected by using objects used or touched by an infected person, such as a pen or pencil, toothbrush, eating utensils, or clothing. Sharing a needle used by a person infected with HIV to inject drugs, to pierce ears or other body parts, or to get a tattoo, can result in HIV infection.

Through contact with animals and insects

A person can become infected with pathogens when bitten by an animal or an insect. Some animals, such as dogs, cats, raccoons, and bats, might carry the rabies virus. Mosquitos carry the virus that causes encephalitis, an infection of the brain. They also carry the pathogen that causes malaria. Both insects and animals might carry pathogens from one place to another. An insect can pick up a pathogen when it lands on sewage and deposit it on food. People might eat the food and become infected.

Contact with contaminated food and water

People who prepare or serve food are required by law to wash their hands with soap and water after using the restroom. Washing hands removes pathogens that might have come in contact with feces or urine. This helps prevent pathogens from being spread to food. Water might be contaminated with feces, urine, and pathogens. It is safe to drink tap water, but it is not safe to drink water from streams before it is purified. Pathogens also grow in foods and cause foodborne illnesses. Ways to prevent foodborne illnesses were covered in Lesson 18.

How the Body Defends Itself Against Disease

Your body has many ways to defend itself against disease. Some body functions are designed to protect the body from disease.

Skin

Unbroken skin prevents pathogens from entering the body. The outer layer of skin, the dead cells, is removed when you bathe. Bathing rids the body of the pathogens that were on the outer layer of the skin.

Mucous Membranes

Mucous membranes are the tissues that line the body openings and secrete mucus. **Mucus** is a thick secretion that coats the mucous membranes. Mucus from the nose and throat collects in the throat and combines with saliva from the mouth. Pathogens are trapped and destroyed.

Tears, Saliva, and Perspiration

Tears, saliva, and perspiration contain chemicals that kill pathogens.

Stomach Acids

When a person puts fingers or hands in the mouth, pathogens might enter. Some of the pathogens are destroyed by saliva. But, most pathogens are swallowed and killed by stomach acids.

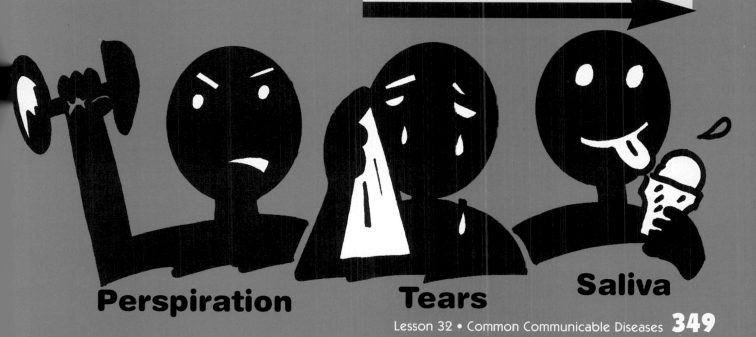

Perspiration   **Tears**   **Saliva**

Fever

A **fever** is an increase in the body temperature from 98.6°F. An increase of one or two degrees in body temperature changes the environment in the body. Many pathogens cannot live at a higher body temperature. Therefore, fever may be helpful in fighting certain infections.

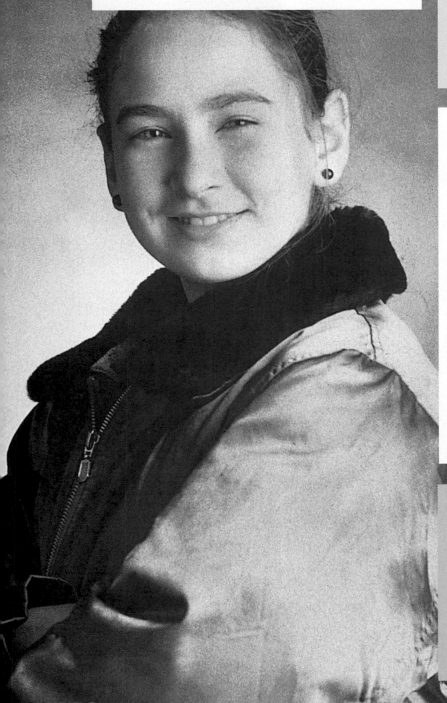

Immune System Response

The **immune system** is the body system that contains cells and organs that fight disease. **T cells** are white blood cells that regulate the action of the immune system. **Phagocytes** are white blood cells that surround and kill pathogens by ingesting them. **B cells** are cells that produce antibodies. An **antibody** is a protein that helps fight infection.

Active Immunity

Immunity (i·MYOO·nuh·tee) is a resistance to disease. **Active immunity** is a resistance to disease due to the production of antibodies. You develop active immunity from having a disease or from being given a vaccine. A **vaccine** (vak·SEEN) is dead or weakened pathogens that are introduced into the body to give a person more immunity. A vaccine is given orally or by injection. The vaccine causes the body to make antibodies for a specific pathogen. When these pathogens enter the body again, the antibodies destroy them. Examples of vaccines are those protecting people from measles, mumps, polio, and typhoid.

Passive Immunity

Passive immunity is immunity that results from introducing antibodies into the bloodstream. The antibodies might be those from another person's blood. This type of immunity is short-term. It is used when the risk of developing a disease is immediate.

Choose Behaviors to Keep the Immune System Healthy

Your immune system is your partner in fighting disease. Choose behaviors that keep your immune system healthy.

1. **Avoid alcohol, tobacco, and other drugs.** Harmful drugs lower the number of T cells and phagocytes.

2. **Practice stress management skills.** Too much stress lowers the number of T cells and phagocytes.

3. **Get plenty of rest.** Too little sleep can depress your immune system.

4. **Get plenty of vitamin C in your diet.** Foods and beverages that contain vitamin C help keep the immune system strong.

5. **Get appropriate vaccines.** Vaccines cause the immune system to produce antibodies against specific pathogens.

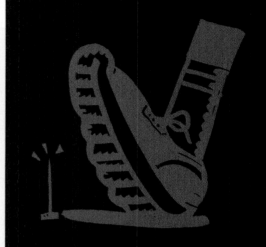

Warning: A Puncture Wound Can Be Dangerous!

Have you ever stepped on a nail? Have you cut your finger on a can of soda pop? When an object punctures the skin, pathogens that cause tetanus can enter the blood. **Tetanus,** or **lockjaw,** is a bacteria that grows in the body and produces a strong poison that affects the nervous system and muscles. It can cause death. A person with a puncture wound might be given an injection of antibodies to tetanus toxin if the person did not receive all of his or her tetanus vaccines as a child. This is an example of being protected from disease by having passive immunity. A person who has received all of his or her tetanus vaccines as a child might get a "booster." The booster is an example of active immunity.

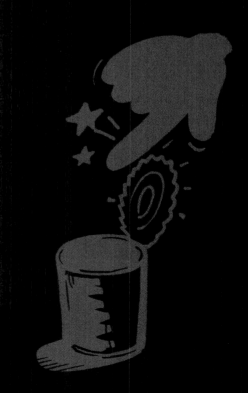

Activity

Defensive Line

Life Skill I will choose behaviors to reduce my risk of infection with communicable diseases.

Materials: Index cards, pen or pencil, football

Directions: Play Defensive Line to help you think of ways to prevent the spread of pathogens.

1. **Your teacher will assign you one way pathogens are spread and give you two index cards.**

2. **Refer to page 348 and to pages 356–357.** On one of the index cards, write a behavior that would prevent the spread of pathogens in the way you have been assigned. On the other index card, write a behavior that would spread pathogens. Suppose your teacher assigned you "Contact with contaminated objects." On one card you might write, "Do not use injecting drugs." On the other card you might write, "Share a needle to inject drugs."

3. **Your teacher will collect the cards and shuffle them.**

4. **Students on one side of the class will be one team, students on the other side the second team.** Your teacher will decide who goes first and give a student on that team a football.

5. **The student with the football draws an index card and reads it.** If the statement prevents the spread of pathogens, the student will pass the football to the next student. If the statement spreads pathogens, the student must think of an opposite behavior that would prevent the spread. Suppose the statement on the card reads, "Sneeze on the person beside you." The student might say, "Use a tissue to cover your mouth and nose when you sneeze." Then the student passes the football to the next student. If the student cannot think of a way to prevent the spread of pathogens, the football goes to the other team.

6. **Pass the football to a different student each time.** The first team on which everyone has held the football is the winner.

Common Communicable Diseases

The chart, Common Communicable Diseases, on the following pages includes facts about diseases that might infect you and others. Study this chart carefully to learn the following facts: types of communicable diseases, how they spread, symptoms, diagnosis and treatment, and prevention. You need to know the following words. A **symptom** is a change in body function or behavior from the usual pattern. The **diagnosis** is the act of finding out what is wrong by having a physical examination, studying symptoms, and having tests. An **antibiotic** (an·ti·by·AH·tik) is a substance that kills bacteria or slows the growth of bacteria.

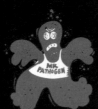

Common Communicable Diseases

Type of Disease and Cause	How It Spreads
The common cold is a respiratory infection caused by any of 200 different viruses.	Direct contact with an infected person Contact with pathogens in the air Contact with contaminated objects
Strep throat is a bacterial infection in the throat.	Direct contact with an infected person Contact with pathogens in the air Contact with contaminated objects
Pneumonia is an infection in the lungs caused by a bacteria or virus.	Direct contact with an infected person Contact with pathogens in the air Contact with contaminated objects
Influenza is a viral infection of the respiratory tract.	Direct contact with an infected person Contact with pathogens in the air Contact with contaminated objects
Mononucleosis is a viral infection that causes extreme tiredness.	Direct contact with an infected person Contact with contaminated objects
Hepatitis is a viral disease that causes serious damage to the liver. Three of the most common are Types A, B, and C hepatitis virus.	Type A—Contact with food or water contaminated with feces Type B—Direct contact with body fluids from an infected person (sharing a needle for injecting drug use; having sexual intercourse) Type C—Same as Type B
Tuberculosis (TB) is a bacterial infection that affects the lungs.	Contact with pathogens in the air

Diagnosis and Treatment

Symptoms

Runny and stuffy nose

Watery eyes

Coughing and sneezing

OTC drugs to relieve symptoms

Bed rest, fluids

Prevention

Avoid direct contact with an infected person and contact with contaminated objects.

Wash hands often.

Sore throat when swallowing

Fever

Muscle soreness

Throat culture for diagnosis

Antibiotics to prevent permanent heart damage

Bed rest, fluids

Avoid direct contact with an infected person and contact with contaminated objects.

Wash hands often.

Cough

Chest pain

Chills and fever

Difficulty breathing

Shortness of breath

Physical examination

Chest X-ray

Antibiotics for bacterial pneumonia; viral pneumonia is difficult to treat

Bed rest, fluids

Avoid direct contact with an infected person and contact with contaminated objects.

Wash hands often.

Get treatment for respiratory infections and allergies.

Runny nose, sneezing

Sore throat, headaches

Muscle aches, fatigue

Rarely nausea and vomiting

High fever

Physical examination

OTC drugs to relieve symptoms

Antibiotics for secondary infections

Bed rest, fluids

Avoid direct contact with an infected person and contact with contaminated objects.

Wash hands often.

Get flu vaccine.

Extreme tiredness

Loss of appetite, weight loss

Sore throat

Fever

Blood test to confirm diagnosis

OTC drugs to relieve symptoms

Antibiotics

Bed rest, fluids

Avoid direct contact with an infected person and contact with contaminated objects.

Wash hands often.

Often no symptoms

Nausea and vomiting

Dark-colored urine

Abdominal pain

Jaundice

Blood test to confirm diagnosis

Injections of antibodies

Bed rest, fluids

Type A—Wash hands frequently.

Type B—Get vaccine.

Type C—Avoid injecting drugs.

Antibiotics are given to those who are infected.

Extreme tiredness

Coughing

Night sweats

Weight loss

Chest X-ray for diagnosis

Long term use of antibiotics

Bed rest, fluids

Avoid direct contact with an infected person.

Have a chest X-ray.

Reducing the Risk of Communicable Diseases

The following behaviors help you and others reduce the risk of being infected with communicable diseases:

- Avoid being with people who are ill.
- Stay home from school when you are ill with a communicable disease.
- Practice abstinence.
- Do not touch ulcers or sores on another person's body.
- Follow universal precautions when exposed to body fluids from another person (see Lesson 34).
- Cover the mouth and nose with a tissue when coughing or sneezing.
- Do not share personal items, such as towels, toothbrushes, and eating utensils.
- Do not use injecting drugs. (This will keep you from sharing an infected needle.)
- Do not share a needle for ear or body piercing. Have permission from parents or guardian before piercing ears or body parts.

- Check with your physician if you are bitten by an animal.
- Keep animals and insects away from foods.
- Wash your hands with soap and water after using the restroom.
- Wash your hands with soap and water before eating.
- Keep fingers and hands away from the nose, eyes, and mouth.
- Drink tap water, bottled water, or water that has been purified.
- Follow precautions to prevent foodborne illnesses (see Lesson 18).
- Get appropriate vaccines.
- Bathe or shower each day.
- Choose behaviors that keep the immune system healthy.

Lesson 32

Review

Vocabulary

Write a separate sentence using each of the vocabulary words listed on page 346.

Health Content

Write responses to the following:

1. What is the difference between a communicable and a noncommunicable disease? **page 346**

2. What is an example of a communicable disease? **page 346**

3. What is an example of a noncommunicable disease? **page 346**

4. What are five different kinds of pathogens and an example of a disease caused by each? **page 347**

5. What are five ways pathogens can be spread? **page 348**

6. What are eight ways the body defends itself against disease? **pages 349–350**

7. What are five behaviors that keep the immune system healthy? **page 351**

8. Why might a tetanus shot be given? **page 351**

9. Identify the causes, symptoms, diagnosis and treatment, and prevention for the following communicable diseases: common cold, strep throat, pneumonia, influenza, mononucleosis, hepatitis, and tuberculosis. **pages 354–355**

10. What are 19 behaviors that reduce the risk of being infected with communicable diseases? **pages 356–357**

Sexually Transmitted Diseases

Vocabulary

sexually transmitted disease (STD)

chlamydial infection

sterile

gonorrhea

nongonococcal urethritis (NGU)

pelvic inflammatory disease (PID)

syphilis

spirochete

chancre

congenital syphilis

genital herpes

genital warts

candidiasis

trichomoniasis

pubic lice

Life Skill

• **I will choose behaviors to reduce my risk of infection with sexually transmitted diseases.**

A **sexually transmitted disease (STD)** is a disease caused by pathogens that are transmitted from an infected person to an uninfected person during intimate sexual contact. STDs can be serious and life threatening. For some STDs, there is no cure. Once infected with these STDs, a person will always be infected. Fortunately, STDs can be prevented. *You can decide to choose abstinence and then stick to your decision.*

The Lesson Objectives

• Discuss the cause, symptoms, and treatment for these STDs: chlamydial infection, gonorrhea, nongonococcal urethritis, syphilis, genital herpes, genital warts, candidiasis, trichomoniasis, pubic lice.

• List ten reasons to avoid infection with STDs.

Chlamydia

Chlamydial (kluh·MI·dee·uhl) **infection** is an STD caused by a bacterium that produces inflammation of the reproductive organs. The reproductive organs also are discussed in Lesson 12. In the male, there is an inflammation of the epididymis and urethra. A clear, thin mucus discharge is present, often in the morning. There might be a burning feeling during urination.

In the female, there is inflammation of the vagina and cervix. There might be an unusual discharge from the vagina. Many infected females do not experience signs and symptoms. Yet, they are infected.

Chlamydia can be detected by a physician. A cotton swab is used to collect the discharge. The discharge is examined at a lab. Antibiotics are used to treat this STD. Treatment usually lasts from two to three weeks. If left untreated, *Chlamydia* can cause sterility. To be **sterile** means that a person is unable to produce children.

Chlamydia is spread by having intimate sexual contact with an infected person. A baby born to an infected female can become infected during childbirth if the pathogen enters the eyes or lungs. If not treated, the baby can become blind or develop pneumonia.

Gonorrhea

Gonorrhea (gah·nuh·REE·uh) is an STD caused by bacteria that produce a discharge from the urethra and/or vagina. Signs in males include a white, milky discharge from the urethra two to nine days after infection. Females might have a discharge from the vagina. Both males and females might experience a burning sensation during urination. Sometimes, females have no signs of infection.

Diagnosis of gonorrhea in males is made by examining the discharge under a microscope. In females, cultures are taken from the vagina and grown in the lab. Antibiotics are used to treat gonorrhea. Some strains of gonorrhea are resistant to antibiotics, making treatment difficult. If left untreated, gonorrhea can cause sterility in both males and females.

Gonorrhea is spread by having intimate sexual contact with an infected person. A baby born to an infected female can become infected during childbirth if the pathogen enters the eyes. If not treated, the baby can become blind.

Nongonococcal Urethritis

Nongonococcal (nahn·gahn·uh·KAH·kuhl) **urethritis (NGU)** is an STD that produces an infection and inflammation of the urethra. Many cases of NGU are caused by bacteria. The cause of some cases is unknown. Today, NGU is more common than gonorrhea.

Symptoms of NGU in males are similar to those of *Chlamydia.* There is painful and frequent urination with a discharge. These symptoms may disappear for a while without treatment. However, the pathogens are still in the body and a male can infect others although he has no symptoms.

Many females have no symptoms. When symptoms occur, they are usually mild. There is itching and burning during urination. If left untreated, a female can develop PID. **Pelvic inflammatory disease (PID)** is an infection of the internal female reproductive organs.

Diagnosis of NGU is through a culture of the discharge. A lab test is needed so that correct treatment is prescribed. Treatment is with antibiotics if the NGU is caused by bacteria.

NGU is spread by having intimate sexual contact with an infected person. This STD also can be spread from a mother to her baby during vaginal delivery.

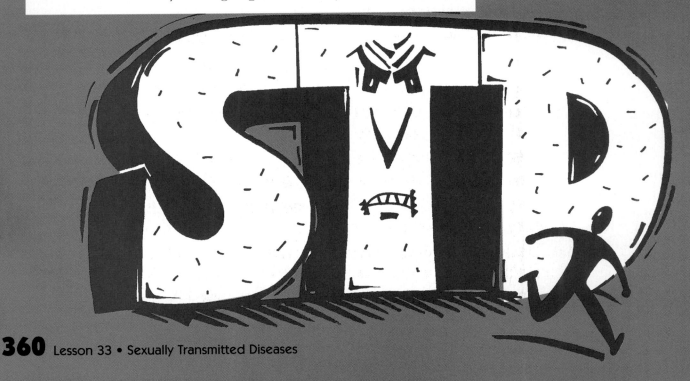

Syphilis

Syphilis (SI·fuh·lis) is an STD caused by spirochetes that produce a chancre, skin rash, and damage to body organs. A **spirochete** (SPY·roh·keet) is a spiral-shaped bacterium. Untreated syphilis passes through several stages. In the first stage of syphilis, a chancre appears. A **chancre** (SHAN·ker) is a hard, round, painless sore. It usually appears several weeks after infection at the place where the spirochetes entered the body. This might be on the genitals or in the mouth. The chancre might heal on its own in three to six weeks. However, if syphilis is untreated, the pathogens remain in the body. A person can then infect others.

From a month to a year later, the secondary stage of syphilis appears. The person continues to be contagious in this stage. A rash of small, round patches covers the whole body. The rash might or might not itch. There also might be fever, headache, and loss of weight and hair. Again, these symptoms will disappear without treatment after a few weeks. Syphilis then progresses to a latent or hidden stage. Symptoms might appear and disappear several times. The spirochete affects tissues and organs.

If left untreated, syphilis goes into the final stage. In the final stage, the spirochetes damage body organs. The heart and nervous system are damaged. Blindness, paralysis, liver damage, and mental problems might occur. People often seek medical help when these symptoms appear. However, damage to body organs cannot be reversed.

A blood test will detect the presence of syphilis in any stage. Once detected, syphilis can be treated with antibiotics.

Syphilis is spread by having intimate sexual contact with an infected person. It can be spread by having a blood transfusion. The spirochete can also be transmitted from a pregnant female to her fetus. **Congenital** (kuhn·JEN·uh·tuhl) **syphilis** is syphilis that is transmitted to a fetus from an infected pregnant female. It causes mental retardation and other birth defects.

I will choose behaviors to reduce my risk of infection with sexually transmitted diseases.

Genital Herpes

Genital herpes is an STD caused by a virus that produces cold sores or fever blisters in the genital area and/or mouth. Symptoms of genital herpes occur within a week after contact with an infected person. Clusters of small, painful blisters appear in the genital area. After a few days, the blisters break and form red, painful, open sores. A person is highly contagious at this time. Other symptoms include tiredness, fever, headache, and pain and swelling in the lymph nodes. There might be burning during urination. The symptoms can last from two to four weeks and then disappear. In some people, these symptoms reappear during times of stress or illness. In other people, the symptoms never recur.

Diagnosis of genital herpes is made by special lab tests. There is no known cure for genital herpes. However, there is a drug that helps relieve symptoms on a short-term basis.

The consequences of being infected with genital herpes are serious. An infected person must always be cautious because this STD can be transmitted when there are no symptoms. Males and females who are infected are at increased risk for being infected with HIV. HIV is the virus that causes AIDS. HIV can enter the body through the broken blisters.

Genital herpes is spread by having intimate sexual contact with an infected person. A person who is infected can spread the blisters to other areas of the body through touch. A person might have lesions in the mouth and place the fingers in the mouth and then touch the genitals. The virus is spread from the mouth to the genitals. If the person puts fingers in the eyes, the virus can get into the eyes. People infected with herpes must keep their hands very clean. An infected pregnant female can infect her baby during vaginal delivery. An infected baby can develop a brain infection that causes brain damage.

Genital Warts

Genital warts are dry, wartlike growths that are caused by a virus. The warts are often soft, red or pink, and resemble a small cauliflower. Sometimes the warts are hard and yellow-gray. Genital warts are spread by having intimate sexual contact with an infected person.

Genital warts appear three to eight months after infection. They should be treated promptly. A physician inspects the warts to make a diagnosis. The Centers for Disease Control and Prevention reports that there is no treatment to completely get rid of genital warts. Medication is available that can be placed on warts. Laser surgery is a means of removing warts by burning them away. Warts may be frozen and removed by using liquid nitrogen. None of these treatments will completely get rid of warts because the virus remains in the body. Genital warts may recur. Studies have linked them to the development of cervical cancer.

Candidiasis

Candidiasis (kan·duh·DY·uh·suhs) is an STD caused by fungi that produce itching and burning. In females, there is a white, foul-smelling discharge and itching. In males, there might be itching and burning during urination. A physician makes a diagnosis based on observation and a lab test. Special creams, tablets, and suppositories are used for treatment. Candidiasis is spread by having intimate sexual contact with an infected person.

Trichomoniasis

Trichomoniasis (trik·oh·moh·NY·uh·sis) is an STD caused by protozoa that infect the vagina, urethra, or prostate. This STD affects about 10 to 15 percent of people who are sexually active. About half of all infected females have no symptoms. When symptoms appear, there is a greenish-yellow vaginal discharge that has an odor. There might be itching, pain, or burning during urination. Most males have no symptoms. If a male does have symptoms, there is pain and burning during urination.

A smear of the discharge is examined under a microscope to make a diagnosis. A special prescription drug is given for treatment.

Trichomoniasis is spread by having intimate sexual contact with an infected person. Much less commonly, it can be transmitted nonsexually by sharing contaminated towels.

Pubic Lice

Pubic lice is an infestation with pubic, or crab, lice. Lice are insects that are yellowish-gray in color and about the size of a pinhead. The lice attach themselves to pubic hairs and burrow into the skin where they feed on blood. Little black spots, which are lice, might be visible on body parts that have dense hair growth. In addition, a person will feel intense itching where the lice are attached.

A physician examines the body to find the lice. A prescription drug is used as a lotion to kill lice. Over-the-counter preparations also are used.

Pubic lice are spread from one person to another usually through intimate sexual contact. Lice can live outside the body for as long as a day. It is possible for a person to become infested by sleeping on infested sheets or wearing infested clothing.

Ten Reasons to Avoid Infection with STDs

Because I like myself and believe myself to be of value:

1. I want to live a long, productive, and healthful life.

2. I want to keep my body healthy.

3. I want my reproductive organs to function as they should.

4. I want to keep my body free of recurring symptoms of STDs.

5. I want to maintain self-respect.

6. I want to avoid unnecessary medical expenses.

7. I want to be able to tell a future marriage partner that I have never been infected with an STD.

8. I want to have a healthful marriage without recurring symptoms of an STD.

9. I want to remain fertile so that I have the option of being a parent.

10. I do not want to infect my offspring with an STD.

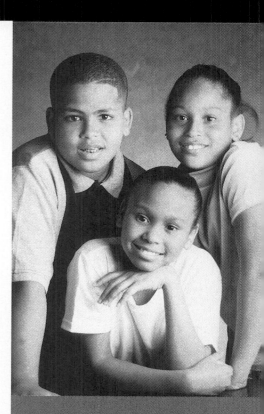

Grapevine Fact or Fiction

Activity

 Life Skill I will choose behaviors to reduce my risk of infection with sexually transmitted diseases.

Materials: Green construction paper, twist ties or yarn, scissors, hole puncher, markers, plastic or silk garland attached to classroom wall

Directions: Information spread "through the grapevine" is usually rumor or gossip. In this activity, you will determine whether the information you get from the grapevine is true or false.

1. **Draw and cut out two leaves from construction paper.**

2. **Choose any statement about an STD from this lesson.** Write the statement on one of the leaves. For example, you might write, "Most males with trichomoniasis have no symptoms." On the other leaf, create and write a statement about STDs that is not true. It does not have to be about the same STD you chose for the first leaf. You might write, "A person with pubic lice has no symptoms."

3. **Punch a hole in one end of each leaf.** Attach the leaf to the garland with a twist tie or yarn.

4. **Have everyone in the class remove two leaves from the garland.** The leaves cannot be the ones they wrote.

5. **Use your book to determine whether the statement is true.** If the statement is false, decide how the statement could be changed to make it true. For example, suppose you got the statement, "Antibiotics will cure genital herpes." You could change the statement to "There is no cure for genital herpes" or "Antibiotics do not work against viruses."

6. **Take turns sharing the statements on your leaves.** Tell the class why your statement is true or false. If it is false, tell them how you changed it.

Apply...

The Responsible Decision-Making Model™

A friend has become sexually active. (S)he tells you, "I'm not worried about getting an STD. I know my (girl)boyfriend will not have sex with anyone but me."

Answer the following questions on a separate sheet of paper. Write "Does not apply" if a question does not apply to this situation.

1. Is it healthful for your friend to be sexually active? Why or why not?

2. Is it safe for your friend to be sexually active? Why or why not?

3. Is it legal for your friend to be sexually active? Why or why not?

4. Does your friend show respect for herself or himself by being sexually active? Why or why not?

5. Would your friend's parents or guardian approve of your friend being sexually active? Why or why not?

6. Does your friend demonstrate good character by being sexually active? Why or why not?

What is the responsible decision for your friend to make?

What should you tell your friend?

Lesson 33

Review

Vocabulary

Write a separate sentence using each of the vocabulary words listed on page 358.

Health Content

Write responses to the following:

What are the causes, symptoms, and treatments for

1. chlamydial infection? **page 359**
2. gonorrhea? **page 359**
3. nongonococcal urethritis? **page 360**
4. syphilis? **page 361**
5. genital herpes? **page 362**
6. genital warts? **page 363**
7. candidiasis? **page 363**
8. trichomoniasis? **page 364**
9. pubic lice? **page 364**
10. What are ten reasons to avoid infection with STDs? **page 365**

HIV Infection and AIDS

Vocabulary

human immunodeficiency virus (HIV)

Acquired Immune Deficiency Syndrome (AIDS)

opportunistic infection

ELISA

Western blot

thrush

oral hairy leukoplakia

pneumocystis carinii pneumonia (PCP)

Kaposi's sarcoma (KS)

AIDS dementia complex

AZT

DDI

compassion

abstinence

Life Skill

• **I will choose behaviors to reduce my risk of HIV infection.**

You already know some facts about AIDS. The disease known as AIDS is being discussed on the radio and television, and in newspapers and magazines. You should learn all you can about AIDS. AIDS is a dangerous and fatal disease. AIDS is caused by a virus. Protecting yourself from infection with the virus that causes AIDS is your responsibility.

The Lesson Objectives

• Explain how HIV destroys the immune system.

• Describe seven risk behaviors for HIV infection.

• Discuss tests, signs, and treatment for HIV infection and AIDS.

• State ways to express compassion for people living with HIV and AIDS.

• Outline six responsible behaviors that prevent infection with HIV and AIDS.

HIV and the Immune System

The **human immunodeficiency** (IM·yoo·noh·di·FI·shuhn·see) **virus (HIV)** is a pathogen that destroys infection-fighting T cells in the body. HIV causes AIDS. **Acquired Immune Deficiency Syndrome (AIDS)** is a condition that results when infection with HIV causes a breakdown of the body's ability to fight other infections. Being infected with HIV and having AIDS are two different conditions.

A person is infected with HIV as soon as the virus enters the blood. When HIV enters the blood, the virus attaches to helper T cells. HIV reproduces its genetic material in these cells. HIV can then take control of the cell, produce new viral parts, and infect other cells. HIV attacks, multiplies in, and finally destroys the invaded helper T cells. The number of helper T cells is lowered. The immune system is less able to fight pathogens, and infections develop.

A person is said to have AIDS when opportunistic infections and noncommunicable diseases are present and other symptoms develop. An **opportunistic infection** is an infection that develops in a person with a weak immune system. Opportunistic infections are difficult to treat and can cause death in people who have AIDS.

I will choose behaviors to reduce my risk of HIV infection.

I will choose behaviors to reduce my risk of HIV infection.

I will choose behaviors to reduce my risk of HIV infection.

How HIV Is Spread

People who are infected with HIV have HIV in their body fluids. HIV is spread from infected people to others by contact with certain body fluids. These body fluids are:

- Blood
- Semen
- Vaginal secretions
- Breast milk (a few cases)
- Other body fluids that might contain blood (such as wound secretions)

Traces of HIV have been found in saliva, sweat, and tears; however, to date, there have been no documented cases of HIV transmission through saliva, sweat, or tears.

HIV is transmitted when a person engages in specific risk behaviors.

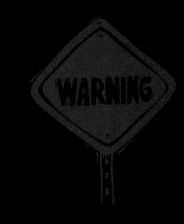

Warning:

Any person, regardless of gender, age, race, or sexual orientation, can become infected with HIV by engaging in specific risk behaviors.

Risk Behaviors

Having sexual contact with an infected person During sexual contact, HIV from an infected person might enter the blood of an uninfected person through exposed blood vessels in small cuts or tiny cracks in mucous membranes.

Sharing needles or syringes to inject drugs A person infected with HIV who uses a needle to inject drugs might leave a small amount of his or her blood containing HIV on or in the needle. If the needle is used by another person, this second person can become infected with HIV. The infected blood from the needle can get into his or her blood.

Sharing needles for tattooing, ear-piercing, or piercing other body parts A person infected with HIV who uses a needle for tattooing, ear-piercing, or piercing other body parts might leave a small amount of his or her blood containing HIV on or in the needle. If the needle is used by another person, this second person can become infected. The infected blood from the needle can get into his or her blood.

Having contact with the blood or other body fluids, mucous membranes, or broken skin of an infected person If a person handles the body fluids of an infected person, HIV might enter the body through small cuts or tears on the skin or through splash into the eyes. If a person touches the mucous membranes or broken skin of an infected person, there might be contact with exposed blood vessels. HIV-infected blood can enter the person's body through small cuts and tears on the skin.

Having a blood transfusion with infected blood or blood products Currently in the United States, because of blood screening, there is little chance of infection with HIV through a blood transfusion. A person cannot become infected with HIV from giving blood at a blood bank. Only sterile needles are used. They are destroyed after one use.

Having an organ transplant Transmission of HIV has occurred through organ transplants in the past. However, new testing procedures have made this form of transmission highly unlikely.

Being born to a female infected with HIV A female infected with HIV can spread the virus to her baby during pregnancy, while giving birth, or when breast-feeding. If a female is infected before or during pregnancy, her child has about one chance in three of being born with HIV infection.

Once HIV enters a person's blood, the person is infected with HIV. Health officials believe that once infected with HIV, a person will always be infected.

Warning:

WARNING

A person can become infected with HIV from having sex with an infected person, even though it is only one time.

A person can become infected with HIV by injecting anabolic steroids with a contaminated needle used by an infected person.

You cannot tell if a person is infected with HIV by the way the person looks. Someone who is infected with HIV might look and feel healthy. This person might or might not have symptoms. But, (s)he can still spread the virus to others.

You can become infected with HIV by having contact with blood. Suppose someone you know has a nosebleed or is cut while playing sports. There is no way to know for certain if this person is infected with HIV. If you help the person, wear latex gloves. Latex gloves reduce the risk that you will get blood through small cuts and scratches on your hands. Dispose of the used gloves in a trash container. Wash your hands with soap and water.

How HIV Is Not Spread

There are many myths about how HIV is spread. Knowing how HIV is not spread keeps people informed. The Centers for Disease Control and Prevention states that, to date, HIV is not spread in the following ways:

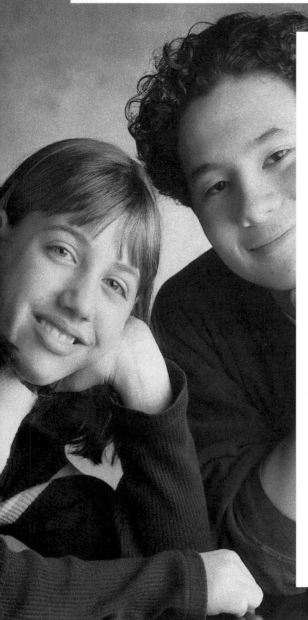

- **hugging;**
- **closed mouth kissing;**
- **touching, holding, or shaking hands;**
- **coughing or sneezing;**
- **sharing food or eating utensils;**
- **sharing towels or combs;**
- **having casual contact with friends;**
- **sharing bathroom facilities or water fountains;**
- **sharing a pen or pencil;**
- **being bitten by insects;**
- **donating blood;**
- **eating food prepared or served by someone else;**
- **attending school;**
- **using a telephone or computer used by someone else;**
- **swimming in a pool;**
- **using sports and gym equipment.**

Testing for HIV Infection

Any person who has chosen a risk behavior for HIV should be tested for HIV infection. A person should not wait for signs and symptoms. The only way for a person to know if (s)he is infected with HIV is to be tested. The tests available to detect HIV are among the most accurate medical tests known.

When a person becomes infected with HIV, the body makes antibodies. These HIV antibodies usually show up in the blood within three months after infection. Almost all people who are infected with HIV will show antibodies within six months. **ELISA** is a blood test used to check for antibodies for HIV. **Western blot** is a blood test used to check for the presence and size of antibodies for HIV. When used together, these tests are correct more than 99.9 percent of the time.

A negative HIV test means that no antibodies were found and that a person is probably not infected with HIV. This means either the person is not infected with HIV or the antibody level was not high enough yet to be detected by the ELISA test. (A Western blot test is normally used only to confirm a positive ELISA.) If a person engaged in a risk behavior, the person must be retested in a few months.

HIV Status

A person is HIV positive when antibodies for HIV are detected during a blood test. A person is HIV negative when antibodies for HIV have not been detected during a blood test. A person can be infected with HIV and test HIV negative. This is because the antibody level was not yet high enough to be tested.

I will choose behaviors to reduce my risk of HIV infection.

I will choose behaviors to reduce my risk of HIV infection.

Signs of HIV Infection and AIDS

Once a person is infected with HIV, this person will always be infected. Some people do not know they are infected with HIV because signs and symptoms do not appear right away. These people appear healthy, but they can infect others.

The signs of HIV infection might appear right away or take 12 years or more to occur. These signs usually include tiredness, fever, swollen glands, rash, headaches, and flu-like symptoms. They come and go, depending on the helper T cell count. During times when there are no symptoms, HIV continues to destroy the immune system.

The helper T cell count continues to drop. Many infections develop. Two of these infections are thrush and oral hairy leukoplakia. **Thrush** is a fungal infection of the mucous membranes of the tongue and mouth. White spots and ulcers cover the infection. **Oral hairy leukoplakia** (loo·koh·PLAK·ee·uh) is an infection in which fuzzy white patches are found on the tongue.

When opportunistic infections develop, a person is diagnosed as having AIDS. There are many opportunistic infections.

Pneumocystis (noo·muh·SIS·tus) **carinii pneumonia (PCP)** is a form of pneumonia often found in people who have AIDS. It is one of the causes of death for people who have AIDS. Symptoms of PCP include a dry cough, fever, and difficulty breathing.

Kaposi's (KA·poh·seez) **sarcoma (KS)** is a type of cancer in people who have AIDS. KS causes purplish lesions and tumors on the skin and in the linings of the internal organs. These lesions spread to most of the linings of the body.

AIDS dementia complex is a loss of brain function caused by HIV infection. There is a gradual loss of a person's ability to think and move. The person has forgetfulness, personality changes, and loss of coordination. The disorder worsens. The person feels more confused and has severe memory loss. A person might be unable to do usual tasks.

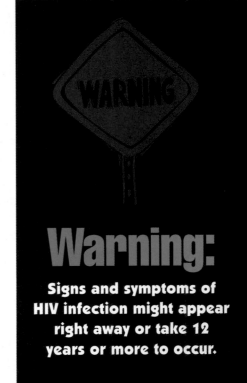

Warning:

Signs and symptoms of HIV infection might appear right away or take 12 years or more to occur.

Treatment for HIV and AIDS

There is no cure for HIV infection or AIDS. Treatment focuses on making the immune system strong. **AZT** is a drug that slows the multiplication of HIV. **DDI** is another drug that slows the multiplication of HIV. These drugs need to be given as soon as possible after a person tests HIV positive. By slowing the multiplication of HIV, a person will stay healthier longer.

Protease inhibitors are antiviral drugs that decrease the amount of HIV in the blood and increase the helper T cell count. Protease inhibitors are newer and more effective against HIV than some other drugs. Some people who have used them have had the amount of HIV in the blood drop to a level where it cannot be detected. Researchers believe they still have HIV in their bodies. If they stop taking this drug, HIV will multiply again. Research is being conducted to find out where HIV hides in the body when the level drops. Researchers also are studying why these drugs do not work the same in all people.

There are other ways to help the immune system. Some people who are infected with HIV get transfusions of healthy white blood cells. Some have bone marrow transplants. People who are infected with HIV can choose habits that protect the immune system. They should not smoke or use tobacco products. They should avoid alcohol and other drugs. These habits depress the immune system. People who are infected with HIV need to have a healthful diet. They need to get the nutrients needed for optimal health.

Researchers are currently working on a number of vaccines and drugs to prevent and cure HIV and AIDS. People infected with HIV who practice healthful habits and who get early treatment will delay the development of AIDS. This might give them more time to live.

Compassion for People Living with HIV and AIDS

Compassion is showing concern and a desire to be helpful. You can have compassion for people living with HIV and AIDS. They have the same needs as others do. They need friendship and support. They want to live their lives in the most productive ways possible. They need encouragement. Remember, you cannot become infected by being a friend.

Preventing HIV Infection and AIDS

HIV infection can be prevented. You can avoid risk behaviors. There are responsible behaviors you and others can choose.

Practice abstinence.

Abstinence is choosing not to be sexually active. Practicing abstinence until marriage is a way to prevent the spread of HIV. Both partners must enter the marriage uninfected and have sex only with each other. By practicing abstinence, you avoid HIV infection, unwanted pregnancy, and infection with other STDs. You follow parents' guidelines. You promote your health and that of your friends.

Change your behavior if you have been sexually active.

If you have been sexually active, you can stop. Choose abstinence beginning today. Talk to a trusted adult about being tested for HIV. If you are not infected and you stop being sexually active, HIV infection will not occur.

Choose not to use drugs.

Drugs change the way you think and act. If you use drugs, you make a wrong decision. You might not stick to responsible decisions. For example, you might choose to become sexually active or use injecting drugs.

Sharing a needle to inject drugs is risky. Sharing a needle to inject anabolic steroids is risky. Protect your health and safety by avoiding illegal drug use. Choose friends who do not use drugs.

Seek treatment if you are addicted to harmful drugs.

If you are dependent upon drugs, you have a serious problem. To protect your health and the decisions you make, you must get treatment. Talk to a trusted adult, such as your parents or guardian. They can help you get the help you need.

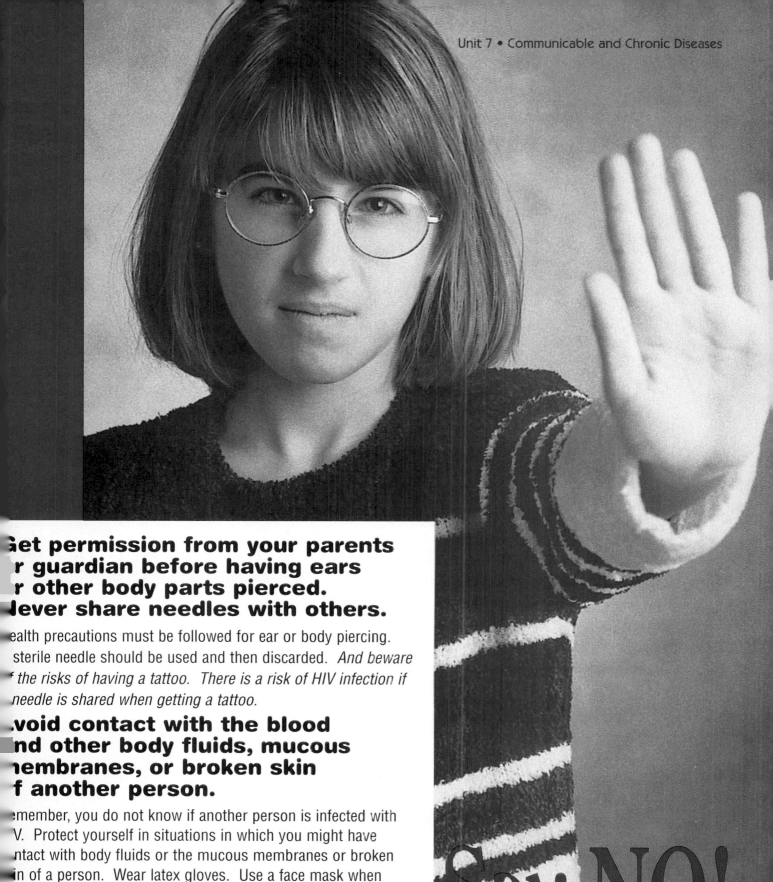

Get permission from your parents or guardian before having ears or other body parts pierced. Never share needles with others.

Health precautions must be followed for ear or body piercing. A sterile needle should be used and then discarded. *And beware of the risks of having a tattoo. There is a risk of HIV infection if a needle is shared when getting a tattoo.*

Avoid contact with the blood and other body fluids, mucous membranes, or broken skin of another person.

Remember, you do not know if another person is infected with HIV. Protect yourself in situations in which you might have contact with body fluids or the mucous membranes or broken skin of a person. Wear latex gloves. Use a face mask when giving first aid for breathing. Do not share toothbrushes, tweezers, nail cutters, razors, dental floss, or other personal items that might have blood on them.

Say NO!

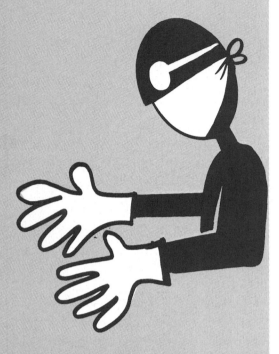

Protection for Health Care Workers

Health care workers are at special risk for having contact with the blood and other body fluids, mucous membranes, and broken skin of others. Health care workers should do the following:

- **Wear latex gloves when handling blood and certain body fluids.**
- **Wear masks and protective eyewear when splash is possible.**
- **Wear a gown or apron when splash on clothing is possible.**
- **Wash immediately if contaminated with blood or body fluids.**
- **Dispose of used syringes and needles immediately and properly.**
- **Use face masks or resuscitation bags when needed.**

Apply...

The Responsible Decision-Making Model™

A friend invites you and some other friends to his house. His older brother has AIDS. One of the friends who was invited says, "I'm not going. His brother's a freak and I don't want to catch HIV." This friend tries to persuade everyone who was invited not to go.

Answer the following questions on a separate sheet of paper. Write "Does not apply" if a question does not apply to this situation.

1. Is it healthful for you to turn down your friend because his brother has AIDS? Why or why not?

2. Is it safe for you to turn down your friend because his brother has AIDS? Why or why not?

3. Is it legal for you to turn down your friend because his brother has AIDS? Why or why not?

4. Will you show respect for yourself and others if you turn down your friend because his brother has AIDS? Why or why not?

5. Will your parents or guardian approve if you turn down your friend because his brother has AIDS? Why or why not?

6. Will you demonstrate good character if you turn down your friend because his brother has AIDS? Why or why not?

What is the responsible decision to make in this situation?

Know the Facts About HIV

Many people believe they cannot become infected with HIV. They might think that HIV infects only certain groups of people. They might think teens cannot become infected. They might think having sex or injecting drugs just one time cannot result in infection; however,

- **You know you can become infected with HIV if you choose a risk behavior known to cause HIV infection.**

- **You know that HIV can infect all groups of people.**

- **You know that teens can become infected. More than one-fourth of people with AIDS were infected as teens.**

- **You know that having sex or taking drugs, even just one time, can result in HIV infection.**

Avoiding infection with HIV and AIDS is up to you. Assume responsibility for your life as you make decisions regarding your health and relationships. Realize that the decisions you make now have an impact on your future. Continue to learn the latest facts about HIV and AIDS.

Lesson 34

Review

Vocabulary

Write a separate sentence using each of the vocabulary words listed on page 368.

Health Content

Write responses to the following:

1. How does HIV destroy the immune system? **page 369**

2. What body fluids can spread HIV? **page 370**

3. What are seven risk behaviors for HIV infection? **pages 370–371**

4. What are 16 ways HIV is not known to be spread (to date)? **page 372**

5. What are two tests for HIV infection? **page 373**

6. Why might a person who has a negative test for HIV need to be retested? **page 373**

7. What are signs of HIV infection? What are opportunistic infections in a person with HIV? **page 374**

8. What is treatment for HIV and AIDS? **page 375**

9. What are ways to express compassion for people living with HIV and AIDS? **page 375**

10. What are six responsible behaviors that prevent infection with HIV and AIDS? **pages 376–377**

Cardiovascular Diseases

Vocabulary

cardiovascular diseases

arrhythmia

heart attack

arteriosclerosis

atherosclerosis

stroke

hypertension

angina pectoris

risk factors

premature heart attack

stress management skills

antioxidants

essential hypertension

secondary hypertension

electrocardiogram (EKG)

diabetes

personal health record

beta-blockers

bypass surgery

Life Skills

- **I will choose behaviors to reduce my risk of cardiovascular diseases.**
- **I will keep a personal health record.**

  Cardiovascular (KAR·dee·oh·VAS·kyoo·ler) **diseases** are diseases of the heart and blood vessels. They are referred to as "lifestyle diseases." The lifestyle you choose and the habits you develop can prevent or delay the development of cardiovascular diseases. This lesson will help you make a plan to keep your heart and blood vessels in good condition.

The Lesson Objectives

- Identify seven types of cardiovascular diseases.
- List risk factors for cardiovascular diseases.
- Describe ways to prevent cardiovascular diseases.
- Identify tips for starting and keeping a personal health record.
- Discuss treatments for cardiovascular diseases.

Types of Cardiovascular Diseases

There are many different types of cardiovascular diseases.

Arrhythmia (ay·RITH·mee·uh) is a heart condition in which the heartbeat is abnormal and irregular. The heart may beat very slowly or very fast for no apparent reason.

Stroke is a condition caused by a blocked or broken blood vessel in the brain. A stroke can result in paralysis or death.

Heart attack is the death of part of the heart muscle caused by a lack of blood flow to the heart. A heart attack can result in disability or death.

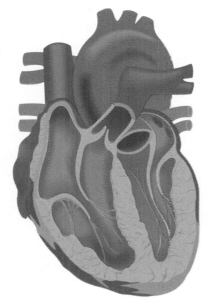

Hypertension is a condition in which the pressure exerted by the blood on the artery walls when the heart beats is above normal for a long period of time; also called high blood pressure.

Arteriosclerosis (ahr·tee·ree·oh·skluh·ROH·sis) is a general term used to describe several conditions that cause hardening and thickening of the arteries.

Angina pectoris (an·JY·nuh PEK·tuhr·is) is a chest pain that results from narrowed blood vessels in the heart. If the blockage is severe enough, heart attack can occur.

Atherosclerosis (A·thuh·ROH·skluh·ROH·sis) is a disease in which fat deposits on artery walls.

Preventing Cardiovascular Diseases

Risk factors are ways that a person might behave and characteristics of the environment in which a person lives that threaten health, safety, and well-being. There are specific risk factors for cardiovascular diseases. You cannot control some of these risk factors, such as your blood relatives, race, age, and sex. Other risk factors, such as smoking, being overweight, being stressed, having a high fat diet, being out of condition, and failing to get medical checkups, can be controlled.

Obtain information about your family history.

Knowing about your blood relatives is important. If your blood relatives are African American, you have a 45 percent greater risk of having high blood pressure. If a parent, brother, or sister had a premature heart attack, you are more at risk. A **premature heart attack** is one that occurs before age 55 in males and before age 65 in females.

Recognize how age and sex increase risk.

Your risk of developing heart disease increases with age. About 80 percent of people who develop heart disease do so after age 65. Males have a higher risk of developing cardiovascular diseases than do females until the age of 40. But once a female reaches the age of 65, heart disease becomes the number one cause of death.

Choose to be tobacco-free.

As early as 1964, the U.S. Surgeon General stated that cigarette smoking was the greatest risk factor in the development of cardiovascular diseases. The more a person smokes, the greater the risk for developing a heart attack or a stroke. In fact, the risk is 70 percent higher for a smoker than for a nonsmoker. Tobacco products contain nicotine. Nicotine causes the heart to pump more often than it should. It increases resting blood pressure. The carbon monoxide in smoke takes the place of oxygen in the bloodstream. The heart is denied adequate amounts of oxygen. If you use tobacco products, refer to the tobacco cessation programs described in Lesson 28.

Practice stress management skills.

Being stressed causes the heart to pump more often than it should. It increases resting blood pressure. You become tired, but might not be able to sleep well. Your heart does not get the rest it needs. **Stress management skills** are techniques to cope with the body changes produced by stress. To protect your heart and blood vessels, practice the stress management skills described in Lesson 5.

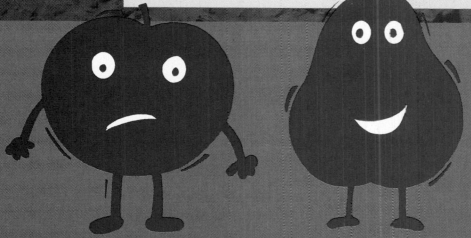

Apple or Pear?

Another important risk factor for cardiovascular disease is how weight is distributed in the body. People who carry fat around the waist in a "pot-bellied" or "apple-shaped" manner have a greater risk than those who are "pear-shaped" and carry weight on their hips.

Choose a diet low in fat, saturated fat, and cholesterol.

Diets high in saturated fat and cholesterol increase the risk of heart disease. Too much cholesterol can stick to the inner linings of blood vessel walls and form plaque. This leads to atherosclerosis. Lesson 17 presents guidelines for reducing the amount of fat, saturated fat, and cholesterol in your diet.

Include foods with antioxidants in your diet.

Antioxidants (an·tee·AHK·suh·duhnts) are substances that protect cells from being damaged by oxidation. A balanced diet containing antioxidants might lower the risk of heart disease. Vitamins C and E and beta-carotene are antioxidants. Carrots, sweet potatoes, oranges, broccoli, whole grain breads, and green leafy vegetables are good sources.

Maintain your desirable weight.

The heart must work harder to pump blood to body cells if a person is overweight. Being overweight also increases the risk for high blood cholesterol, high blood pressure, and diabetes. Tips for weight management are included in Lesson 19.

Participate in regular physical activity.

Physical activity helps you maintain desirable weight and lowers your percentage of body fat. It helps clear fat from the blood, reduces the effects of stress, and lowers blood pressure. Aerobic exercise reduces the risk of cardiovascular diseases. Even physical activity such as walking, cutting grass, and raking leaves, if done regularly and long-term, can keep the heart and blood vessels healthy. Refer to Lesson 24 and make a physical fitness plan.

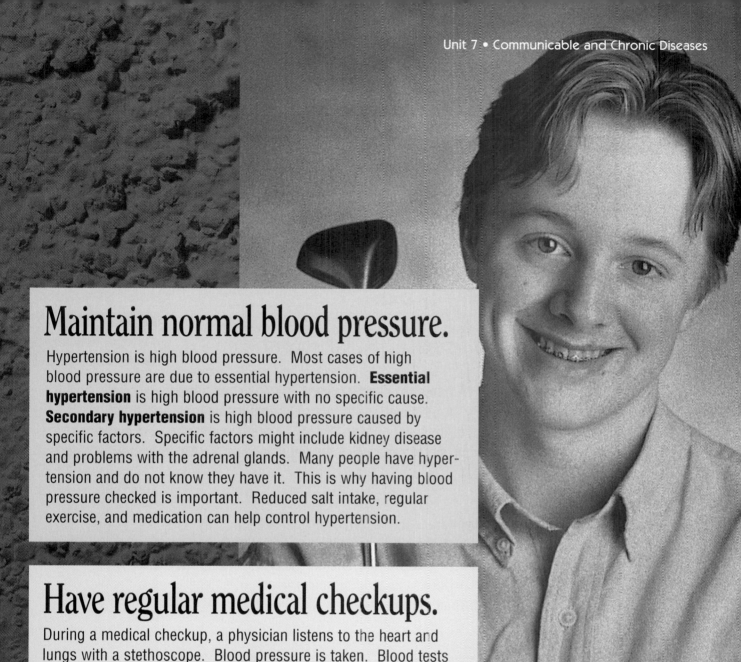

Maintain normal blood pressure.

Hypertension is high blood pressure. Most cases of high blood pressure are due to essential hypertension. **Essential hypertension** is high blood pressure with no specific cause. **Secondary hypertension** is high blood pressure caused by specific factors. Specific factors might include kidney disease and problems with the adrenal glands. Many people have hypertension and do not know they have it. This is why having blood pressure checked is important. Reduced salt intake, regular exercise, and medication can help control hypertension.

Have regular medical checkups.

During a medical checkup, a physician listens to the heart and lungs with a stethoscope. Blood pressure is taken. Blood tests and an electrocardiogram also might be taken. An **electrocardiogram (EKG)** is a measure of the electrical activity of the heart.

A physican checks for other conditions that can affect the heart and blood vessels. **Diabetes** is a disease in which the body produces little or no insulin or cannot use insulin. Insulin is a hormone that enables the body to use sugar from foods. People who have diabetes might have an increase in blood fat levels. They might suffer from damaged small blood vessels. Through medication, diet, and exercise, diabetes can be managed. There is no known cure for diabetes.

Follow a...

Health Behavior Contract

Copy the health behavior contract on a separate sheet of paper.

DO NOT WRITE IN THIS BOOK.

Name:_____ **Date:**_____

Life Skill: I will keep a personal health record.

Effect On My Health: A **personal health record** is a record of a person's health, health care, and health care providers. A personal health record should include my health habits. It should include information about my family health history. I can take my personal health record with me to my physician. My physician can review my habits and family health history and help me make a plan for my health.

My Plan: I will include information about cardiovascular health in my personal health record. I will list each of the risk factors for cardiovascular diseases that I can control. I will discuss whether or not I practice behaviors to reduce these risk factors. I will ask my parent or guardian to share information about the cardiovascular health of at least four of my blood relatives. I will record this information, too.

Tips for Starting and Keeping a Personal Health Record

- **Discuss your plan to create a personal health record with your parents or guardian.**

- **Get a folder and label it.**

- **Keep your personal health record in a place where you can find it easily.**

- **Include additional information. Record the dates of vaccinations, illnesses you have had, and medications you have taken or take now.**

How My Plan Worked: Write down the recommendations of your physician in your personal health record (after your next visit to your physician).

Treatment for Cardiovascular Diseases

People who have cardiovascular diseases can often be treated successfully.

- Drugs can lower blood pressure and control arrhythmia. **Beta-blockers** are drugs that slow the heartbeat rate and reduce the force of the heart's contractions.

- Surgery is effective in opening or bypassing blocked arteries. **Bypass surgery** is surgery to create a detour around a narrowed artery or vein so that blood can reach and leave the heart.

- Lifestyle changes can improve the condition of the heart and blood vessels.

Lesson 35

Review

Vocabulary

Write a separate sentence using each of the vocabulary words listed on page 380.

Health Content

Write responses to the following:

1. What are seven types of cardiovascular diseases? **page 381**
2. What are four risk factors for cardiovascular diseases that cannot be controlled? **page 382**
3. What are six risk factors for cardiovascular disease that can be controlled? **page 382**
4. Describe ten ways to prevent cardiovascular diseases. **pages 382–385**
5. What are three treatments for cardiovascular diseases? **page 387**

Cancer

Vocabulary

cancer

carcinomas

metastasis

tumor

sarcomas

lymphomas

leukemia

carcinogen

malignant melanoma

radon

radiation therapy

chemotherapy

immunotherapy

biological therapy

Life Skill

- **I will choose behaviors to reduce my risk of cancer.**

Cancer is a group of diseases in which cells divide in an uncontrolled manner. It is a leading cause of death. Many people are fearful of cancer. Yet many types of cancer can be prevented or successfully treated if detected early enough. This lesson will help you learn how to avoid risk factors for cancer.

The Lesson Objectives

- Explain how cancers are classified.
- Describe ways to reduce your risk of developing cancer.
- Discuss different treatments for cancer.

Types of Cancer

What are your first thoughts when you hear the word "cancer"? Some people think of the progression of the disease. They think of a specific stage of the disease. Some people think of a specific kind of cancer. They might think of breast cancer, leukemia, or liver cancer. Some people think of a family member or friend who has had cancer. When you hear the word "cancer," try to think of education and prevention. These two words are keys to reducing the incidence of cancer.

How much do you know about cancer? Did you know that the term cancer does not apply to a single disease? Cancer is any number of diseases that result in abnormal cell growth. Cancers are classified into four categories. The categories have to do with where the cancer grows.

Carcinomas (kar·si·NOH·muhs) are cancers of tissues that cover the body surfaces and linings of body organs. Growths on the skin and lungs are types of carcinomas. These types of cancers invade the body by metastasis. **Metastasis** (muh·TAS·tuh·sis) is the spreading of cancer cells to other body parts from an original source. Cancer cells often metastasize through the circulatory system. When they attach to other body parts, they can form tumors. A **tumor** is a growth of cells that form a lump. Most tumors found in the body are not cancerous. These tumors do not spread through the body or cause disease.

Sarcomas (sar·KOH·muhs) are cancers that form in middle tissues such as bones and muscles. Sarcomas metastasize through the blood.

Lymphomas (lim·FOH·muhs) are cancers that develop and metastasize in the lymph system. Hodgkin's disease is a lymphoma.

Leukemia (loo·KEE·mee·uh) is a cancer of the blood-forming parts of the body. A person with leukemia will have a higher than usual number of white blood cells.

Carcinomas

Metastasis

Sarcomas

Lymphomas

Leukemia

Preventing Cancer

Why a normal cell develops into a cancerous cell is not completely known. Many factors can be involved. Some cancers are associated with specific carcinogens. A **carcinogen** (kar·SIN·uh·juhn) is a substance that causes cancer. Cancers are associated with viruses, chemicals, radiation, and heredity.

Most cancers, however, are associated with choices over which you have control. There are things you can do to help reduce your cancer risk.

1. **Know the warning signs of cancer.** Detecting cancer in an early stage increases the chances that it can be successfully treated. The American Cancer Society recommends that people learn seven early warning signs of cancer. The beginning letter of each warning sign corresponds to a letter in the word CAUTION:

Change in bowel or bladder habits

A sore that does not heal

Unusual bleeding or discharge

Thickening or lump in a breast or elsewhere

Indigestion or difficulty in swallowing

Obvious change in a wart or mole

Nagging cough or hoarseness

CAUTION

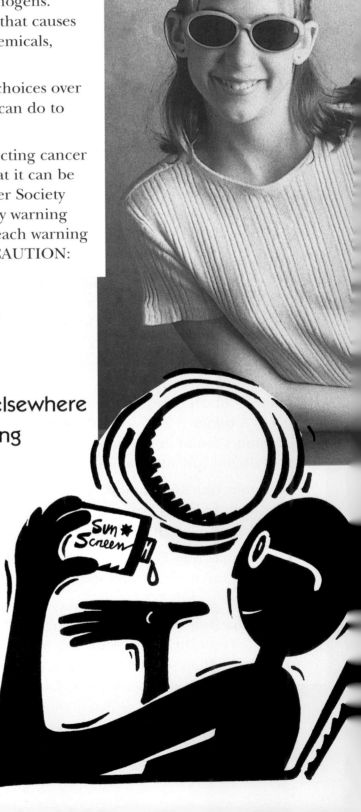

2. **Choose to be tobacco-free.** Smoking is the most important risk factor you can control. Cases of lung cancer would be greatly reduced if people would never begin to smoke. Teens who begin to smoke will have difficulty stopping later. And smoking as a teen can increase the likelihood that some cancers will develop later in life. Other tobacco products also increase cancer risk. Smokeless tobacco increases the risk of cancers of the mouth, gums, and throat. These cancers can develop within a few years of first use. If you use tobacco products, quit today. Review the tobacco cessation programs described in Lesson 28.

3. **Protect yourself from the sun and avoid tanning booths and lamps.** The number of cases of skin cancer, including malignant melanoma, has increased dramatically. **Malignant melanoma** (muh·LIG·nuhnt mel·uh·NOH·muh) is a form of skin cancer that is often fatal. The sun's harmful rays are most powerful between 10:00 a.m. and 3:00 p.m. Try to avoid being in the sun during these hours. If you are in the sun, cover exposed body parts. Wear a sunscreen lotion containing a sun protection factor (SPF) of at least 15. Never use a tanning booth or lamp. Check your skin regularly. If you notice any growths on your skin that appear abnormal, get medical help. Red or brown blotches or moles that grow should be checked by a physician. Skin cancer can be cured if treated early.

4. **Maintain your desirable weight.** People who are overweight are more at risk for developing cancer. Exercise regularly and manage your weight. Tips for weight management are included in Lesson 19.

5. **Eat at least five servings of fruits and vegetables each day.** Fruits and vegetables play a protective role in reducing the risk of cancers of the stomach, colon, bladder, pancreas, mouth, larnyx, cervix, ovary, and breast. They contain antioxidants, such as vitamins A, C, and E. A diet rich in vitamin A might reduce the risk of lung, gastrointestinal, and bladder cancers. Vitamins C and E are helpful in reducing cancer growths. These vitamins can be obtained from the foods you eat or from a standard multivitamin product. Be cautious that your vitamin A intake does not become excessively high.

6. **Eat more high-fiber foods.** Foods rich in fiber play a protective role against colon cancer. Consuming foods in the cabbage family might reduce your risk of developing colon and rectal cancers. Cauliflower, broccoli, and brussels sprouts are in the cabbage family.

7. **Reduce your intake of foods containing nitrates.** Cut down on foods such as ham, bacon, bologna, and hot dogs. These foods contain chemicals that keep food from spoiling, but they increase cancer risk.

8. **Reduce your intake of fat, saturated fat, and cholesterol.** A high-fat diet is linked to breast, colon, and prostate cancers. Follow the suggestions for reducing fat, saturated fat, and cholesterol in Lesson 17.

9. **Avoid alcoholic beverages.** Drinking alcohol increases the risk of developing cancers of the mouth, esophagus, larynx, and liver. Your chances of cancer are multiplied further if you drink alcohol and smoke cigarettes or marijuana.

10. **Avoid exposure to harmful chemicals and airborne fibers.** Wear rubber gloves and a mask when exposed to chemicals, such as those found in insect sprays for the garden or lawn. Wear protective clothing if you will be exposed to airborne fibers, such as asbestos.

11. **Avoid air pollutants.** Many carcinogens are found in polluted air. Try not to inhale the exhaust from cars, buses, and trucks. Have your home tested for radon. **Radon** is an odorless, colorless radioactive gas that is given off by rocks and soil. It can collect and be trapped in basements. Breathing radon can cause lung cancer.

Treatment for Cancer

People who have cancer can often be treated successfully. In some instances, the cancer can be cured. In other instances, the progress of the cancer can be slowed, life can be prolonged, and quality of life can be improved.

- Surgery is the most common treatment. If tumors are confined to a particular site, surgery can remove cancerous tissue from the body.
- **Radiation therapy** is treatment of cancer with high-energy rays to kill or damage cancer cells. This treatment can come from a machine or from materials placed in or near the cancer. Radiation therapy does not make the patient radioactive.
- **Chemotherapy** is treatment with anti-cancer drugs. These drugs kill cancer cells inside the body.
- **Immunotherapy** is a process in which the immune system is stimulated to fight cancer cells.
- **Biological therapy** is treatment to improve the ability of immune cells to fight infection and disease.

Side Effects of Chemotherapy

Chemotherapy works mainly on the cancer cells. However, healthy cells can be harmed as well. This can cause unwanted side effects, and almost all people taking chemotherapy will have side effects. Most side effects do not last long and will gradually go away. If you know someone who is having chemotherapy, this person might have nausea, vomiting, and hair loss.

When chemotherapy acts on normal cells in the stomach and the rest of the digestive tract, it can cause nausea and vomiting. Nausea and vomiting usually stop a day or two after each chemotherapy treatment. Temporary hair loss is another common side effect. Sometimes the hair falls out all at once, and other times it slowly thins out. There is no way to know whether the hair will come out or if some parts of the body will lose more hair than others. Even if hair is lost, it usually grows back after treatment has stopped. Some people wear a wig, cap, or scarf until their hair grows back.

When Someone in Your Family Has Cancer. National Cancer Institute, NIH Publication No. 94-2685. Revised March 1994.

When a Family Member Has Cancer

When someone in your family has cancer, it might mean many things to you. Other teens who have had a family member with cancer say it was confusing, scary, and lonely. You might find that you have feelings that are hard to understand and sometimes hard to share. Talking with a trusted adult family member, relative, doctor or nurse can be helpful.

The unexpected is what makes most teens afraid. When you ask questions, you are prepared. You know what to expect. You also know ways you can help. Then you do not feel as afraid or helpless. You also might not know what to say to the family member who has cancer. It is normal to be uneasy.

Learning About a Family Member's Cancer

- What kind of cancer is it?
- Where is the cancer?
- Will my family member get better?
- What is the best kind of treatment for this type of cancer? Will more than one kind of treatment be used?
- How will my family member feel when (s)he receives this treatment? Does the treatment hurt?
- How often is this treatment given?
- Does the treatment change how my family member will look, feel, or act? If so, how?

- How long do treatments last—a morning, a week? Can I visit?
- Where are treatments given? What is it like? Can I come along?
- What will happen to me during these treatments?
- Can my family member go back to school or work right away? Is it better for him or her to stay at home?
- Can my family member eat the same foods as everyone else? If not, what special foods or diets are needed?
- What can I do to help?

When Someone in Your Family Has Cancer. National Cancer Institute, NIH Publication No. 94-2685. Revised March 1994.

Apply...
The Responsible Decision-Making Model™

You are cleaning the bathroom using a commercial spray cleaner for bathrooms. You are wearing rubber gloves and a mask. Your brother comes in and says, "You look like a dork."

Answer the following questions on a separate sheet of paper. Write "Does not apply" if a question does not apply to this situation.

1. Is it healthful for you to wear a mask and gloves when using household cleaners? Why or why not?

2. Is it safe for you to wear a mask and gloves when using household cleaners? Why or why not?

3. Is it legal for you to wear a mask and gloves when using household cleaners? Why or why not?

4. Will you show respect for yourself if you wear a mask and gloves when using household cleaners? Why or why not?

5. Will your parents or guardian approve if you wear a mask and gloves when using household cleaners? Why or why not?

6. Will you demonstrate good character if you wear a mask and gloves when using household cleaners? Why or why not?

What is the responsible decision to make in this situation?

Lesson 36

Review

Vocabulary

Write a separate sentence using each of the vocabulary words listed on page 388.

Health Content

Write responses to the following:

1. What are the four categories of cancer? **page 389**

2. Discuss 11 ways to reduce your risk of developing cancer. **pages 390–392**

3. What are the warning signs that correspond to each of the letters in CAUTION? **page 390**

4. What are ways to protect against the sun's rays? **page 391**

5. What are antioxidants that protect against cancer? **page 391**

6. What are some foods rich in fiber that protect against colon and rectal cancer? **page 392**

7. What are some foods containing nitrates that increase the risk of developing cancer? **page 392**

8. Discuss five different treatments for cancer. **page 393**

9. What are some side effects from chemotherapy? **page 393**

10. What are some questions teens who have a family member with cancer might ask? **page 394**

Chronic Health Conditions

Vocabulary

chronic health conditions

allergy

allergen

arthritis

asthma

cerebral palsy

chronic fatigue syndrome
(CFS)

diabetes

epilepsy

seizure

petit mal

grand mal

headache

tension headache

migraine headache

multiple sclerosis (MS)

sickle-cell anemia

systemic lupus
erythematosus (SLE)

Life Skills

- **I will recognize ways to manage chronic health conditions.**
- **I will recognize ways to manage asthma and allergies.**
- **I will choose behaviors to reduce my risk of diabetes.**

Chronic health conditions are recurring or persistent conditions. These conditions often develop over time. If untreated, they can progressively harm body parts and functions. While many chronic health conditions do not cause death, they can cause great suffering. You need to know about chronic health conditions. It is estimated that 5 to 15 percent of young people have chronic health conditions.

The Lesson Objectives

- Discuss the definition, symptoms, and treatments for allergies, arthritis, asthma, cerebral palsy, chronic fatigue syndrome, diabetes, epilepsy, headaches, multiple sclerosis, sickle-cell anemia, and systemic lupus erythematosus.

ENCYCLOPEDIA OF CHRONIC HEALTH CONDITIONS

An Encyclopedia of Chronic Health Conditions

Allergies

An **allergy** is the reaction of the body to certain substances. An **allergen** is a substance that causes an allergic reaction. Common food allergens are milk, strawberries, wheat, eggs, corn, nuts, citrus fruits, and shellfish. Airborne allergens include pollen, dust, molds, grass, and cigarette smoke. Medications, such as antibiotics and aspirin, are allergens for some people. Bee stings also can cause an allergic reaction. Some people have severe reactions to allergens. Symptoms of a reaction might include dizziness, nausea, skin rash, drop in blood pressure, and difficulty breathing. People with severe allergies might carry special medications with them.

Asthma

Asthma is a condition in which the bronchial tubes constrict, making breathing difficult. Symptoms of asthma include coughing, wheezing, and shortness of breath. Asthma attacks often occur at night because a person is lying down. This position can cause mucus to build up in the air passages. Most attacks are mild. In a severe attack, a person will struggle to breathe. An asthma attack can be brought on by triggers in the environment. Triggers might include allergies, dust, very cold or humid air, cigarette smoke, or strenuous exercise. Stressful situations can also bring on an asthma attack. Medicines are used to control asthma. Some people with asthma use an inhaler to get medicine into the lower part of the respiratory system.

Arthritis

Arthritis is the painful inflammation of joints in the body. One kind of arthritis is the wearing down of the moving parts of a joint. This can be caused by heredity, sports injuries, or being overweight. Treatment consists of pain relievers and exercise to improve movement of the joint area. Sometimes surgery is performed to replace joints. A second kind of arthritis involves joint deformity and loss of joint function. Medicine is prescribed to reduce swelling and pain. A regular program of exercise must be followed to prevent loss of joint function.

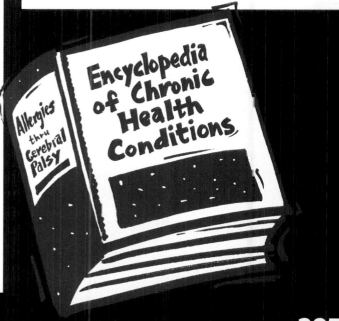

ENCYCLOPEDIA OF CHRONIC HEALTH CONDITIONS

Cerebral Palsy

Cerebral palsy is a nervous system disorder that interferes with muscle coordination. The cause might be a head injury, too much pressure on the head during childbirth, lead poisoning, accidental injury, and certain illnesses. A person with cerebral palsy might stand and walk in an awkward manner. The person might have difficulty speaking, hearing, and seeing. These symptoms remain throughout life. Mental skills are seldom affected. Treatment includes physical therapy and speech therapy. Surgery might be of benefit in some cases.

Chronic Fatigue Syndrome

Chronic fatigue syndrome (CFS) is a condition in which severe tiredness recurs and makes it difficult for a person to function in normal ways. The symptoms include headache, sore throat, low-grade fever, fatigue, and weakness. There also might be tender lymph glands, muscle and joint aches, and inability to concentrate. Unlike the flu that goes away in a few weeks, CFS symptoms recur frequently for more than six months. The cause of CFS is unknown. In teens, CFS might follow mononucleosis. CFS might begin during periods of high stress. There is no treatment for CFS. Health experts recommend that people with CFS maintain a healthful lifestyle and eat a balanced diet, exercise, and get plenty of rest.

Diabetes

Diabetes is a disease in which the body produces little or no insulin or cannot use insulin. The pancreas may not produce enough insulin to break down the sugar for use. The body may be unable to use insulin. The result is excess sugar in the bloodstream. The symptoms of diabetes are frequent urination, abnormal thirst, weakness, and blurred vision. The hands and feet may feel tingly and numb. Cuts heal slowly. Young people who have diabetes are given injections of insulin. Diabetes is usually controlled with oral medications and diet or diet alone in older people. Of particular concern is untreated diabetes. Untreated diabetes can lead to heart disease, blindness, and death.

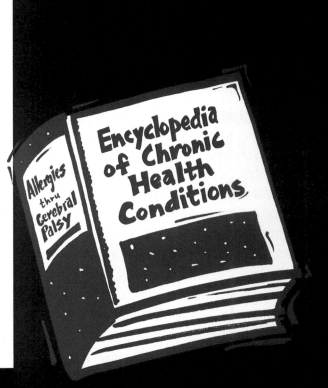

ENCYCLOPEDIA OF CHRONIC HEALTH CONDITIONS

Epilepsy

Epilepsy is a disorder in which abnormal electrical activity in the brain causes a temporary loss of control of the mind and body. A person with epilepsy might have a seizure. A **seizure** is the period in which a person loses control over mind and body. **Petit mal** is a small seizure in which a person loses consciousness for a few seconds. There might be a rolling of the eyes. **Grand mal** is a major seizure in which a person might have a convulsion. During a convulsion, the body stiffens and twitching might occur. You can help a person who experiences a major seizure. Remove any objects that might cause injury to the person. Do not put anything in the person's mouth. Seizures can often be controlled with medication.

Multiple Sclerosis

Multiple sclerosis (MS) is a disease in which the protective covering of nerve fibers in the brain and spinal cord is destroyed. It is believed that the immune system attacks the protective covering. This results in scarring of the nerve fibers. Symptoms might include tingling and numbness in the body. There might be tiredness and dizziness. These symptoms might last several weeks to several months. Relapses might follow illness or periods of stress. Some people with MS are not able to walk or care for themselves. There is no cure for MS. Physical therapy helps to strengthen muscles.

Headaches

A **headache** is a pain in the head. A **tension headache** is pain that results from muscle contractions in the neck or head. These muscle contractions might be caused by actual strain placed on the neck or head muscles. The strain might be due to stress. It might last a few minutes or several days or weeks. Treatment involves relieving the strain by relaxing the muscles. A warm bath and sleep are helpful. A **migraine headache** is severe head pain that is caused by dilation of blood vessels in the brain. The symptoms might include severe throbbing, visual disturbances, nausea, and vomiting. In some cases, the pain is so severe that a person cannot work. People with migraine headaches should be treated by a physician. Other causes of headache are hypertension and colds. Treating these conditions will relieve the headache.

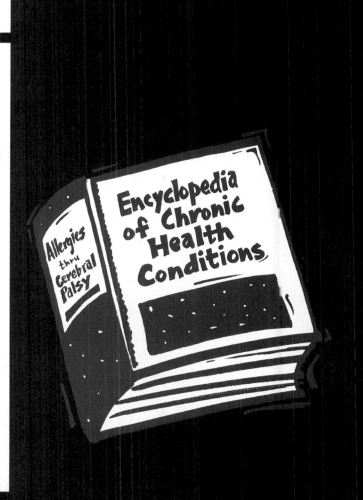

ENCYCLOPEDIA OF CHRONIC HEALTH CONDITIONS

Sickle-Cell Anemia

Sickle-cell anemia is an inherited blood disease in which the red blood cells have less oxygen. Sickle-cell anemia occurs primarily in African Americans. When a person has sickle-cell anemia, the red blood cells are S, or sickle, shaped. As a result, they are fragile and easily destroyed. They have difficulty passing through tiny blood vessels because of their shape. The symptoms of sickle-cell anemia first appear after six months of age. Symptoms include fatigue, headache, and shortness of breath. Children with sickle-cell anemia are at increased risk for developing pneumonia. They are also at increased risk for blood infections. There is no cure. Affected children are given protective vaccines. Teens with sickle-cell anemia might take penicillin to guard against blood infections.

Systemic Lupus Erythematosus

Systemic lupus erythematosus (er·i·THEE·muh·toh·sis) **(SLE)** is a chronic disease that causes inflammation of the connective tissue. SLE affects the skin, kidneys, joints, muscles, and central nervous system. There might be bleeding in the central nervous system, kidney failure, or heart failure. SLE most often occurs during the teen years and is more common in females than males. SLE runs in families. Treatment varies according to the body tissues involved. Medicines are used to reduce inflammation. Long-term use of these medicines can cause bone disease and loss of muscle. A person might be short in stature.

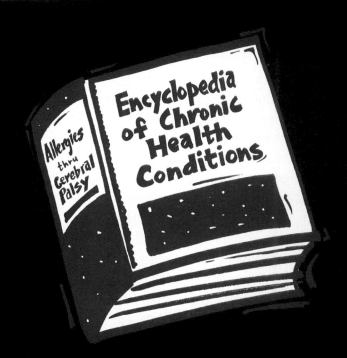

Think Chronic!

Activity

Life Skill I will recognize ways to manage chronic health conditions.

Materials: None

Directions: Play Think Chronic! to review your knowledge of chronic diseases.

1. **Your class will be divided into two teams.**

2. **One student starts the game.** This student says, "I'm thinking of a chronic disease." Then (s)he states one fact about that disease and chooses a student on his or her team to name the disease. A different student must be chosen each time to give every student a chance to answer.

3. **The team wins a point if the student answers correctly.** That student names a fact next and calls on another student. If the student answers incorrectly, play goes to the other team. All students may use their health textbooks.

4. **Play continues until every student has a chance to answer.** The team with the most points wins.

Lesson 37

Review

Vocabulary

Write a separate sentence using each of the vocabulary words listed on page 396.

Health Content

Write responses to the following:

1. Describe chronic health conditions. **page 396**

2. Discuss the definition, symptoms, and treatments for allergies. For arthritis. For asthma. **page 397**

3. Discuss the definition, symptoms, and treatments for cerebral palsy. For chronic fatigue syndrome. For diabetes. **page 398**

4. Discuss the definition, symptoms, and treatments for epilepsy. For headaches. For multiple sclerosis. **page 399**

5. Discuss the definition, symptoms, and treatments for sickle-cell anemia. For systemic lupus erythematosus. **page 400**

Unit 7 Review

Health Content

Review your answers for each Lesson Review in this unit. Then write answers to each of the following questions.

1. How does the body defend itself against disease? **Lesson 32 pages 349–350**

2. How can you keep your immune system healthy? **Lesson 32 page 351**

3. What are symptoms and treatment for chlamydial infection? **Lesson 33 page 359**

4. What are symptoms and treatment for pubic lice? **Lesson 33 page 364**

5. How is HIV not spread? **Lesson 34 page 372**

6. How can you prevent infection with HIV? **Lesson 34 pages 376–377**

7. How can cardiovascular diseases be treated? **Lesson 35 page 387**

8. How can you reduce your risk of skin cancer? **Lesson 36 pages 390–392**

9. What is chemotherapy and what are possible side effects? **Lesson 36 pages 393–394**

10. How is arthritis caused and treated? **Lesson 37 page 397**

Vocabulary

Number a sheet of paper from 1–10. Select the correct vocabulary word. Write it next to the corresponding number. DO NOT WRITE IN THIS BOOK.

antioxidants	DDI
B cells	ELISA
candidiasis	stroke
carcinogen	syphilis
cerebral palsy	viruses

1. _____ are the smallest pathogens. **Lesson 32**

2. A(n) _____ is a condition caused by a blocked or broken blood vessel in the brain. **Lesson 35**

3. _____ are substances that protect cells from being damaged by oxidation. **Lesson 35**

4. _____ is a drug that slows the multiplication of HIV. **Lesson 34**

5. _____ is a blood test used to check for antibodies for HIV. **Lesson 34**

6. _____ is a nervous system disorder that interferes with muscle coordination. **Lesson 37**

7. _____ is an STD caused by fungi that produce itching and burning. **Lesson 33**

8. A _____ is a substance that causes cancer. **Lesson 36**

9. _____ are cells that produce antibodies. **Lesson 32**

10. _____ is an STD caused by spirochetes that produce a chancre, skin rash, and damage to body organs. **Lesson 33**

The Responsible Decision-Making Model™

During a neighborhood softball game, a player is injured and begins to bleed from the nose and mouth. A friend hands you some tissues to try to stop the bleeding. Answer the following questions on a separate sheet of paper. Write "Does not apply" if a question does not apply to this situation.

1. Is it healthful to have contact with another person's blood without wearing gloves? Why or why not?

2. Is it safe to have contact with another person's blood without wearing gloves? Why or why not?

3. Is it legal to have contact with another person's blood without wearing gloves? Why or why not?

4. Will you show respect for yourself if you have contact with another person's blood without wearing gloves? Why or why not?

5. Will your parents or guardian approve if you have contact with another person's blood without wearing gloves? Why or why not?

6. Will you demonstrate good character if you have contact with another person's blood without wearing gloves? Why or why not?

What is the responsible decision to make in this situation?

Multicultural Health

Research the leading causes of death for another country. Compare them to those of your country. What might account for similarities and differences?

Health Literacy

Effective Communication

Design a crossword puzzle for your school newspaper. Include names of communicable and chronic diseases and their descriptions.

Self-Directed Learning

Search the Internet for the following: American Heart Association, American Cancer Society, American Lung Association. Write three new things you learn from each site.

Critical Thinking

Search the Internet for the site of the Centers for Disease Control and Prevention. Find the rate of teen deaths from AIDS in the past five years. Is the rate increasing or decreasing? What might account for changes in rate?

Responsible Citizenship

Write a pamphlet on HIV/AIDS using information from Lesson 34. Ask the school nurse or guidance counselor to make copies to distribute to students.

Family Involvement

Share with your family ways to keep your immune system healthy. Ask them for additional suggestions.

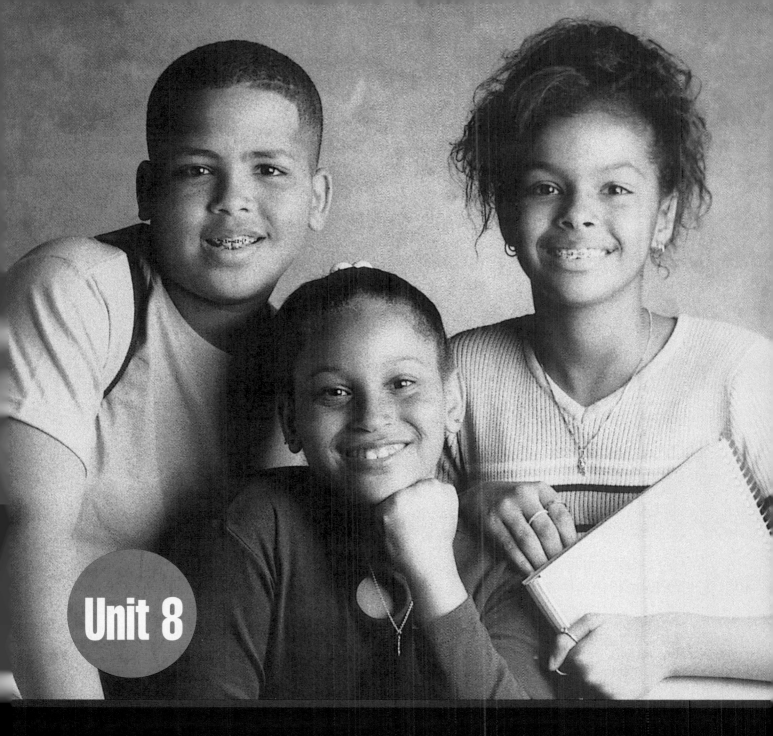

Unit 8

Consumer and Community Health

Being an Informed Consumer

Vocabulary*

consumer

products

services

consumerism

*A complete listing of vocabulary words appears at the end of the lesson.

 Life Skill

• **I will evaluate sources of health information.**

A **consumer** (kuhn·SOO·mer) is a person who chooses sources of health-related information and buys or uses health products and services. **Products** are material goods, such as food, medicine, and clothing, that are made for consumers to purchase. **Services** are work that is provided by people. **Consumerism** is the practice of choosing reliable and tested products, services, and information. You practice consumerism when you evaluate health-related information and make informed choices about what to buy and believe.

The Lesson Objectives

• Explain how to evaluate sources of health-related information.

• Identify organizations that are reliable sources of information.

• Describe ways you can use your computer to obtain health-related information.

• State safety tips you should use when online.

Evaluating Sources of Health-Related Information

Reliable health information is based solely on scientific research and information. It does not attempt to influence your decisions about what to buy. You can evaluate health information by asking questions. The next time you read or hear something about health, use The Consumer's Guide to Evaluating Health-Related Information.

The Consumer's Guide to Evaluating Health-Related Information

1. **What is the source of the information?**

2. **What are the qualifications of the researcher, author, speaker, organization, or group providing the information?**

3. **Is the information based on current research and scientific knowledge or is it the opinion of certain individuals or groups?**

4. **Have reputable health care professionals evaluated the information and accepted it?**

5. **Is the purpose of sharing the information to inform you or to convince you that you need to buy a specific product or service?**

6. **Is the information provided in a way that educates you without trying to appeal to your emotions?**

7. **Are you able to get additional information if you request it?**

8. **Does the information make realistic claims?**

The Directory of Agencies, Associations, and Organizations That Promote Health

Professional Associations

American Dental Association (ADA):
an organization that sets standards for the education and conduct of dentists.

American Medical Association (AMA):
an organization that sets standards for the education and conduct of medical physicians. It is the world's largest publisher of scientific and medical information.

American Public Health Association (APHA):
an organization that establishes standards for scientific procedures in public health, conducts research, and makes policies in the public health field.

Association for the Advancement of Health Education (AAHE):
an organization for health educators that provides support, training, grants, and publications.

National School Health Education Coalition (NaSHEC):
an organization for health educators that distributes health information through publications and other resources.

Society of Public Health Education (SOPHE):
an organization for public health educators that focuses on promoting health and preventing disease.

Private Organizations

Council of Better Business Bureaus:
a nonprofit organization that monitors consumer complaints and advertising and selling practices. It provides listings to the public of businesses that have received consumer complaints.

Consumers' Research:
an organization that tests products and provides ratings for consumers to make comparisons with regard to products' performance and safety.

Consumers' Union:
an organization that tests products and publishes a magazine which provides ratings for consumers to make comparisons with regard to products' performance and safety.

The Directory of Agencies, Associations, and Organizations That Promote Health

Community Organizations

Alzheimer's Association:
an organization that focuses on the prevention of Alzheimer's disease and the care and treatment of patients and families with Alzheimer's disease.

American Cancer Society:
an organization that focuses on educating the public and health care professionals about cancer, provides cancer research, and offers services for patients and families dealing with cancer.

American Diabetes Association:
an organization established to prevent and cure diabetes and to improve the life of people affected by diabetes.

American Heart Association:
an organization devoted to reducing disability and death from cardiovascular diseases and stroke.

American Lung Association:
an organization that focuses on the prevention and cure of lung disease.

American Red Cross:
an organization that provides relief to victims of disaster and helps people prevent, prepare for, and respond to emergencies. Its services also include first aid training, CPR training, blood services, and HIV/AIDS education.

The Asthma and Allergy Foundation of America:
an organization dedicated to finding a cure for and controlling asthma and allergic diseases through research, public education programs, and support groups.

National Safety Council:
an organization that focuses on the prevention of accidental deaths, injuries, and preventable illnesses through training programs and publications.

World Health Organization (WHO):
an agency of the United Nations that focuses on improving the quality of health by coordinating health services throughout the world.

The Directory of Agencies, Associations, and Organizations That Promote Health

Federal Government Agencies

Centers for Disease Control and Prevention (CDC):
an agency within the United States Public Health Service responsible for tracking diseases, coordinating disease control and prevention efforts, and taking action in response to epidemics and natural disasters.

Consumer Product Safety Commission (CPSC):
an agency that establishes and enforces product safety standards and receives consumer complaints about the safety of products.

Food and Drug Administration (FDA):
an agency within the Department of Health and Human Services that monitors the safety and effectiveness of new drugs, medical devices, and the safety of cosmetics and food.

Federal Trade Commission (FTC):
an organization that monitors trade practices; the advertising of foods, drugs, and cosmetics; and advertising that appears on television.

Federal Communications Commission (FCC):
an agency charged with regulating interstate and international communications by radio, television, wire, satellite, and cable.

National Health Information Center (NHIC):
a health information referral agency that sponsors a toll-free hotline which refers consumers to organizations that can provide health-related information.

National Institutes of Health (NIH):
an agency within the Public Health Service that supports and conducts research into the causes and prevention of diseases and provides information to the public.

National Institutes on Drug Abuse (NIDA):
an agency that focuses on improving the understanding, treatment, and prevention of drug abuse and addiction through research, training, and community programs.

United States Department of Agriculture (USDA):
an agency that enforces standards to ensure that food is processed safely, and that oversees the distribution of food information to the public.

United States Office of Consumer Affairs:
an organization that coordinates federal consumer complaints, coordinates research, and provides information to the public on consumer issues.

The Directory of Agencies, Associations, and Organizations That Promote Health

United States Postal Service (USPS): an organization that offers postal services throughout the country and protects the public when products and services are sold through the mail.

United States Public Health Service: an agency within the Department of Health and Human Services that consists of many smaller agencies which promote the protection and advancement of physical and mental health.

State and Local Agencies

State health department: the official agency that has responsibility for the health services and programs for people living within the state. Responsibilities include investigating consumer complaints, collecting and distributing health information, and preventing and controlling disease.

Local health department: the official agency that has responsibility for providing health services and programs for people living within a community. Responsibilities include: investigating consumer complaints, collecting and distributing health statistics, maternal and child care programs, alcohol and other drug abuse programs, communicable disease control, and health education.

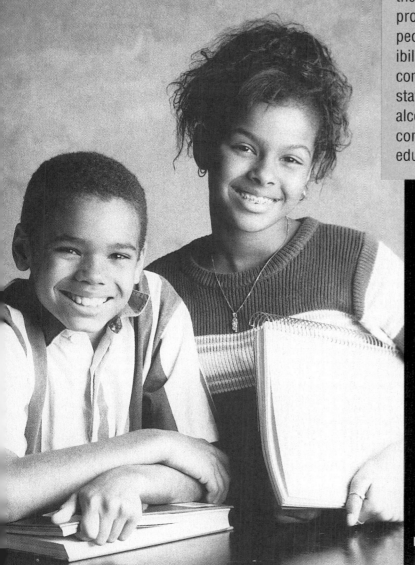

Going Online

You can gain health-related information by using computers online. **Online** is the interactive use of computers using telecommunications technology. The "information highway" and "cyberspace" are names for the "world" you are in when you are online. Millions of people have used online services in the past decade. The **Internet** is a worldwide collection of networks that connect millions of people worldwide. To go online, you need a personal computer, modem, communications software (such as one from a commercial service) and a telephone line. A **modem** is a device that allows a computer to talk to another computer over the telephone lines. **E-mail,** or electronic mail, is a message delivered quickly from one computer to another.

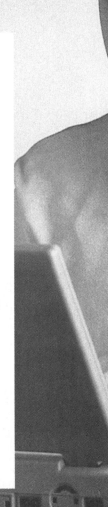

World Wide Web (WWW)

The **World Wide Web (WWW),** or Web, is a computer system that allows a person to view information as text and/or graphics. On the Web, it is possible to search for information and then be "linked" to many other sources of related information just by clicking on the screen. For example, if you searched for the words "American Red Cross," you would find the organization's home page. A home page is the starting page the Web would show. A menu allows you to find more information, just by clicking on a word or graphic on the screen. On the American Red Cross page, you might select a listing of the first aid courses available in your area. Organizations and individuals can make their own pages on the Web for anyone to access. It is important to remember this when you look for health-related information on the Web. Any person, whether (s)he is a medical expert or health professional, can post health-related information on the Web. It is important to determine whether or not the person or organization who sponsors the Web site is a reliable source of information.

Health-related agencies you can find on the WWW include:

- **The Centers for Disease Control and Prevention (CDC)**
- **The American Red Cross**
- **The Environmental Protection Agency (EPA)**
- **The National Institutes of Health (NIH)**
- **The Department of Health and Human Services**
- **The Department of Education**
- **The American Cancer Society**
- **The American Heart Association**
- **The Food and Drug Administration (FDA)**
- **The United States Department of Agriculture (USDA)**

Using CD-ROM and Laser Discs

Another way to gain health-related information is by using CD-ROM and laser discs. A **CD-ROM** is a computer disc that stores computer programs, text, graphics, music, and animation. CD-ROM stands for Compact Disc Read-Only Memory. One CD-ROM can store a vast amount of information. An entire encyclopedia can fit on one CD-ROM! A CD-ROM is played on a personal computer that has a special CD-ROM drive. If your computer has a CD-ROM drive installed, you can use CD-ROMs to gain health-related information.

A **laser disc** is a disc that presents computer programs, text, images, music and animation onto a television or computer monitor. A laser disc is capable of playing video to a large audience. The user can immediately access any frame or chapter on the disc using a remote control.

Sources of Health-Related Information Online

The following list provides examples of reliable sources of health-related information online.

Libraries
From your local library to the Library of Congress, you can search online books and resources to help you learn about any health topic.

Government Agencies
Most federal and many state and local government agencies offer information online.

Nonprofit Organizations
Many nonprofit organizations provide information online about their organizations, the services they provide, and the organizations' areas of focus.

Magazines, Newspapers, and Journals
Many magazines, newspapers, and journals offer information online. Many can be searched. For example, if you wanted articles about violence prevention, you could search for words such as violence, gangs, or weapons. Articles on those topics would be listed for you to read.

Medical Information Services
Medical reference services, such as Medline, are available to the public online. **Medline** is a bibliographic medical data base created by the National Institutes of Health. Medline consists of articles from thousands of medical journals.

The Business Directory Section of the Telephone Book
You can look up the telephone number of any business from any telephone book.

Encyclopedias, Dictionaries, and Reference Guides
You can search through a variety of reference materials, including medical dictionaries, online.

Weather Services
You can find information about the weather any place in the world from weather services such as the National Weather Service. Safety tips from organizations such as the National Hurricane Center also can be located.

Time Tracker

Life Skill I will evaluate sources of health information.

Materials: Paper, pen or pencil

Directions: Read the information below. Then follow the steps to create a plan to keep track of time when you are online.

You might find that it is easy to lose track of time when you are online. Most services charge a fee based on the amount of time you use. After you use up the free time most services offer each month, extra charges are added!

1. Discuss with your parents or guardian what is an appropriate length of time for you to use the computer.

2. Decide whether to set an alarm clock, watch, or a kitchen timer to go off after a certain period of time.

3. Design a time log to write down how much time you are on the computer each time you use it.

Activity

Ways to Use an Online Service

You might go online to explore health topics of interest to you. For example, by searching through topics on health, you might discover the latest facts on smoking and cancer, or read an article from the latest medical journal.

Many people go online for research. You might do research for a school project, find health terms in a medical dictionary, access the American Red Cross to find out what courses are being offered, or e-mail a health professional.

Many students go online for homework assistance. Many services offer assistance from teachers and professors to help students with questions about their schoolwork.

Many teens go online to "chat," or talk online, with other people. They might have e-mail pen pals from all over the world, or enter discussion groups in which other teens discuss interesting health topics. Entire classes might have a group chat with another class from another part of the world. There also are support groups online, including groups for teens with disabilities, diseases, and illnesses.

Safety Tips When Online

1. **Always discuss the use of online services with your parents or guardian.** Your parents or guardian might tell you about ways that it is appropriate for you to use the services. They also might use a device called a parental control, which can block out all areas online except those specifically designed for teens and children.

2. **Do not give out personal information.** Do not give your last name, your address, your telephone number, your school name—any information that might help a stranger identify you. Never give out your online password to anyone you do not know. Remember that you cannot be sure to whom you might be sending e-mails or with whom you are chatting. Just because a person claims to be someone, does not mean (s)he is that person. Anyone online can claim to be a teen, an adult, a male, a female, or a celebrity. There have been reports of people posing as someone else to meet teens. Some people who have arranged to meet teens in person or have called them on the telephone have turned out to be dangerous.

3. **Always consider the source of the information you find online.** Refer to The Consumer's Guide to Evaluating Health-Related Information on page 407. Information that is distributed by a government agency, such as the Centers for Disease Control and Prevention, can be considered reliable. However, information distributed by other groups might in fact be a form of advertising. People who post health-related information might not have the knowledge or training to give out accurate information. An appropriate way to think about online information is to compare it to word-of-mouth conversations. Would you believe something a friend of a friend told you? You would be cautious about the source before believing what you heard.

4. **Do not purchase any products online without permission from your parents or guardian.** Many reputable stores now sell products online. However, there also are many people selling products online using quackery. Do not give out your credit card number. Be cautious when considering buying products sold online.

Lesson 38

Review

Vocabulary

Write separate sentences using twenty of the vocabulary words listed below.

Health Content

Write responses to the following:

1. What are the eight questions you should ask yourself to evaluate sources of health information? **page 407**

2. What are reliable sources of health-related information that are professional organizations? Private organizations? Community organizations? Government agencies? **pages 408–411**

3. What are ways to gain health-related information when using a computer? **pages 412–413**

4. What are reliable sources of health-related information online? **page 414**

5. What are four safety tips to follow when using an online service? **page 416**

consumer
products
services
consumerism
American Dental Association (ADA)
American Medical Association (AMA)
American Public Health Association (APHA)
Association for the Advancement of Health Education (AAHE)
National School Health Education Coalition (NaSHEC)
Society of Public Health Education (SOPHE)
Council of Better Business Bureaus
Consumers' Research
Consumers' Union
Alzheimer's Association

American Cancer Society
American Diabetes Association
American Heart Association
American Lung Association
American Red Cross
The Asthma and Allergy Foundation of America
National Safety Council
World Health Organization (WHO)
Centers for Disease Control and Prevention (CDC)
Consumer Product Safety Commission (CPSC)
Food and Drug Administration (FDA)
Federal Trade Commission (FTC)
Federal Communications Commission (FCC)
National Health Information Center (NHIC)

National Institutes of Health (NIH)
National Institutes on Drug Abuse (NIDA)
United States Department of Agriculture (USDA)
United States Office of Consumer Affairs
United States Postal Service (USPS)
United States Public Health Service
State health department
Local health department
online
Internet
modem
e-mail
World Wide Web (WWW)
CD-ROM
laser disc
Medline

Being a Cautious Consumer

Vocabulary

comparison shopping
price
brand name
generic name
coupon
discount store
catalog store
warranty
convenience
features
quality
healthful entertainment
advertising
advertisement
commercial
media
bandwagon appeal
brand loyalty appeal
false image appeal
glittering generality appeal
humor appeal
progress appeal
reward appeal
scientific evidence appeal
testimonial appeal
sex appeal
media literacy
fad
quackery

- **I will recognize my rights as a consumer.**
- **I will choose healthful entertainment.**
- **I will develop media literacy.**
- **I will take action if my consumer rights are violated.**

Open a magazine and you might see an ad trying to convince you to wear a particular brand of jeans. Ride in an automobile and you might notice billboards trying to convince you to listen to a particular radio station. Shop with a friend and the friend might try to influence what you buy. Your consumer choices can be influenced in many different ways. But the choice is still up to you and your family. Take responsibility and be a cautious consumer.

The Lesson Objectives

- Discuss criteria to use when you comparison shop.
- List guidelines for choosing healthful entertainment.
- Describe appeals used in advertisements.
- State ways peers and salespeople influence your shopping decisions.
- List ways you can recognize quackery.
- Describe how to make a consumer complaint.

Comparison Shopping

Many different products and services are available from which you can choose. As a cautious consumer, you will want to have some objective criteria to use when you make choices. Using objective criteria keeps you from making choices based on your emotions alone. **Comparison** (kuhm·PEHR·i·suhn) **shopping** is evaluating products and services using objective criteria, such as price, convenience, features, quality, and warranty.

Price

The **price** is the cost of a product or service. A **brand name** is a product or service made by a certain company or manufacturer. A **generic** (jeh·NEHR·ik) **name** is a product or service that meets certain standards, but does not have fancy packaging. Generic name products and services are usually lower in price than those with brand names. A **coupon** (KOO·pahn) is a ticket that can be used to reduce the price of something a person plans to buy. However, it is not wise to buy something you do not need just because you have a coupon for a product or service. A **discount store** is a store that sells products and services lower than the regular price. A **catalog store** is a store that sells products and services from a book containing pictures, descriptions, and prices.

Warranty

A **warranty** is a written assurance that a product or service will be replaced or repaired if it is not satisfactory. What is the length of time that the warranty is in effect? How convenient will it be to have the product or service replaced or repaired?

Convenience

Convenience is anything that saves time or effort. Consider convenience when you shop for a particular product or service. You might save time but pay more if you buy a product at a store near your home. Shipping costs are usually added when you purchase something from a catalog store out of town. But you might save time and effort.

Features

The **features** are the important or outstanding characteristics of a product or service. When comparison shopping, you must compare each feature. For example, the price for two computers might be the same, but the features might differ. Knowing what features you need helps you compare products and services.

Quality

The **quality** is the degree of excellence of a product or service. How thorough is the service? What is the length of time for which the service is provided? How well is the product made? How does the product perform? How long will the product last?

Choosing Healthful Entertainment

Healthful entertainment is entertainment that promotes physical, mental, or social health. Healthful entertainment influences your thoughts in a positive way. Positive thinking causes biochemical changes in your body that help build your immune system. You are less likely to become ill. Healthful entertainment influences you to make responsible decisions. You choose decisions that are healthy, are safe, are legal, demonstrate respect for yourself and others, are approved by your parents or guardian, and demonstrate good character. Healthful entertainment influences your value system in a positive way. You see, hear, and do things that are consistent with your value system.

Guidelines for Choosing Healthful Entertainment

- Entertainment should be approved for your age group.
- Entertainment should be approved by your parents or guardian.
- Entertainment should not present harmful drug use as acceptable behavior.
- Entertainment should not present violence as acceptable behavior.
- Entertainment should not lead you to believe sex outside of marriage is acceptable behavior.

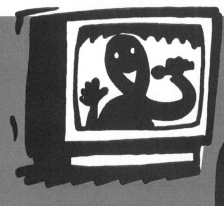

The Power of Advertising

You are less likely to be influenced by advertising if you are skilled in comparison shopping. **Advertising** is a form of selling that provides information about products and services. An **advertisement,** or ad, is a paid announcement about a product or service. A **commercial** is an advertisement on television or radio. Unlike reliable health-related information, advertisements and commercials are designed to influence you. Someone pays money for an advertisement or commercial. It might be paid by an individual, a company, or a manufacturer.

Much money is spent placing advertisements in the media. **Media** are the various forms of mass communication. Examples of media are television, radio, magazines, billboards, and newspapers. Advertisers think carefully about when and where to place their ads. Ads are placed where they will have the greatest influence. For example, commercials for children's cereals are often shown during Saturday morning cartoons. Commercials for cars and beer often appear during televised football and basketball games. Ads for clothes for teens are placed in teen magazines and other places where you will see them.

Advertisements are designed to influence your choices. Many talented and creative people work on the ads. They develop ads that appeal to your wants and needs. Examine the Ten Tempting Advertising Appeals on the next page. These appeals usually get an emotional response from consumers. Think about your wants and needs. Do certain appeals cause you to respond in an emotional way instead of being objective?

Recognizing appeals is one way to lessen the effects ads and commercials will have on you. Suppose you see an ad or commercial you like. You know why the ad or commercial appeals to you. You know it is the appeal that hooks you and not the product being promoted. Then you do not have to rush out and buy something you do not need. You do not rush out and buy something that is not healthful for you.

Who's Who in TV Commercials?

Make a list of five commercials in which a famous person appears. Next to each person you list, write the product, food, or beverage that was promoted. How might the person be linked to the product, food, or beverage? For example, an Olympic athlete might appear in a commercial for cereal. Why might an Olympic athlete be chosen for the commercial? Suppose you were making a commercial for teens. Think of a hot product, food, or beverage that teens want. Who would you have appear in the commercial? Why?

Ten Tempting Advertising Appeals

BEWARE!

1. **Bandwagon appeal** is an advertising appeal that tries to convince a person that everybody is using a particular product or service and (s)he should, too. These ads often show a group of people at a party. The product or service is helping them enjoy one another and have a good time. These ads say that you, too, can "jump on the bandwagon" and join the crowd if you buy the product or service.

2. **Brand loyalty appeal** is an advertising appeal that tries to convince a person that one brand is better than the rest. A brand is a product made by a certain company. Think about the popularity of clothing with logos. Some teens feel they must wear clothes to show the logo of a specific brand to be really "in."

3. **False image appeal** is an advertising appeal that tries to convince a person that (s)he will have a certain image if (s)he buys a specific product or service. There might be a person or people in the ad who are very attractive and appear to be sophisticated and very popular. You might want to be like these people. These ads are false and misleading. Having a particular product or service is no guarantee that you will have the same image as the person or people in the ad.

4. **Glittering generality appeal** is an advertising appeal that includes a general statement that is exaggerated to appeal to the emotions. Usually these ads are designed to appeal to people with specific concerns. An ad might claim to "clear up ALL acne" or "give your hair 24-hour hold." Teens who have a specific concern might feel that they can buy a product or service that will take care of their needs.

5. **Humor appeal** is an advertising appeal that contains a catchy slogan, jingle, or cartoon that grabs attention. It is easy to remember certain words or the tune used in the ad. You are so attracted to the ad that you become attracted to the product or service.

6. **Progress appeal** is an advertising appeal that emphasizes that a product is "new and improved." They imply that a product or service is a step ahead of other products and services with which you are already familiar. They appeal to your desire to have the "latest" and the "best."

7. **Reward appeal** is an advertising appeal that offers a special prize, gift, or coupon when a specific product or service is purchased. When you are comparing two different products or services, there is an additional reason to choose the one mentioned in the ad. You might not be as objective when you are comparing products and services if you like the prize, gift, or coupon.

8. **Scientific evidence appeal** is an advertising appeal that includes the results of surveys and laboratory tests. These ads might say, "Laboratory tests show that...," "More dentists recommend...," or "Nine out of ten doctors use..." Statements such as these are designed to make you feel confident that you are making the best choice.

9. **Testimonial appeal** is an advertising appeal that focuses on a person who gives a statement about the benefits of a specific product or service. The person might be someone who is well known, such as a movie star or athlete. Sometimes the person is not well known. Consumers watching the ad identify with the person in some way. The ad tries to convince you that you will be as pleased with the product or service as the person in the ad is.

10. **Sex appeal** is an advertising appeal that tries to convince a person that others will find him or her irresistible if a specific product or service is used.

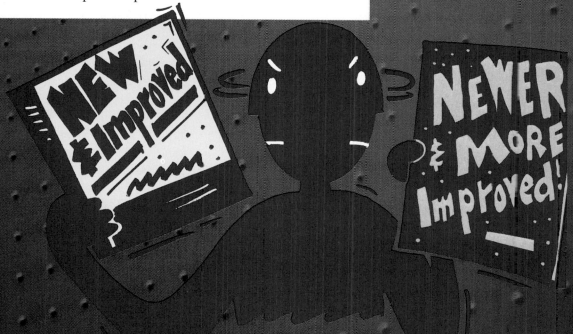

Activity

How Do You Want to Be Today?

Life Skill

I will develop media literacy.

Materials: Paper, pen or pencil

Directions: **Media literacy** is the ability to recognize and evaluate the messages in media. Completing this activity will help you gain skill in evaluating advertisement or ads.

Eight Ways Teens Want to Be

I want to be **athletic**. Ads use sports heroes and feature sports activities, particularly risky ones.

I want to be **older.** Ads use teens or adults who are older than the audience they want to reach.

I want to be **attractive**. Ads use attractive people and imply that you will look a certain way if you use the product.

I want to be **rich** and **famous**. Ads use famous people, especially sports heroes and movie stars.

I want to be **cool**. Ads try to convince you that you will be "in" if you buy the product.

I want to be **smart**. Ads use results of surveys or laboratory tests or people who appear knowledgeable.

I want to be **excited**. Ads use fastpaced action, appealing backgrounds, appealing music, and people engaged in risky activities, such as skydiving.

I want to be **special.** Ads make their products appear to be the best. The products might be sold only in exclusive stores.

1. **Watch or listen to five ads, one from each type of media.**

2. **Evaluate the ad.** Use the questions below. Write your answers on a separate sheet of paper.

Questions to Evaluate Media Messages™.

1. What is the purpose of the message?

2. Who is the target audience for the message?

3. Who will profit if members of the target audience are influenced by the message?

4. Does the message encourage members of the target audience to choose responsible behavior? How?

5. What techniques are used to make the message appealing to the target audience? Why?

6. What information is missing from the message? Why?

7. Is this message consistent with messages found in other media on the same subject? How?

3. **Choose a way the ad is trying to make you be from the box to the left.** Think of three ways you can be that way without buying anything. Choose a responsible behavior. For example, if you want to be older, you might write "Do my chores without being reminded."

Persuasion from Peers and Salespeople

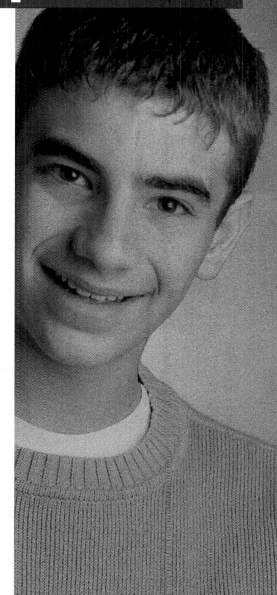

There are other influences on your consumer choices. Stop for a moment and think about ways peers influence each other. For example, peers can begin a fad and expect you to join the fad. A **fad** is something that is very popular for a short period of time. Some of your peers might begin to have haircuts similar to the haircut of a popular star on television. Soon, many of your peers have the same haircut. You might think about having your hair cut in a similar way, even though it is not the best haircut for you.

Peers might wear specific brands of clothes. Another brand might be of better quality and be a better fit for you. Are you tempted to wear the same brands of clothing as your peers?

Your consumer choices might say something about your self-confidence. Be self-confident and decide for yourself how to have your hair cut, what clothing to wear, where to shop, and what to buy. You can ask for the opinions of others, as long as you take responsibility for your choices. Of course, it is important to respect the advice of your parents or guardian. Develop your own style and feel good about yourself.

Feel confident when you are shopping and are approached by salespeople. Some salespeople can be very pushy. Some salespeople will offer false opinions. They might say clothing fits you or flatters you when it does not. Recognize that salespeople are working to make a sale. Although some salespeople are objective, others are not. Rely on yourself to determine how the product or service will benefit you. Never feel like you have to buy something.

Beware of Quackery

Have you ever seen an advertisement for something that seemed too good to be true? Then it probably was. Some people try to sell products, services, and information that are not reliable. **Quackery** is consumer fraud, or deception that involves the practice of promoting or selling useless products or services. A quack is a person who markets inaccurate health-related information, unreliable health care, or useless products and services. Much of quackery is health-related. Three kinds of health-related quackery include:

- **Weight loss and diet scams**
- **Unproven medical treatments**
- **Unproven medical products**

Health-related quackery is extremely dangerous. A health condition might go untreated while a person is using unproven medical treatments or products. The cost of the treatments or products might deplete health-related savings. Following an unproven weight loss plan might actually harm health. As a cautious consumer, you cannot afford to be a victim of quackery. Read the Ten Ways to Recognize a Quack. Then you will know how to recognize quackery.

Ten Ways to Recognize a Quack

1. A quack promises quick cures, miracles, and unknown or secret formulas.

2. A quack often sells door-to-door or by telephone.

3. A quack might use testimonials from people who use the product (often celebrities) and claim to have experienced miracles.

4. A quack often claims that the medical profession does not recognize a product or service.

5. A quack might promote products without labels that provide indications, directions, or cautions about use.

6. A quack often claims that traditional medical treatment is more harmful than healthful.

7. A quack might sell products that only can be ordered through a post office box number.

8. A quack might use a person or group of people to promote products or services about whom little or nothing is known.

9. A quack might advertise in the back pages of magazines, over the telephone, by direct mail, in newspaper ads that look like articles, or in television infomercials.

10. A quack often tries to appeal to your fears or emotions.

How to Make a Consumer Complaint

Many consumers are joining together to protect themselves and others from misleading and inaccurate advertising and selling. You can be responsible and involved in consumer protection. You might have a complaint about an ad, or a product or service you have purchased. The National Consumers' League suggests you take the following actions.

1. Talk to your parents or guardian and agree on a plan of action.

2. Keep records including sales slips, receipts, and cancelled checks.

3. Begin by making a complaint to someone where the purchase was made.

4. If unsuccessful, write a letter explaining your complaint and send it to the president of the company. Type the letter, date it, and keep a file copy. Send the letter by certified mail with a return receipt requested.

5. If you are not satisfied with the response you get, make photocopies of the letter and send it to city, county, or state voluntary consumer groups, the state's attorney general, the local Better Business Bureau, the state's consumer affairs office, a senator, or a member of Congress.

6. If the company is involved in interstate commerce, send a copy of your complaint to the FTC or the FDA.

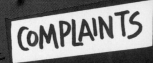

7. Advise the original company that you have notified groups responsible for consumer protection.

8. If the company has a misleading or deceptive ad in the local news media, tell the station or newspaper involved and encourage them to stop running the ad.

9. If these steps do not work, contact a local voluntary consumer organization. Some voluntary groups will write letters and make visits to the business on your behalf. Government agencies often send out investigators and will take action if it is justified.

10. Finally, you and your family can sue the business in a small claims court. This court will process suits to recover moderate amounts of money. The fee to the consumer is kept at a minimum.

Lesson 39

Review

Vocabulary

Write a separate sentence using each of the vocabulary words listed on page 418.

Health Content

Write responses to the following:

1. What are five objective criteria to use for comparison shopping? **pages 419**

2. What are five guidelines for choosing healthful entertainment? **page 420**

3. What are five kinds of media in which you can find ads? **page 421**

4. How do advertisers decide when and where to place their advertisements? **page 421**

5. What are ten tempting appeals used in ads? **pages 422–423**

6. What are six questions you can ask to evaluate the appeal of an advertisement? **page 424**

7. Why should a person take responsibility for his or her shopping decisions? **page 425**

8. What are three kinds of health-related quackery? **page 426**

9. What are ten ways to recognize a quack? **page 427**

10. What are ten actions to take when making a consumer complaint? **pages 428–429**

Spending Time and Money

Vocabulary

time management plan

budget

income

expenses

savings

balanced budget

credit card

interest

debt

shopping addiction

entertainment addiction

desensitization

 Life Skill • **I will make a plan to manage time and money.**

Your time is very precious. If you are like most people, your money is limited. You cannot afford to waste time or money. A totally awesome teen has a budget and a time management plan.

The Lesson Objectives

* Explain how to make a time management plan.
* Describe how to make a budget.
* State how to recognize shopping addiction.
* Discuss how to recognize entertainment addiction.

Making a Time Management Plan

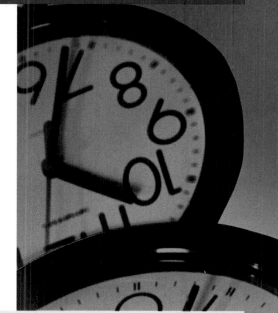

A **time management plan** is a plan that shows how a person will set aside time for activities done regularly and leisure activities. As a consumer, you must decide what is quality time. This means examining your values and deciding what is important to you. For example, you might value your family relationships. This means that setting aside time to be with family members is a priority. You might value education. This means that making time to study is a priority.

As a consumer, you make choices about how to use time. These choices help determine the quality of your life. Do you have a time management plan? A time management plan is a plan that shows how a person will set aside time for activities done regularly and for leisure activities.

A time management plan can help you in different ways.

You can check to see if you honor your priorities. A priority is something that is very important to you. Some of your priorities might be family members, grades, and your health. As you make your plan, you set aside time for your priorities first. Without a plan, you might neglect priorities.

You are less stressed. Right now you are very busy. You have a lot of homework and school activities. There are family responsibilities. You might have a job such as childsitting for a neighbor. Thinking about how busy you are without planning for action will stress you. When you have a plan, you can focus on what is planned for that moment. You are relaxed because you know you have set aside time for the other things you must do.

You can plan time for yourself. Suppose you do not have a plan and you get busy. What usually happens? You probably will skip time for yourself. But, alone time is necessary for optimal health. You need time to reflect or think back on your day. You will feel more in control of your life. Plan to take a walk, read a book, or write in your journal. You deserve it!

You will get better grades. You will get better grades if you have a plan. Set aside time to do homework. Set aside time to review each subject each day. Regular review helps you retain what you learn.

You can add variety to your social life. Have you ever felt like you keep doing the same old thing? If you do, you will get bored. You can plan for variety if you plan ahead. You can check out what movies or plays are in town. You can think about new sports to try with friends.

Making a Budget

A **budget** is a plan for spending and saving money. The first thing to do when you make a monthly or weekly budget is to list your income. Your **income** is money received from different sources. Your income might include an allowance, money for jobs such as child care or delivering newspapers, and any gifts of money that you receive. The next thing to do is to list your expenses. Your **expenses** are the amounts of money needed to buy or do something. Perhaps you contribute some of the money you earn from odd jobs to your family. You might spend money on clothes, snacks, or entertainment. You might put money into a savings account. **Savings** is money set aside for future use. You might be saving money for college or vocational school.

Making a Weekly Budget

A sample budget appears below. The sample budget is for someone your age. The list of income and expenses might be similar or very different from yours. On a separate sheet of paper, design your own budget. List and total the income that you receive for one week. Then list and total the expenses you expect to have for one week. Compare the two numbers.

Income		**Expenses**	
Allowance:	$10	Food:	$ 5
Paper route:	$20	Entertainment:	$15
		Sports league:	$ 5
		Family savings:	$ 5

Your Budget

Look at the budget you made. Your budget can tell much about your ability to manage money. A **balanced budget** is a plan in which income is equal to expenses. It is difficult to have a balanced budget if you do not keep track of your income and expenses. You have savings when you have more income than expenses. It is smart to get into the habit of saving. You might have to give up some of the things you want to have savings. It might not be possible for you to save. You might need to contribute any extra money you have to your family.

Some people spend more money than they have. They might charge expenses on a credit card. A **credit card** is a card used for payment in which the owner of the card agrees to pay later. Each month a statement of expenses charged on the credit card is sent to the owner of the card. The bill is paid in full or in part. If only part of the bill is paid, interest is charged on the remaining balance. **Interest** is money that is paid for the use of a larger sum of money.

Credit cards are convenient, but they should be used with caution. It is not smart to have more charges on your credit card than you can pay off in one month. You can go into debt if you make a habit of charging more than you can pay off each month. **Debt** (DET) is the condition of owing.

You can learn about yourself from reviewing your budget. How often do you spend money on entertainment? How much money do you spend on clothing? How much money do you earn? How much money can you contribute to your family? Are you able to save money for the future?

Review your budget with your parents or guardian. Remember, it is important for you to learn to manage money wisely.

Shopping Addiction

Have you ever heard someone say, "Money burns a hole in my pocket?" Do you know what this saying means? Some teens have shopping addiction. **Shopping addiction** is the uncontrollable urge to shop and buy. Teens with shopping addiction buy on impulse, over and over again. These teens go on shopping sprees even when they do not need anything.

They get a temporary "high" from shopping that might relieve their boredom, loneliness, or insecure feelings. They feel better for a short time and then the uncomfortable feelings come back again. Of course, shopping will not really solve teens' problems. Shopping addiction is similar to drug addiction. There is only temporary relief from emotional pain. Teens with shopping addiction need help. Shopping addiction can continue into adulthood and lead to debt.

Entertainment Addiction

Have you ever known anyone that appeared to be "glued to the tube?" Some teens have what is known as entertainment addiction. **Entertainment addiction** is a strong desire to be amused or interested in something at the expense of mental-emotional, family-social, and physical health. Teens with entertainment addiction might spend most of their time watching television, going to movies, listening to music, or playing computer games. They spend so much time being entertained that there is not much time to be involved in other healthful activities. Their relationships with family and friends suffer. They might put off doing homework and completing chores. There is not enough time to exercise or to learn to play a musical instrument. Teens with entertainment addiction might watch television, go to the movies, play computer games, or listen to music as a way of dealing with loneliness, depression, and anxiety.

Entertainment addiction is very risky when teens are addicted to certain television programs. These teens might think that things in life happen the way they do on a television program. For example, soap operas and popular teen programs often portray life in an unrealistic way. Teens on television programs might get into difficult situations, such as unwed parenthood or drug use, and then find simple solutions. In real life, the solutions are not as simple as those presented on television programs.

There are many television programs and movies that include violence. Teens who become addicted to violent programs are at risk for being desensitized to violence. **Desensitization** (dee·sen·suh·tuh·ZAY·shun) is the effect of reacting less and less to the exposure to something. Teens who are addicted to violence begin to see violence as a way of life.

Some teens spend time using computers as a way of dealing with loneliness, depression, and anxiety. These teens might find it easier to talk with others by computer than to have relationships with people in person. E-mail friends should never be a substitute for healthful relationships with family and friends.

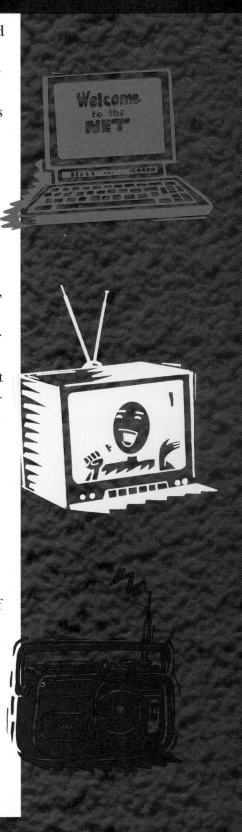

Apply...

The Responsible Decision-Making Model™

Your class is planning a trip to Washington, D.C. in the spring. Your parents have told you to make a budget and start saving money. Your friends want to come to your house tonight and watch a movie. Renting a video tonight is not in your budget.

Answer the following questions on a separate sheet of paper. Write "Does not apply" if a question does not apply to this situation.

1. Is it healthful to rent a video? Why or why not?
2. Is it safe to rent a video? Why or why not?
3. Is it legal to rent a video? Why or why not?
4. Will you respect yourself if you rent a video? Why or why not?
5. Will your parents or guardian approve if you rent a video? Why or why not?
6. Will you demonstrate good character if you rent a video? Why or why not?

What is the responsible decision to make in this situation?

Lesson 40

Review

Vocabulary

Write a separate sentence using each of the vocabulary words listed on page 430.

Health Content

Write responses to the following:

1. How do you make a time management plan? **page 431**
2. How do you make a budget? **page 432**
3. Why is it important to be cautious when charging products and services on a credit card? **page 433**
4. Describe behaviors that indicate shopping addiction. **page 433**
5. Describe behaviors that indicate entertainment addiction. **page 434**

Planning for Health Care

Vocabulary*

health care system

health care provider

primary care provider

specialist

health care practitioner

allied health professional

health care facility

health insurance policy

*A complete listing of vocabulary words appears at the end of the lesson.

Life Skills

- **I will make responsible choices about health care providers and facilities.**
- **I will evaluate ways to pay for health care.**

The **health care system** is a system that includes health care providers, health care facilities, and payment for health care. You can learn how to choose health care providers. You can become familiar with health care facilities in your community. Knowing how to plan for paying for health care also is important.

The Lesson Objectives

- List ten questions to ask when choosing a health care provider.
- Give examples of medical specialists and allied health professionals.
- Identify health care facilities.
- Explain ways to pay for health care.

Choosing Health Care Providers

A **health care provider** is a professional who helps people obtain optimal health. The best time to choose health care providers is before health care is needed. What are some ways to locate competent health care providers?

The local chapters of the American Medical Association and the American Dental Association keep lists of their members. Your family can call for a recommendation. These associations usually provide three names. Hospitals also keep names of physicians they believe to be competent. Your family might ask a trusted health care provider to recommend other health care providers. Your family also might have a health care plan that includes certain health care providers.

Your relationship with a health care provider is important.

Plan a meeting with the health care provider that your family is considering. Get answers to the following questions.

- What are the credentials of the health care provider?
- What hospital(s) affiliations does the health care provider have?
- What arrangements can be made for weekend or after hours care?
- How long do you have to wait to get an appointment?
- Are telephone calls returned promptly?
- Does the health care provider emphasize a prevention plan?
- How much are fees?
- How are fees paid?
- Is this health care provider eligible for payment if your family has a health care plan?
- Are you comfortable speaking with the health care provider?

The Who's Who
of Health Care Providers

There are many different health care providers. A **physician** (fuh·ZI·shun) is a professional who is licensed to practice medicine and, with special training, surgery in all branches of medicine. A **medical doctor** is a physician who is trained in a medical school and who has a doctor of medicine degree (MD). An **osteopath** (AH·stee·oh·path) is a physician trained in a college of osteopathic medicine who has a doctor of osteopathy degree (DO).

Physicians can either be primary care providers or specialists. A **primary care provider** is a physician or other health care provider who provides general care. A **specialist** is a physician who has additional training in a particular aspect of health care.

A **health care practitioner** is a professional whose practice is restricted to a specific area of the body. Examples of health care practitioners include podiatrists, optometrists, and dentists. A **podiatrist** (puh·DY·uh·trist) is a doctor of podiatric medicine (DPM) who specializes in problems of the feet. An **optometrist** (ahp·TAHM·uh·trist) is a doctor of optometry (OD) who specializes in examining the eyes and prescribing lenses. An optometrist cannot perform surgery or prescribe drugs. A **dentist** is either a doctor of dental surgery (DDS) or a doctor of medical dentistry (DMD) who specializes in the treatment of teeth.

An **allied health professional** is a trained practitioner who practices under some degree of supervision. There are over 70 different types of allied health professionals.

Medical Specialists

- An **anesthesiologist** (a·nuhs·thee·zee·AH·loh·jist) is a physician who specializes in the administration of drugs to prevent pain and induce unconsciousness during surgery.

- A **cardiologist** (kar·dee·AH·luh·jist) is a physician who specializes in the treatment of disorders of the heart and blood vessels.

- A **dermatologist** (duhr·muh·TAH·luh·jist) is a physician who specializes in the care of the skin.

- A **gastroenterologist** (gas·tro·en·tuh·RAH·luh·jist) is a physician who specializes in disorders of the digestive tract.

- A **geriatrician** (jer·ee·uh·TRI·shun) is a physician who specializes in medical care for the elderly.

- A **gynecologist** (gy·nuh·KAH·luh·jist) is a physician who specializes in treatment of the disorders of the female reproductive tract.

- A **neurologist** (nu·RAH·luh·jist) is a physician who specializes in the diagnosis and treatment of diseases of the brain, spinal cord, and nerves.

- An **obstetrician** (ahb·stuh·TRI·shun) is a physician who specializes in the care of a mother-to-be and her developing baby.

- An **ophthalmologist** (ahf·thuhl·MAHL·uh·jist) is a physician who specializes in the medical and surgical treatment of the eyes.

- An **orthopedist** (or·thuh·PEE·dist) is a physician who specializes in the surgical care of muscle, bone, and joint injuries and disorders.

- A **pediatrician** (pee·dee·uh·TRI·shuhn) is a physician who specializes in the care of children and adolescents.

- A **plastic surgeon** (SUHR·juhn) is a physician who specializes in surgery to correct, repair, or improve body features.

- A **psychiatrist** (sy·KY·uh·trist) is a physician who specializes in the diagnosis and treatment of mental and emotional problems.

- A **urologist** (yur·AH·luh·jist) is a physician who specializes in the treatment of urinary disorders and the male reproductive system.

Allied Health Professionals

- A **registered nurse** is a nurse who is certified for general practice or for any one or more of several nurse specialties.

- A **nurse practitioner** is a specially trained registered nurse who can function as a primary care provider in some states.

- A **dental hygienist** is an allied health professional who provides oral health services, such as cleaning teeth and educating others about proper care of teeth.

- An **audiologist** (aw·dee·AH·luh·jist) is an allied health professional who screens people for hearing problems and makes recommendations for hearing devices.

- A **pharmacist** is an allied health professional who dispenses medications prescribed by physicians.

- A **physical therapist** is an allied health professional who works with people who have physical disabilities and are in need of rehabilitation.

- A **registered dietitian** is an allied health professional who counsels people about healthful dietary principles and designs special diets.

- An **occupational therapist** is an allied health professional who helps people with disabilities learn to adapt to their disabilities.

- A **speech pathologist** (pa·THAH·luh·jist) is an allied health care professional who helps people overcome speech disorders.

- A **respiratory therapist** is an allied health professional who tests for and treats breathing disorders according to a physician's orders.

Using Health Care Facilities

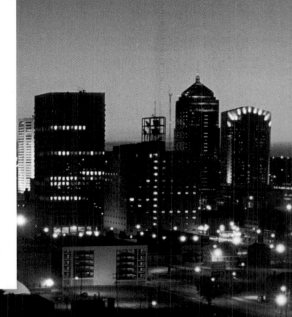

A **health care facility** is a place where people receive health care. A **hospital** is a health care facility where people can receive medical care, diagnosis, and treatment on an inpatient or outpatient basis. An **inpatient** is a person who stays at the hospital while receiving health care. An **outpatient** is a person who comes to the hospital or other health care facility for treatment, but does not stay overnight.

There are many different health care facilities in most communities. You and your family should be aware of where these facilities are located. You also will want to know the hours the facilities are open, the services provided, and the fees charged.

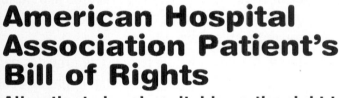

American Hospital Association Patient's Bill of Rights

All patients in a hospital have the right to...

- **receive respectful care;**
- **be given complete information regarding diagnosis, treatment, and prognosis;**
- **receive information necessary for consent prior to any procedure;**
- **refuse treatment;**
- **enjoy privacy regarding care and records;**
- **be granted requests for services within reason;**
- **be advised of any experimental procedure;**
- **expect continuity of care;**
- **receive explanation of the bill;**
- **know hospital regulations.**

Health Care Facilities

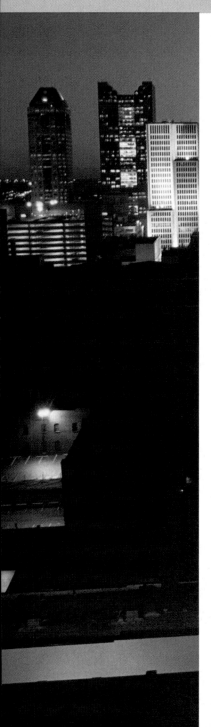

- **Convalescent** (kahn·vuh·LE·sent) **home**—a facility where people can recover from illness or surgery; similar to a hospital, but that does not provide intensive care, surgical, and emergency treatment facilities.

- **Emergency room**—a facility within a hospital where emergency services are provided without an appointment; used at night or on weekends when other care is not available.

- **Extended care facility**—a facility that provides nursing, personal, and residential care; also provides care for people who need assistance in daily living.

- **Government hospital**—a hospital run by the federal government for the benefit of a specific population, such as veterans.

- **Health center**—a facility that provides routine health care to a special population, such as low income families.

- **Health department clinic**—a facility in most state and local health departments that keeps records and performs services, such as immunizations and testing for sexually transmitted diseases.

- **Mental health clinic**—a facility that provides services for people having difficulty coping; might be open daily for 24 hours to help with crises.

- **Private hospital**—a hospital owned by private individuals; operates as a profit-making business.

- **Teaching hospital**—a hospital that is associated with a medical school and/or school of nursing; provides training in addition to the regular services of most hospitals.

- **Voluntary hospital**—a hospital owned by a community and not operated for profit.

- **Urgent care center** or **trauma center**—a facility separate from a hospital that offers immediate care; more expensive than a private physician and less expensive than an emergency room.

- **Walk-in surgery center**—a facility where surgery is performed on an outpatient basis.

Paying for Health Care

A **health insurance** (in·SHUR·ens) **policy** is a plan that helps pay the cost of health care. Health insurance policies are issued by private insurance companies, nonprofit insurance companies, and the federal government.

A policy with a private insurance company is paid for by the individual, by the company where the individual works, or by a combination of both. A **premium** is the required amount of money that will guarantee that an insurance company will help pay for health services.

The chart, Coverage in Health Insurance Policies, shows different kinds of coverage from insurance policies. Some policies pay the entire cost of medical care while others pay only a portion. A **deductible** is a specific amount that must be paid by the individual when insurance payments are needed.

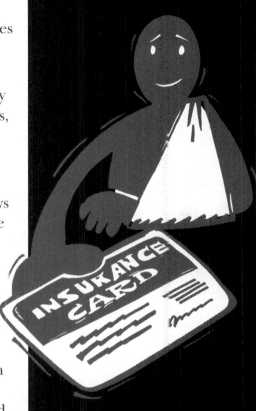

Some insurance companies require people who own a health insurance policy to go to a preferred provider. A **preferred provider** is a health care provider who appears on the approved list for payments from the health insurance company. Patients who use the physicians of the approved list pay lower rates than if they use other physicians. The insurance company contracts with preferred providers and offers managed care. **Managed care** is an organized system of health care services designed to control health care costs. The insurance company controls types of health care that policy owners receive and limits reimbursements for specific kinds of health care.

One type of managed care is a health maintenance organization (HMO). A **health maintenance** (MAYN·te·nuhns) **organization (HMO)** is a business that organizes health care services for its members. Consumers who belong to an HMO are not surprised by large medical bills because they have paid in advance. HMOs try to provide health care at a reduced cost. However, consumers belonging to an HMO must use preferred providers who also belong to the HMO. An HMO encourages regular checkups for preventive health care.

The federal government also is involved in payment for health care for some individuals. **Medicare** (MED·i·kehr) is a government health insurance plan for people 65 years of age and older and people who receive Social Security disability benefits for more than two years. People who are eligible for Medicare pay for part of their health care and the government pays the rest.

The state and federal government also are involved in payment for health care for certain individuals. **Medicaid** (MED·i·kayd) is a health insurance plan for the needy that is managed and paid for by the state and federal government. The state pays a portion of health care costs and the federal government pays the rest, or another portion. People who are poor and have dependent children or have a disability may qualify for Medicaid.

Coverage in Health Insurance Policies

- **Accident insurance** is insurance that pays hospitalization, medical, and surgical expenses that result from accidents.

- **Disability insurance** is insurance that replaces lost income should a person have an accident or illness requiring a period of recovery.

- **Hospitalization insurance** is insurance that pays the cost of a hospital stay.

- **Major medical insurance** is insurance that pays for extra expenses not covered by other insurance policies. Major medical insurance might cover treatment for diseases, such as cancer.

- **Medical insurance** is insurance that pays physicians' fees, laboratory fees from outside the hospital, and fees for prescription drugs.

- **Surgical insurance** is insurance that pays surgeons' fees.

Lesson 41

Review

Health Content

Write responses to the following:

1. What are ten questions to ask when choosing a health care provider? **page 437**
2. What are three examples of medical specialists? **page 439**
3. What are three examples of allied health professionals? **page 440**
4. Choose three health care facilities and describe their services. **page 442**
5. Describe ways to pay for health care. **page 443**

Vocabulary

Make a health care dictionary using each of the vocabulary words listed below and on page 436. Place them in alphabetical order and write the definition for each.

physician

medical doctor

osteopath

podiatrist

optometrist

dentist

anesthesiologist

cardiologist

dermatologist

gastroenterologist

geriatrician

gynecologist

neurologist

obstetrician

ophthalmologist

orthopedist

pediatrician

plastic surgeon

psychiatrist

urologist

registered nurse

nurse practitioner

dental hygienist

audiologist

pharmacist

physical therapist

registered dietitian

occupational therapist

speech pathologist

respiratory therapist

hospital

inpatient

outpatient

convalescent home

emergency room

extended care facility

government hospital

health center

health department clinic

mental health clinic

private hospital

teaching hospital

voluntary hospital

urgent care center

trauma center

walk-in surgery center

premium

deductible

preferred provider

managed care

health maintenance organization (HMO)

Medicare

Medicaid

accident insurance

disability insurance

hospitalization insurance

major medical insurance

medical insurance

surgical insurance

Volunteering for Health Causes

Vocabulary

volunteer

service learning

shadowing

mentor

license

credentials

Life Skills

- **I will be a health advocate by being a volunteer.**
- **I will investigate health careers.**

One of the best things you can do for your health is to help someone else. Helping others might be just as important to your health as eating healthfully and exercising regularly. You do not have to be wealthy to be a volunteer. Your time and caring are precious gifts to another person.

The Lesson Objectives

- Explain steps to get you started as a volunteer.
- Identify ways you can volunteer in your community.
- Discuss possible health careers.

Exploring Volunteer Opportunities

"I coach a group of younger boys and girls in softball—I really look forward to it!" "I planted trees one Saturday with other people in my town and I felt I was doing something good for the environment." "I can't wait to go to the senior center on Sundays—I feel so needed." These comments all came from teens who have discovered the benefits of being a volunteer. A **volunteer** is a person who provides a service without pay. When you give your time to helping others, you get several benefits. You increase your self-respect. You feel connected to others. You boost your immune system because you are having positive thoughts.

You might feel you do not have time to volunteer or you do not how to get started. But helping others does not require a huge time commitment. And it is easy to get started. Here are three steps.

- **List your skills, talents, and interests.** You will enjoy being a volunteer if your abilities and interests match your activities. If you enjoy playing piano, you might play for senior citizens. If you enjoy working with children, you might tutor them.

- **Ask your teacher or guidance counselor about opportunities to participate in service learning. Service learning** is an educational experience that combines learning with community service without pay.

- **Call or visit organizations for which you would like to volunteer.** Get permission from your parents or guardian. Find out what the organizations do and how you can volunteer. Ask if any training is needed, whether you will be supervised, and how many hours you are expected to work.

Consider volunteering for organizations that have careers in which you are interested. You can learn a lot by shadowing a mentor. **Shadowing** is spending time with a mentor as (s)he performs work activities. A **mentor** is a responsible, trusted person who guides and helps a younger person. You will find descriptions of some health careers beginning on page 448.

Ways to Volunteer

- **Serve food in a homeless shelter.**
- **Visit people in a senior citizens center.**
- **Tutor younger children in a school.**
- **Childsit for a neighbor who needs a break.**
- **Walk in a walk-a-thon for a good cause.**

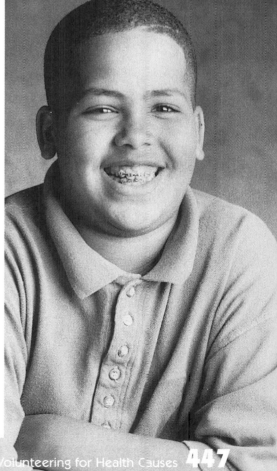

Health Career Guide

EEG Technologist

EEG technologists operate instruments (electroencephalographs) that record the brain's electrical activity or brain waves. The information gathered by these instruments helps physicians diagnose and treat injuries and diseases of the brain.

Responsibilities

- Obtaining a medical history from the patient
- Preparing the patient for the procedure
- Operating and maintaining the electroencephalograph

Qualifications

- High school diploma and specialized training
- Registration or certification required by some employers

Dialysis Technician

Dialysis technicians care for patients who need hemodialysis. Hemodialysis is a procedure in which a machine removes normal waste products from the blood of a person whose kidneys are unable to filter wastes.

Responsibilities

- Preparing the patient for hemodialysis
- Maintaining, repairing, and operating the machine
- Educating the patient about dialysis

Qualifications

- High school diploma and specialized training
- Certification required by some employers

Meteorologist

Meteorologists study Earth's atmosphere and the atmosphere's effects on the environment. They use computer models, weather satellites, weather radar, and remote sensors in many parts of the world to forecast the weather.

Responsibilities

- Forecasting the weather and warning the public about dangerous weather conditions
- Applying information about the weather to air-pollution control, agriculture, and air and sea transportation
- Conducting research on the atmosphere's properties and factors that affect weather

Qualifications

- Bachelor's or master's degree
- Specialized training

Federal Drug Enforcement Agent

Federal drug enforcement agents conduct investigations of illegal drug activity. They help prevent or stop the sale, use, possession, or manufacture of illegal drugs.

Responsibilities

- Gathering facts and collecting evidence by conducting interviews, examining records, and observing the activities of suspects
- Participating in raids or arrests
- Preparing reports and giving testimony in court

Qualifications

- Four-year degree
- One year experience in conducting criminal investigations
- Special training at the FBI Academy

Occupational Safety and Health Worker

Occupational safety and health workers inspect places of employment for unhealthful or unsafe working conditions. They help protect employees from diseases and unintentional injuries.

Responsibilities

- Visiting work sites and looking for work practices, equipment, machinery, and conditions that are unsafe
- Discussing findings and ways to improve work site conditions with employers
- Enforcing compliance with laws governing safe work conditions

Qualifications

- Bachelor's or master's degree
- Specialized training

Pharmacologist

Pharmacologists develop and test drugs and other chemicals. They study the effects of drugs and other chemicals on living things. They develop new drugs.

Responsibilities

- Developing and testing new drugs for use in medicine and determining side effects
- Testing chemicals, pollutants, and poisons to determine how they affect humans, animals, and the environment
- Identifying poisons and other substances

Qualifications

- Doctoral degree
- Specialized training
- Medical degree to conduct testing on humans

Pediatrician

Pediatricians specialize in the care and treatment of infants, children, and teens. Some pediatricians receive further specialization. For example, a pediatric oncologist specializes in cancer in children.

Responsibilities

- Examining patients, obtaining medical histories, and diagnosing diseases
- Providing treatment for patients with an injury or disease
- Counseling patients on diet, injury prevention, and other health issues

Qualifications

- Medical degree
- Specialized training in pediatrics

Physician Assistant

Physician assistants provide health care services to patients. Physician assistants work under the supervision of physicians. They carry out routine tasks that were previously performed by physicians.

Responsibilities

- Obtaining medical histories, performing physical exams, and making preliminary diagnoses
- Performing minor surgical procedures and giving first aid
- Ordering lab tests and giving injections

Qualifications

- Bachelor's degree
- Certification required by most states

Range Manager

Range managers oversee the use and conservation of rangelands. Rangelands are areas for livestock grazing, wildlife habitat, and recreational facilities. Range managers try to maintain resources without damaging the environment.

Responsibilities

- Researching ways to improve and increase the production of plants, wildlife, and livestock without hurting the environment
- Restoring rangelands that have been destroyed by fire or pests
- Developing plans for preventing erosion

Qualifications

- Bachelor's degree

School Psychologist

School psychologists counsel students and their families. Psychologists use their knowledge of psychology to help people solve their problems. Psychology is the study of the mind and behavior.

Responsibilities

- Evaluating academic skills and learning disabilities and helping students reach academic goals
- Testing to determine students' strengths and career goals
- Helping students deal with peer pressure, depression, difficult family relationships, and stress

Qualifications

- Doctoral degree
- License or certification required by all states

Podiatrist

Podiatrists specialize in the care and treatment of the foot. Podiatrists treat problems such as calluses, warts, ingrown toenails, and athlete's foot. They provide foot care for patients with arthritis and diabetes. People with diabetes might have circulation problems in their feet.

Responsibilities

- Taking X-rays and performing other diagnostic tests
- Treating foot problems by using corrective devices, prescribing medication, or manipulating the foot
- Teaching patients how to care for their feet

Qualifications

- Doctor of Podiatric Medicine (D.P.M.) degree
- License required by all states

Prosthetist

Prosthetists design and make special devices (prostheses) for patients with total or partial loss of limb due to illness or an accident. These devices include braces and artificial limbs. Prosthetists help patients use parts of the body that have been damaged or replace parts that have been lost.

Responsibilities

- Examining and measuring a patient for a device
- Designing and making devices to fit the needs of the patient
- Working with physicians and physical therapists to help patients adjust to their prostheses

Qualifications

- Bachelor's degree
- Certification required by some employers

Is This Career for Me?

Life Skill

I will investigate health careers.

Materials: Books on occupations, print-outs on occupations from the Internet

Directions: You will be more satisfied with a career that matches your interests and abilities. Complete this activity to get more information about a health career that might be a good match for you.

1. **Choose two health careers from this lesson that interest you.**

2. **Research interests and abilities for those careers.** For example, a range manager must like to work outdoors and must be able to work well with people. A pharmacologist must like to be a detective and must enjoy detailed laboratory work. Some careers require a license. A **license** is a document granted by a government agency to a person for the right to practice or to use a certain title. **Credentials** are preparations for performing a certain job. Find out what credentials are needed for the careers you select. Write about your findings.

3. **Research health careers not listed in this lesson that might interest you.** Write about your feelings.

4. **Summarize your findings in a one- to two-page paper.** Describe health careers you might enjoy and why.

Activity

Lesson 42

Review

Vocabulary

Write a separate sentence using each of the vocabulary words listed on page 446.

Health Content

Write responses to the following:

1. What are three benefits of being a volunteer? **page 447**

2. What are three steps to get you started as a volunteer? **page 447**

3. How can you find out about a health career through volunteering? **page 447**

4. What are five ways to volunteer? **page 447**

5. Choose three health careers in this lesson and describe how a person in that career helps others. **pages 448–450**

Unit 8 Review

Health Content

Review your answers for each Lesson Review in this unit. Then write answers to each of the following questions.

1. What are some community organizations that provide reliable health information? **Lesson 38 page 409**

2. How can you find health-related information using a computer? **Lesson 38 pages 412–413**

3. What types of appeals do advertisers use? **Lesson 39 pages 422–423**

4. What are reasons you should make your own shopping decisions? **Lesson 39 page 425**

5. Why should you be cautious when using a credit card? **Lesson 40 page 433**

6. How might a person who has shopping addiction behave? **Lesson 40 page 433**

7. What should you ask a health care provider? **Lesson 41 page 437**

8. What are ways you can pay for health care? **Lesson 41 page 443**

9. How can you get started as a volunteer? **Lesson 42 page 447**

10. What are services you can provide as a volunteer? **Lesson 42 page 447**

Vocabulary

Number a sheet of paper from 1–10. Select the correct vocabulary word. Write it next to the corresponding number. DO NOT WRITE IN THIS BOOK.

consumerism	mentor
debt	premium
e-mail	urgent care center
generic name	quackery
health care facility	savings

1. _____ is a quickly delivered message from one computer to another. **Lesson 38**

2. _____ is deception that involves the practice of promoting or selling useless products or services. **Lesson 39**

3. A(n) _____ is a place where people receive health care. **Lesson 41**

4. A(n) _____ is a facility separate from a hospital that offers immediate care. **Lesson 41**

5. _____ is the money set aside for future use. **Lesson 40**

6. _____ is the practice of choosing reliable and tested products, services, and information. **Lesson 38**

7. _____ is the condition of owing. **Lesson 40**

8. A(n) _____ is a responsible, trusted person who guides and helps a younger person. **Lesson 42**

9. A(n) _____ is a product or service that meets certain standards but does not have fancy packaging. **Lesson 39**

10. A(n) _____ is the required amount of money that will guarantee that an insurance company will help pay for health services. **Lesson 41**

The Responsible Decision-Making Model™

You are online with someone sharing thoughts about shopping. You do not know the person. The person starts asking questions such as "What is your name?" and "Where do you live?" Answer the following questions on a separate sheet of paper. Write "Does not apply" if a question does not apply to this situation.

1. Is it healthful to give personal information online? Why or why not?

2. Is it safe to give personal information online? Why or why not?

3. Is it legal to give personal information online? Why or why not?

4. Will you show respect for yourself if you give personal information online? Why or why not?

5. Will your parents or guardian approve if you give personal information online? Why or why not?

6. Will you demonstrate good character if you give personal information online? Why or why not?

What is the responsible decision to make in this situation?

Health Literacy

Effective Communication

Create an advertisement for a health-related product or service. Use two or three appeals you learned in Lesson 39.

Self-Directed Learning

Search the Internet for the Federal Communications Commission (FCC) home page. Find information relating to ways the FCC regulates communication via radio. Make a printout and share it with your class.

Critical Thinking

Pretend you have purchased headphones that do not work. Write a letter explaining your complaint to the president of the company.

Responsible Citizenship

Look in your local newspaper. Find a list of community organizations that need volunteers. Make a list of these agencies and get permission to post your list in your school.

Multicultural Health

Research the behaviors of people in another culture toward time. Compare them to behaviors in your culture. For example, people in some cultures rush through the day. People in other cultures take more time to eat or take long midday breaks from work.

Family Involvement

Share with your family what you have learned about ways to volunteer. Discuss with your parents or guardian ways you volunteer as a family.

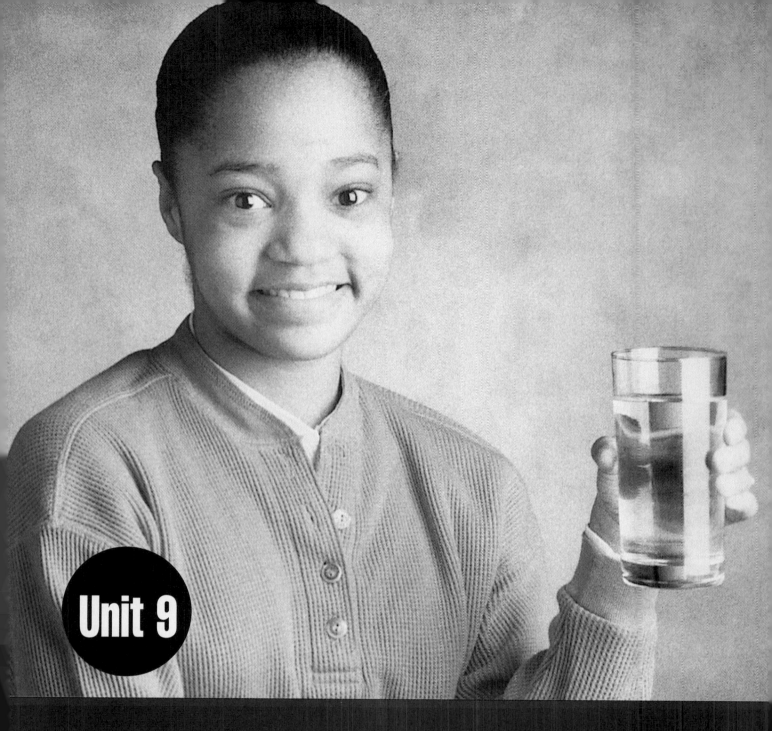

Unit 9

Environmental
Health

Respect for the Environment

Vocabulary

environment
ecosystem
ecology
ecologists
pollution
pollutant
mutagen
teratogen
chlorofluorocarbons
(CFCs)
ozone layer
ozone
malignant melanoma
cataract
greenhouse effect
global warming
rain forest
regulatory agencies
Environmental Protection
Agency (EPA)
Occupational Safety and
Health Administration
(OSHA)
National Institute for
Occupational Safety and
Health (NIOSH)

Life Skills

- **I will stay informed about environmental issues.**
- **I will be a health advocate for the environment.**

The **environment** is everything living and nonliving that is around a person. On a small scale, it is the ground you walk on, the air you breathe, the water you drink, the food you eat, the noise you hear, the places you go, and the people you see. It is your home, your school, and your town. On a larger scale, the environment includes the planet Earth and everything in, on, and around it.

The Lesson Objectives

- Explain how balance is maintained in an ecosystem.
- Name three ways pollutants enter the body.
- Describe how the thinning of the ozone layer affects health.
- Describe effects that might be produced by global warming.
- Discuss ways rain forests help an ecosystem maintain balance.
- List five actions teens living in poverty can take to improve their living environment.
- Name three regulatory agencies that protect the environment.

Maintaining Balance

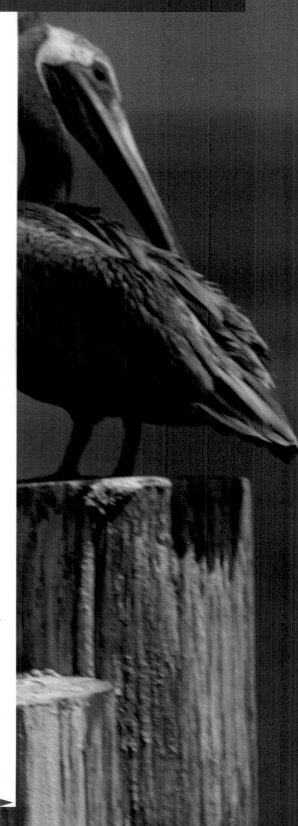

An **ecosystem** is a system made up of living organisms, air, water, soil, and sunlight. Living organisms within an ecosystem can be described as producers, consumers, or decomposers.

Producers are the living organisms that make new food resources. Green plants are producers. Photosynthesis (foh·toh·SIN·thuh·suhs) is the process by which green plants use energy from the sun to change water and carbon dioxide into food. Green plants use some food right away, store some food in their roots, and use the remaining food to grow leaves, stems, and fruits. Animals eat the leaves, stems, and fruits for food. Green plants also produce oxygen during photosynthesis. Other living organisms need this oxygen for survival.

Consumers are living organisms that eat other organisms for food. Some consumers eat producers. Herbivores are living organisms that eat green plants. Some consumers eat other consumers. Carnivores are consumers that eat other consumers; they also are called meat eaters. Omnivores are consumers that eat both green plants and animals.

Decomposers are the living organisms that eat the remains of dead plants and animals. Bacteria, fungi, and earthworms are decomposers. They break down the remains of green plants and animals.

Most living organisms need air, water, soil, and sunlight to survive. Many animals, including humans, breathe air to get oxygen. They exhale carbon dioxide. Green plants use carbon dioxide to produce food and more oxygen. All living organisms need water. Humans need six to eight glasses of water a day for body processes. Water makes up most of the body, including blood. The cells of all living things are mostly water. Green plants obtain nutrients and water from the soil. They also get water from the air. Soil contains minerals, such as salt, phosphorus, and iron. Soil is replenished with nutrients when decomposers break down the remains of plants and animals. Sunlight is used by producers to store energy in food.

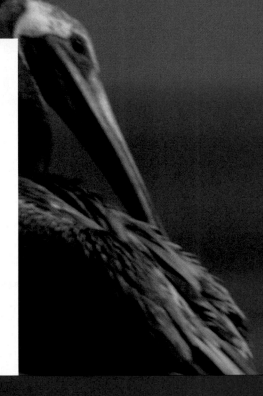

There is interdependence within an ecosystem. Living organisms depend on one another for survival. They also depend on physical factors, such as clean air and water, nutrient-rich soil, and sunlight. The ecosystem is affected when the quality of the air or water, condition of the soil, or amount of sunlight is changed. Balance is destroyed and the health and well-being of people are affected.

Consider the world as an ecosystem. How do people in one country depend on people in another country for survival? How might the quality of the air in one country affect people who live in another part of the world? How might the condition of the soil in one country affect people who live in another part of the world? Why is it important to have all people protect the ecosystem?

Environment Poetry

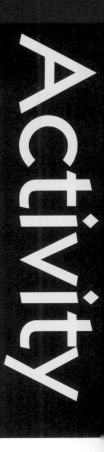

Activity

Life Skill

I will be a health advocate for the environment.

Materials: Pen or pencil; computer (optional); markers or colored pencils

Directions: Write a poem on maintaining balance within an ecosystem.

1. **Write a ten line poem about balance within an ecosystem.**

2. **Use as many of these words as possible:** ecosystem, living organisms, air, water, soil, sunlight, producers, consumers, decomposers, photosynthesis, interdependence.

3. **Use markers or colored pencils.** Make a border to go around the poem.

4. **Put your poem on the bulletin board in your classroom.**

Destroying Balance

Ecology is the study of the relationship between living organisms and the environment. **Ecologists** are people who study ecology. Five ways an ecosystem might be upset or destroyed include:

1. **Pollution**
2. **Changes in the atmosphere**
3. **Changes in the climate**
4. **Depletion of natural resources**
5. **Poverty and overcrowded living conditions**

Pollution

Pollution is any change in the air, water, soil, noise level, or temperature that has a negative effect on life and health. A **pollutant** is something that causes pollution. Natural events, such as smoke from a forest fire, can produce pollutants. Most pollutants, however, are a by-product of people's actions. Cigarette smoke is an example of a pollutant produced by people's actions. Pollutants enter the body in three ways:

1. **Through the skin**
2. **Through the digestive system**
3. **Through the lungs**

Some pollutants are an immediate threat to life and health. Breathing secondhand smoke for several years can cause heart disease and lung cancer. Inhaling smoke from a forest fire can cause someone to suffocate and die. Exposure to pollutants over a period of time also can be a threat to life and health.

Some pollutants alter genes and affect offspring. A **mutagen** is an environmental agent that causes changes in the genetic material of living cells. These changes often increase the risk of cancer. A **teratogen** is an environmental agent that crosses the placenta of a pregnant female and causes miscarriage or birth defects in offspring.

Ways to Reduce Pollution:

Suggestions for ways to reduce a variety of types of pollution will be provided in Lessons 44 and 45.

Changes in Atmosphere: The Ozone Layer

Do you own any aerosol sprays, such as hairsprays or disinfectants? Some contain CFCs. **Chlorofluorocarbons (CFCs)** are a group of gases that are easy to compress and expand. CFCs are used in aerosol sprays, as well as air conditioning units, fire extinguishers, refrigerators, and styrofoam products. In the United States, aerosol sprays that contain CFCs have been banned. When released into the air, CFCs rise into the upper atmosphere and damage the ozone layer. The **ozone layer** is a layer in the upper atmosphere where ozone traps dangerous ultraviolet radiation from the sun and prevents it from reaching Earth's surface. **Ozone** is a form of oxygen created by the energy of sunlight acting upon oxygen.

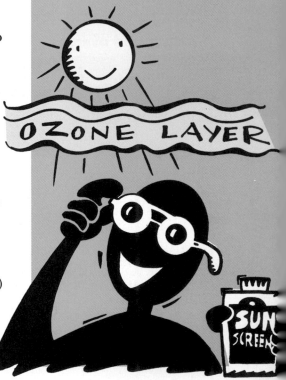

Damage to the ozone layer makes it become thinner, allowing more of the sun's ultraviolet rays to reach Earth's surface. The increased exposure to ultraviolet rays affects the health of human beings. There has been a dramatic increase in skin cancer, including malignant melanoma. **Malignant melanoma** (muh·LIG·nuhnt mel·uh·NOH·muh) is a form of skin cancer that is often fatal. There also has been an increase in the number of people who develop cataracts. A **cataract** is a loss of transparency of the lens of the eye.

Ways to Preserve the Ozone Layer

1. **Avoid using styrofoam products.**
2. **Reduce use of products that release CFCs.**

Protect Yourself from a Thinning Ozone Layer

1. **Wear a sunscreen with a sun protection factor (SPF) of at least 15.**
2. **Wear sunglasses that block the ultraviolet rays from the sun.**

Changes in Climate: The Greenhouse Effect

You might not be upset if the average winter day were a few degrees warmer. However, scientists might be. Scientists all over the world are tracking Earth's average temperature. They are examining the greenhouse effect. The **greenhouse effect** is the trapping of heat from the sun by gases, such as CO_2, in Earth's atmosphere.

Have you ever been in a greenhouse? A greenhouse for plants works the same way. The sun's rays pass through the glass and warm the inside of the greenhouse. However, heat cannot easily escape through the glass. This keeps the greenhouse warm and moist.

If you walk through a greenhouse, you notice how well the plants thrive. Plants are growing in the greenhouse that might not survive anywhere else. This is because the environment is just right for them. They grow best in the correct temperature. Plants need adequate moisture. People who own greenhouses recognize the effects of the environment on plants. They want their plants to thrive so people will want to buy them.

What are the effects of climate on you? How will you thrive best? How can the sun's rays affect you? Is the greenhouse effect on Earth similar to the effect produced by a greenhouse built for plants?

The greenhouse effect is produced in much the same way. There is no glass enclosing Earth. However, some gases in Earth's atmosphere, such as carbon dioxide, water vapor, and other gases, act like the glass roof of a greenhouse. The sun's rays pass through these gases and heat Earth's surface. Much of this heat cannot pass back through the gases. Without the greenhouse effect, the earth would be too cold for most life. However, large amounts of gases from air pollution trap more heat. This might result in global warming.

Global Warming

Global warming is an ongoing increase in Earth's temperature. Some ecologists estimate that the average temperature of Earth might increase by 1°C within 30 years and by 3°C within a hundred years. An increase in Earth's temperature might produce other changes in the environment. The polar ice caps might melt as the temperature rises. This would cause the sea level to rise several feet. Flooding might occur in states at or below sea level, such as Florida and Louisiana. The increase in temperature might also cause rivers and lakes to evaporate. Droughts would become more common. There might be more difficulty raising crops.

The greenhouse effect might be increased by pollutants that are by-products of people's activities. Carbon dioxide is a natural part of the atmosphere. But people are increasing the amounts of carbon dioxide. Carbon dioxide is a waste product produced by burning gasoline and other fossil fuels such as coal, oil, or natural gas. Trees use some of the carbon dioxide from the atmosphere. However, they cannot use all of the extra carbon dioxide being formed by various human activities.

Some scientists think air pollutants will cause changes in the atmosphere that will result in a decrease in temperatures. Others think we cannot predict how the Earth will change. But they all agree that air pollution is changing our climate.

Ways to Reduce the Greenhouse Effect

1. Use less energy, including energy from coal, oil, and natural gas.
2. Car pool to reduce gasoline consumption.
3. Work to save rain forests (trees).

Depletion of Resources: Rain Forests

A **rain forest** is a group of trees and plants covering a warm, wet area. Rain forests cover about 7 percent of Earth's land surface. They provide a place for half of the species on Earth to live. The trees in rain forests absorb carbon dioxide and help maintain the balance of the ecosystem. But rain forests are being destroyed. More than 100 acres of rain forests are cut down each minute. Farmers cut rain forests to make room for more crops. Ranchers clear rain forests to provide pasture. Logging companies cut rain forests for lumber. Changes in the ecosystem will occur as rain forests are depleted or used up. Many species of plants and animals will become extinct. There will be fewer trees to absorb carbon dioxide from the atmosphere. An increase in carbon dioxide in the atmosphere increases the greenhouse effect. Tropical rain forests contain plants that have never been studied. Some plants might contain chemicals to fight disease or be useful for food crops.

Ways to Conserve Rain Forests

1. **Plant a tree.**
2. **Recycle paper.**
3. **Use both sides of paper.**

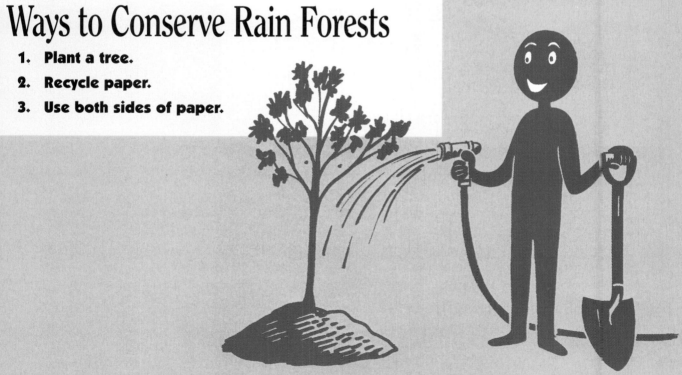

Poverty and Crowded Living Conditions

Another environmental issue of concern focuses on economic and social living conditions. Today, many people live in poverty and have limited access to food, clothing, medical care, and shelter. People who are poor and have crowded living conditions are more likely to:

- **be depressed;**
- **feel hostile toward others;**
- **be stressed;**
- **be malnourished;**
- **have poor health status.**

Teens who live in poverty have a higher risk of doing poorly in school, dropping out, becoming teen parents, and using alcohol and other drugs. Violence and drug use are more common in poor, crowded environments.

Teens who live in poverty must take some actions to improve their living environment. They can:

1. attend school in order to prepare for a career to earn a living and overcome poverty;

2. avoid alcohol, tobacco, and other drug use;

3. stay away from violence;

4. spend time with adults and mentors who behave in healthful ways;

5. avoid teen marriage and parenthood, which continues the cycle of poverty.

Environmental Protection

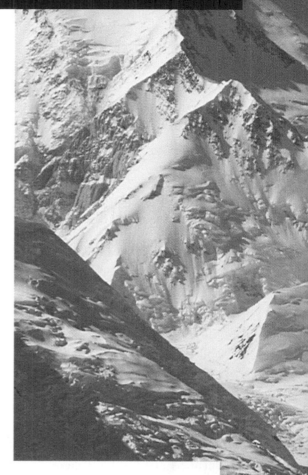

Many agencies focus on protecting and improving the environment. **Regulatory agencies** are government agencies that enforce laws to protect the general public. The **Environmental Protection Agency (EPA)** is a regulatory agency responsible for reducing and controlling environmental pollution. This agency maintains and improves the quality of the environment by setting standards, monitoring conditions, and providing education and research. The EPA deals with safe drinking water, air and water quality, ground water and wetland protection, solid and hazardous waste, pesticides, and radon.

Two government regulatory agencies focus on the environment in the workplace. The **Occupational Safety and Health Administration (OSHA)** is a regulatory agency responsible for the workplace environment. The **National Institute for Occupational Safety and Health (NIOSH)** is an agency that makes recommendations for workplace safety.

Environmental protection agencies exist at the state and local level, too. Contact your local health department to learn the names of the environmental protection agencies in your community.

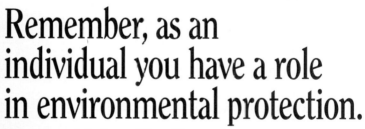

Remember, as an individual you have a role in environmental protection.

You must join with others to:

- **stop pollution;**
- **choose behavior that prevents harmful changes in the atmosphere;**
- **choose behavior that prevents harmful changes in the climate;**
- **conserve natural resources;**
- **improve living conditions for all.**

Follow a...

Health Behavior Contract

Name:_____ **Date:**_____

Copy the health behavior contract on a separate sheet of paper.

DO NOT WRITE IN THIS BOOK.

Life Skill: I will be a health advocate for the environment.

Effect On My Health: A health advocate for the environment chooses actions that protect the environment. When I am a health advocate, I protect my health, too. Suppose I encourage other people to protect the ozone layer. If they do, their actions reduce my risk of being exposed to UV radiation. I am less likely to get skin cancer. Suppose I encourage more people to have a no-smoking policy in their homes. Then I am less likely to develop respiratory diseases. When I am a health advocate, I also am working to protect the health of others.

My Plan: I will choose an action for which I can be a health advocate. For example, I might choose to encourage five families to have a no-smoking policy in their homes. I will list three things I can do as a health advocate. I will get permission from a parent or guardian. Then I will schedule a time to do each task.

The action for which I will be a health advocate is:

The three things I can do as a health advocate:_____

_____

_____

_____

The schedule for doing each task is:_____

_____

How My Plan Worked: I will discuss how effective I was as a health advocate.

Apply...

The Responsible Decision-Making Model™

You have started finding ways to reduce wasting paper. A friend says, "Why bother? The actions of one person can't make any difference."

Answer the following questions on a separate sheet of paper. Write "Does not apply" if a question does not apply to this situation.

1. Is it healthful to waste paper? Why or why not?
2. Is it safe to waste paper? Why or why not?
3. Is it legal to waste paper? Why or why not?
4. Will you show respect for yourself and others if you waste paper? Why or why not?
5. Will your parents or guardian approve if you waste paper? Why or why not?
6. Will you demonstrate good character if you waste paper? Why or why not?

What is the responsible decision to make in this situation?

Lesson 43

Review

Vocabulary

Write a separate sentence using each of the vocabulary words listed on page 456.

Health Content

Write responses to the following:

1. How is balance maintained in an ecosystem? **pages 457–458**
2. What are five ways an ecosystem can be destroyed? **page 459**
3. What are three ways pollutants enter the body? **page 459**
4. How do chlorofluorocarbons affect the ozone layer? **page 460**
5. What are ways to preserve the ozone layer? Ways to protect yourself from the thinning ozone layer? **page 460**
6. How does the greenhouse effect influence Earth's temperature? **page 461**
7. What effects might be produced by global warming? **page 462**
8. What are ways rain forests help an ecosystem maintain balance? Ways to conserve rain forests? **page 463**
9. What are five actions teens living in poverty can take to improve their living environment? **page 464**
10. What are three regulatory agencies that protect the environment? **page 465**

Pollution

Vocabulary

pollution
pollutant
air pollution
carbon monoxide
particulates
motor vehicle emissions
thermal inversion
smog
Environmental Protection
Agency (EPA)
pollutant standard index
(PSI)
sick building syndrome
(SBS)
asbestos
formaldehyde
radon
lead
mercury
secondhand smoke
water pollution
water runoff
sewage
PCBs
dioxins
thermal pollution
trihalomethanes
noise

- **I will help keep the air clean.**
- **I will help keep the water safe.**
- **I will help keep noise at a safe level.**

Pollution is any change in the air, water, soil, noise level, or temperature that has a negative effect on life and health. An environment that is polluted increases your risk of illness. A **pollutant** is something that causes pollution.

The environment not only affects you—you affect the environment. For example, you breathe the air, use water, and make noise. This lesson will focus on air pollution, water pollution, and noise pollution. You will learn ways to keep air clean, water safe, and noise at a safe level.

The Lesson Objectives

- Name five health conditions caused by airborne pollutants.
- State five ways to keep the air clean.
- Explain why it is risky to breathe polluted indoor air.
- Give ways to keep indoor air clean.
- Discuss how water pollution can occur.
- List ways to keep the water safe.
- List ways to keep noise at a safe level.

Keeping the Air Clean

Air pollution is the contamination of air with undesirable gases, particles, dust, smoke, and chemicals. Air pollution is a threat to health and well-being. Health conditions caused by airborne pollutants include: bronchitis, emphysema, lung cancer, asthma, and eye irritation. Sources of air pollution include tobacco smoke, particulates, motor vehicle emissions, thermal inversion and smog, and acid rain.

Breathing Tobacco Smoke

Secondhand tobacco smoke is a common air pollutant. Secondhand tobacco smoke contains carbon monoxide and nitrogen oxides. **Carbon monoxide** (KAR·buhn muh·NAHK·syd) **(CO)** is an odorless, tasteless, colorless, poisonous gas. Carbon monoxide attaches to red blood cells and this reduces the amount of oxygen red blood cells can carry. The heart beats faster to supply oxygen to the body cells. Nitrogen oxides irritate the eyes and respiratory passages. Breathing secondhand smoke increases the risk of lung cancer and asthma.

Breathing Particulates

Particulates are tiny particles in the air. Soot, ashes, dirt, dust, and pollen are examples of particulates. Particulates harm the cilia and surfaces of the respiratory system. When inhaled, particulates can cause a person to have coughing spells or asthma attacks.

Breathing Motor Vehicle Emissions

Motor vehicle emissions are products of the combustion of motor fuels, such as gasoline. These products include carbon monoxide, airborne lead, sulfur oxides, and nitrogen oxides. The switch to unleaded gasoline has lowered the amount of lead in the air. But the amounts of other gases have not been lowered because more automobiles and trucks are on the road. Breathing motor vehicle emissions increases the risk of lung cancer, asthma, and bronchitis.

Breathing Ozone Created from Smog

Thermal inversion is a condition that occurs when a layer of warm air forms above a cooler layer. Air is unable to circulate and pollutants are trapped in the cooler layer. When pollutants cannot escape, smog forms.

Smog is a combination of smoke and fog. In the presence of sunlight, smog combines with motor vehicle emissions and creates harmful gases.

One of the harmful gases in smog is ozone. Ozone in the upper atmosphere promotes health by trapping and preventing UV light from the sun from reaching Earth. However, ozone in the air you breathe irritates the eyes, lungs, and throat. It also produces headaches, coughing, and shortness of breath. Healthy, nonsmoking adults might have inflammation of the lungs and bronchial tubes within two hours of breathing ozone. Teens are at even greater risk when breathing ozone.

The Pollutant Standard Index

The **Environmental Protection Agency (EPA)** is a regulatory agency responsible for reducing and controlling environmental pollution. The EPA measures air quality.

The **pollutant standard index (PSI)** is a measure of air quality based on the sum of the levels of five different pollutants. The EPA warns the public when the PSI is high. It is best not to exercise outdoors when the PSI is high.

Ways to Keep the Air Clean

1. **Do not smoke tobacco products.**
2. **Ask other people not to smoke tobacco products.**
3. **Ask family members who drive to avoid leaded gas and to drive at a reasonable speed.**
4. **Carpool whenever possible.**
5. **Pay attention to the PSI and do not exercise outdoors when it is high.**

Being Healthy Indoors

Most people spend 90 percent of their time indoors. Newer homes and buildings are often made airtight to save energy. There is less air circulation and more indoor air pollution in airtight homes and buildings. **Sick building syndrome (SBS)** is an illness that results from indoor air pollution. The signs of SBS include headaches, irritated eyes, nausea, dizziness, hoarseness, and respiratory conditions. SBS is very risky for the elderly, infants, and people with asthma. SBS usually disappears when people get away from the building and spend some time outdoors.

There are many sources of indoor pollution. Chemicals, asbestos, formaldehyde, carbon monoxide, radon, lead, mercury, and secondhand smoke change the quality of indoor air.

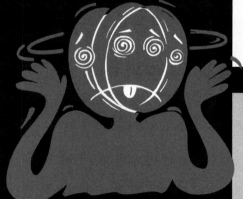

Breathing Chemicals

Cleaning agents and insecticides are dangerous to breathe. Some hobby supplies, such as glue, release toxic fumes into the air. Breathing chemicals can cause respiratory damage. The brain can be affected when toxic fumes are inhaled and enter the blood.

Breathing Asbestos

Asbestos is a heat-resistant mineral that is found in building materials. Today, asbestos use is banned. However, it is present in older buildings and homes. It was once used in heating systems, floor and ceiling tiles, shingles, and insulation around household pipes. Asbestos fibers can get into the air. Breathing asbestos has been linked to lung and gastrointestinal cancer. Your family can have a certified expert check for asbestos at your residence. Asbestos can be removed or sealed in places.

Breathing Formaldehyde

Formaldehyde (for·MAL·duh·hyd) is a colorless gas with a strong odor. It was once used to make plywood, furniture, and other wood products. Many mobile homes have high formaldehyde levels because of the plywood used in them.

Formaldehyde also can be found in insulation, cosmetics, carpets, floor coverings, and household appliances. Cigarette smoke contains this harmful gas. Breathing formaldehyde causes shortness of breath, coughing, dizziness, eye irritation, headaches, nausea, asthma attacks, and cancer.

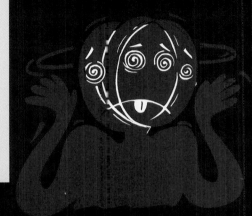

Breathing Carbon Monoxide

Carbon monoxide (CO) is an odorless, tasteless, colorless, poisonous gas. Faulty space heaters, furnaces, and water heaters can release carbon monoxide. Signs of carbon monoxide poisoning include headaches, nausea, vomiting, fatigue, and dizziness. You can become unconscious and die from carbon monoxide poisoning. Your family can install a carbon monoxide detector in your residence.

Breathing Radon

Radon is an odorless, colorless radioactive gas that is given off by rocks and soil. Radon enters homes from cracks in the floors and basement walls, and through drains and sump pumps. One in 12 homes has an unsafe radon level. Breathing radon increases the risk of lung cancer. Smoking cigarettes and breathing radon multiplies the risk of lung cancer. Your family can use a radon testing kit to check the radon level at your residence. Cracks in the floor and basement walls can be sealed and fans can be installed to lower the radon level.

Breathing Lead

Lead is a toxic metal that may be present in air or water. At one time, lead was used to make paint. Many young people have a toxic level of lead in their blood from chewing on objects covered with lead paint. Lead poisoning destroys brain cells, reduces memory, slows reaction time, and causes learning disabilities. High concentrations of lead in the blood can cause sterility, kidney disease, and anemia. The central nervous system can be damaged. Pregnant females who have high levels of lead in their blood can miscarry.

The American Academy of Pediatrics and the Centers for Disease Control and Prevention recommend that children from age six months to six years be screened each year for blood levels of lead. Children who live in older housing need to be screened more often.

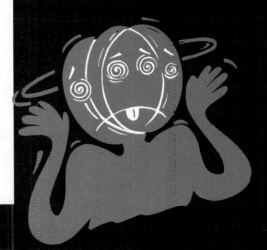

Breathing Mercury

Mercury is a metal contained in some latex paints that might cause poisoning. The risk of mercury poisoning is greatest when painting is being done and shortly after. Signs of mercury poisoning include tremors, fast heartbeat, sweating, aching, kidney disease, skin disorders, and changes in mood.

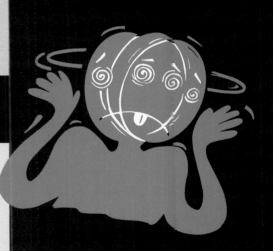

Breathing Secondhand Smoke

Secondhand smoke is exhaled smoke and sidestream smoke. Secondhand cigarette smoke has been identified by the EPA as a known cause of lung cancer. Breathing secondhand smoke increases the risk of respiratory infections and asthma. You and your family should not smoke or allow others to do so in your presence.

Ways to Keep Indoor Air Clean

1. **Limit your use of household cleaners in aerosol containers.**

2. **Use hobby supplies, such as glue, in areas that are well ventilated.**

3. **Check your house for asbestos and have it removed or sealed in place.**

4. **Make sure wood products are sealed to eliminate formaldehyde fumes.**

5. **Check often to see that space heaters, furnaces, and water heaters are working properly.**

6. **Install a carbon monoxide detector in your home.**

7. **Check the radon level in your home. Seal cracks in the floor and basement and install fans to lower the radon level.**

8. **Have family members from ages six months to six years screened each year for blood levels of lead.**

9. **Avoid breathing latex paint containing mercury.**

10. **Do not smoke or allow others to smoke.**

Apply...

The Responsible Decision-Making Model™

Your aunt smokes cigarettes. You have considered asking her politely not to smoke when you visit. You are afraid you will hurt her feelings.

Answer the following questions on a separate sheet of paper. Write "Does not apply" if a question does not apply to this situation.

1. Is it healthful to inhale secondhand smoke? Why or why not?

2. Is it safe to inhale secondhand smoke? Why or why not?

3. Is it legal to inhale secondhand smoke? Why or why not?

4. Will you show respect for yourself if you inhale secondhand smoke? Why or why not?

5. Will your parents or guardian approve if you inhale secondhand smoke? Why or why not?

6. Will you demonstrate good character if you inhale secondhand smoke? Why or why not?

What is the responsible decision to make in this situation?

Keeping the Water Safe

After air, water is the most essential requirement of the human body. Humans can live without water for only a few days. Drinking clean water is essential to health. **Water pollution** is the contamination of water with sewage, waste, gases, or chemicals that harm health. There are many different sources of water pollution.

Water Runoff

When you think of water pollution, you probably think of wastes and chemicals being dumped into the water. But, water runoff is a major source of water pollution. **Water runoff** is water that runs off the land into a body of water, and contains solids and dissolved substances. Farmers water their crops. Only some of the water is absorbed by the crops. Some water flows along the surface of the land until it reaches a stream, lake, or ocean. Some water trickles into the ground until it reaches an underground stream known as groundwater. The water runoff from agriculture might contain fertilizer, pesticides, and insecticides. There is other water runoff. There might be waste or sewage on land that gets into underground water, lakes, and streams when it rains. Chemicals that have been dumped enter water this way also.

Sewage and Waste

Sewage and waste from animals can get into the water. **Sewage** is waste liquids or matter carried off by sewers. Sewage and waste increase the amount of nitrates in the water. Nitrates can accumulate in groundwater and contaminate wells. Infants who drink this water containing nitrates can get blood diseases. Polluted groundwater can cause cancer and other diseases in adults.

Chemicals

PCBs are chemicals containing chlorine. Discarded electrical equipment at dump sites can break down and release PCBs into groundwater. PCBs collect in the fatty tissues of the body and liver. They cause birth defects, reproductive disorders, liver and kidney damage, and cancer. **Dioxins** are a group of chemicals used in insecticides. Chlorine bleaching of pulp and paper at mills produces dioxins. The dioxins get into the water. They are found in fish that live downstream from mills. People who eat fish contaminated with dioxins become very ill.

Thermal Pollution

Thermal pollution is pollution of water with heat. Thermal pollution kills aquatic plants. Heat reduces the amount of oxygen in water. Without enough oxygen or plants for food, fish die. Thermal pollution occurs when heated water used to cool steam turbines in power plants is dumped into nearby bodies of water.

Trihalomethanes

Most water treatment systems use chlorine to purify water. **Trihalomethanes** (try·ha·luh·ME·thaynz) are harmful chemicals that are produced when chlorine attacks pollutants in the water. Any drinking water that contains these chemicals is dangerous. These chemicals increase the risk of bladder and rectal cancer, birth defects, and central nervous system disorders.

Lead

Lead enters the water from lead pipes and water lines in older housing. Lead can affect almost every organ and system in the body. The most sensitive is the central nervous system, particularly in children. Lead also damages kidneys and the immune system. The effects of lead are the same whether it is breathed or swallowed.

Ways to Keep the Water Safe

1. **Do not dump garbage or chemicals into lakes, streams, rivers, or ditches.**

2. **Do not pour or spill harmful chemicals on the ground; they can seep into groundwater supplies.**

3. **Do not pour toxic chemicals down the drain or in the toilet. Dispose of them at a hazardous waste collection center.**

4. **Contact the public health department if drinking water from a faucet has an orange or red hue. It may be unsafe to drink.**

5. **Run the tap a few minutes before taking water for drinking or cooking. This lowers the risk of drinking lead in standing water.**

Keeping Noise at a Safe Level

Noise is sound that produces discomfort or annoyance. Too much noise can cause stress, increase blood pressure, and increase blood cholesterol. Exposure to loud noises causes headaches, tension, sleep disturbances, and anxiety. Exposure to very loud noises can cause permanent loss of hearing.

Ways to Keep Noise at a Safe Level

1. **Keep music low enough to hear someone speaking when listening to music through headphones.**

2. **Sit at a safe distance from performers or speakers when attending a concert.**

3. **Wear hearing protection devices, such as earplugs, when exposed to loud noise.**

4. **Wear earplugs when you cut the grass, use power tools, or use a weed trimmer.**

5. **Press your fingers against your ears if there is a sudden, loud noise.**

6. **Do not drink alcohol. Alcohol intensifies the impact of noise. Drinking alcohol increases the risk of long-term hearing damage.**

7. **Have your hearing checked regularly by a professional.**

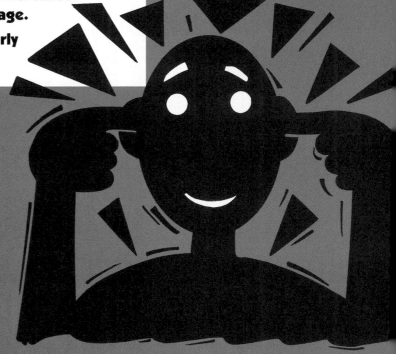

Pollution Rap

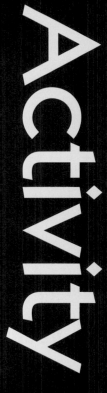

Life Skills

I will help keep the air clean.

I will help keep the water safe.

I will help keep noise at a safe level.

Materials: Paper, pen or pencil, handheld musical instruments

Directions: Create a rap song to share ideas on preventing pollution.

1. Your teacher will arrange your class into small groups.
2. **Your group will create a rap song that is at least 12 lines long.** The song should include ways to keep the air, water, or noise level safe.
3. Perform your rap for the class.

Lesson 44

Review

Vocabulary

Write a separate sentence using each of the vocabulary words listed on page 468.

Health Content

Write responses to the following:

1. What are five health conditions caused by airborne pollutants? **page 469**
2. Why is it risky to breathe tobacco smoke? Particulates? Motor vehicle emissions? Ozone? **pages 469–470**
3. What are five ways to keep the air clean? **page 470**
4. What are signs of sick building syndrome? **page 471**
5. Why is it risky to breathe chemicals? Asbestos? Formaldehyde? Carbon monoxide? Radon? Lead? Mercury? Secondhand smoke? **pages 471–473**
6. What are ten ways to keep the indoor air clean? **page 474**
7. Why is water runoff a major source of pollution? **page 475**
8. Why is it dangerous for water to be polluted with sewage and animal wastes? PCBs and dioxins? Heat from power plants? Trihalomethanes? Lead? **pages 476–477**
9. What are five ways to keep the water safe? **page 477**
10. What are seven ways to keep noise at a safe level? **page 478**

Conserving Resources

Vocabulary

renewable resource

nonrenewable resource

conservation

energy

energy conservation

water conservation

land conservation

landfill

solid waste

toxic waste

radwaste

precycling

recycling

biodegradable

composting

Life Skills

• **I will help conserve energy and natural resources.**

• **I will precycle, recycle, and dispose of waste properly.**

Natural resources are either renewable or nonrenewable. **Renewable resources** are resources that can be replaced. Examples are trees, water, and soil. Though they can be replaced, replacement takes time. These resources must be managed wisely so they are in adequate supply. **Nonrenewable resources** are resources that cannot be replaced once they are used. Examples are minerals and oil. To protect the environment, all resources must be saved. **Conservation** is the saving of resources.

The Lesson Objectives

• List ways to conserve energy.

• List ways to conserve water.

• List ways to conserve land.

Energy Conservation

Energy is the ability to do work. Heat and electrical energy are obtained from resources, such as oil, coal, natural gas, falling water, and nuclear power. **Energy conservation** is actions to save heat and electricity. Most energy comes from the sun. Plant material is buried under rocks and soil in Earth. Heat and pressure convert the plant material into fossil fuels—oil, coal, and natural gas. The energy in fossil fuels originally came from the sun. Energy is released when fossil fuels are burned.

Falling water is another source of energy. After a dam is constructed, the energy from rushing water is converted into electricity.

Another source of energy is radioactive elements. Radioactive elements are one source of nuclear power. Nuclear power gets its energy from the forces that hold together nuclei in atoms. Energy is released when nuclei split. This energy in the form of heat is used to boil water to make steam. The steam is then used to generate electricity.

Oil, coal, natural gas, and radioactive elements are nonrenewable resources. They will eventually be used up. There is a special problem with nuclear power. Nuclear power produces highly radioactive waste material. It is difficult to dispose of this material safely.

Scientists and environmental specialists are working to develop new ways to conserve energy. They are working to develop new sources of energy. For now, energy conservation involves using less heat. Energy conservation also involves using less electricity and water. There are ways you can use less heat. There are ways you can use less electricity and water. The rest of this lesson gives you suggestions. Put the suggestions to practice. Make a health behavior contract. Use this life skill: *I will help conserve energy and natural resources.*

I will help conserve energy and natural resources.

I will help conserve energy and natural resources.

I will help conserve energy and natural resources.

Ways to Conserve Energy

1. Turn off lights when you leave the room.

2. Use fluorescent lights except for reading; they use 75 percent less energy than incandescent (heat) bulbs.

3. Use lamps instead of overhead lights when you read.

4. Use light bulbs with a low wattage except when you read.

5. Turn off electrical appliances, such as televisions, stereos, and radios, when you are not using them.

6. Use manual appliances instead of electrical appliances, such as electric pencil sharpeners.

7. Use batteries that can be recharged instead of disposable ones.

8. Use fans instead of air conditioning to cool your home.

9. Plant fast-growing trees near your home to keep it cooler.

10. Wear warm clothes instead of turning up the heat in cold weather.

11. Install weather stripping around windows and seal air leaks around doors to prevent heat loss from your home.

12. Turn down your thermostat at night and when you are away.

13. Use less hot water.

14. Dry your clothes on a clothesline instead of in a dryer in warm weather.

Water Conservation

Did you know...?

5–7 . . . . **gallons of water are used when you flush the toilet.**

25 . . . . . **gallons of water are used when you take a shower.**

50 . . . . . **gallons of water are used when you bathe.**

You would die within days without clean water. **Water conservation** is actions to save water. You and your family can conserve thousands of gallons of water.

Ways to Conserve Water

1. Install a low-flow shower head.
2. Check faucets and pipes for leaks.
3. Run washing machines and dishwashers only when they are full.
4. Water the lawn at the coolest time of the day; use about one inch of water a week.
5. Keep water in the refrigerator rather than running water to cool it to drink.
6. Take a short shower instead of a bath.
7. Collect rainwater and use it to water flowers and shrubs.
8. Do not let water run when you rinse dishes or brush teeth.
9. Plant trees in your yard; they store water and release it into the ground.

Land Conservation

What are ways you enjoy using land? Perhaps you like to play soccer or other sports on a sports field. Maybe you like to have picnics with your family in a local or state park. You might enjoy hiking and camping in a state or national forest. You might like to watch wild animals in their natural surroundings. These all are ways you enjoy open land.

You use developed land, too. Your home sits on developed land. Your school is built on developed land. If you live in a town or city, you live in a developed area. You shop in stores, shopping centers, and shopping malls. These services all are built on developed land.

People need both developed land and open land. People use both kinds of land for different purposes. People need to keep a balance between the amount of land that is developed and the amount of land that is left open. If too much land is developed, there will not be open spaces to enjoy. Wild animals will not have as many places to live. But if too much land is left open, people might not have the services they need. They might not have enough housing. **Land conservation** is actions to save land. While cities continue to grow, planners realize people's needs for trees, parks, and unspoiled countryside. Gardens, bike trails, and hiking trails add to the quality of the environment.

One threat to land conservation is trash. Anything that is thrown away ends up somewhere. Most trash ends up in landfills. A **landfill** is a place where wastes are dumped and buried. Wastes usually are dumped in layers and covered in soil. Landfills take up space.

People must make less trash to conserve the land used by landfills. This means buying less, keeping things longer, and lending or sharing with others what is not needed. Actions that promote land conservation include:

1. disposing of solid waste properly;
2. precycling;
3. recycling;
4. composting.

Disposing of Solid Waste

Solid waste is discarded solid material such as paper, metals, and yard waste. Most people put solid waste in the proper places, such as garbage cans or junkyards. Sometimes people throw trash on the ground or in water. Litter is a type of pollution.

Most solid waste is dumped in landfills. At one time, any type of waste was disposed of in landfills. In the past few decades, it was discovered that harmful chemicals and other waste that was dangerous were contaminating the water and air. Today, there are stricter laws about what can be in a landfill. However, there is still concern about the odor and appearance of landfills, the danger of harmful substances leaking into nearby water, and disease-carrying organisms in landfills. As more solid waste is being dumped, there also is concern about the lack of space for more landfills.

Solid waste also is disposed of through incinerators. An incinerator (in·SIN·uh·ray·ter) is a furnace that burns waste products. Many countries have successful incinerator programs. However, some people believe that incinerators are harmful to the environment and people. Some incinerators might produce smoke containing harmful pollutants. There is concern that people who live near these incinerators might be at risk.

Waste from industry has created a particular problem. Some industries produce waste that is hazardous to people and the environment. Some of this waste is toxic. **Toxic waste** is waste that is poisonous. Toxic waste can enter the ground, air, or water. Toxic waste can cause illness or death. Some industries produce radwaste. Each kind of toxic waste must be disposed of in a specific way. **Radwaste** is radioactive waste material. Nuclear power plants produce radwaste. Some radwaste continues to give off radiation for tens of thousands of years. It is difficult to dispose of radwaste safely. Some radwaste is currently being stored in vats and underwater barrels. The Environmental Protection Agency (EPA) regulates the disposal of solid waste. The EPA has determined that certain places where toxic waste has been dumped are hazardous. Efforts are being made to clean up these sites.

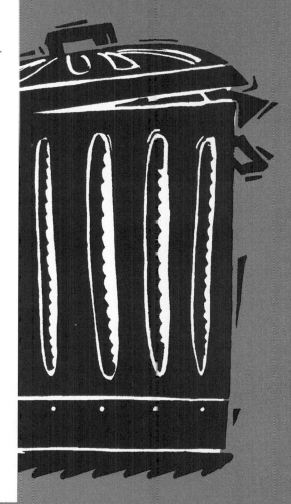

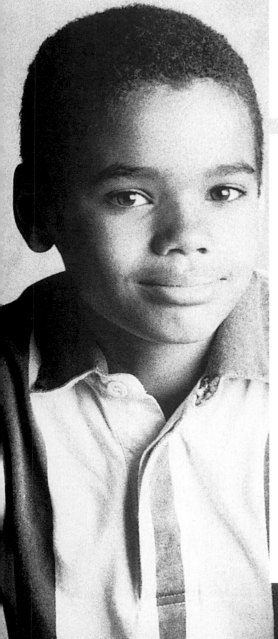

Precycling

Have you ever considered how you might dispose of a product before you bought it? Did you know that one third of what is thrown away is packaging? **Precycling** is the process of reducing waste by:

- **buying recycled products;**
- **buying products in packages or containers that can be recycled;**
- **buying products with less packaging;**
- **repairing products rather than buying new ones.**

Ways to Precycle

1. Purchase beverages and household products in refillable bottles.
2. Use glass and reusable plastic containers rather than aluminum foil or plastic wrap.
3. Bring a cloth bag to the store instead of requesting paper or plastic bags; refuse bags for small purchases.
4. Purchase foods and products in recyclable cardboard packages rather than in plastic or styrofoam.
5. Consider how you will dispose of packaging before purchasing items.
6. Do not buy items that can be used only once when reusable items are available.
7. Do not buy items overpackaged for display purposes.
8. Use reusable eating utensils, plates, cups, and napkins rather than disposable ones.
9. Use both sides of paper.
10. Use a towel instead of paper towels to dry your hands.

Recycling

Recycling is the process of reforming or breaking down waste products so they can be used again. Some materials are biodegradable. **Biodegradable** is having the ability to be broken down by living organisms. Recycling involves collecting reusable material, processing, marketing, and reusing the raw material for a new product. Recycling reduces the amount of energy and water used. It cuts down on the amount of pollution created by normal processing. And recycling helps to save land because there is less solid waste to be dumped in landfills. Recycling one ton of paper preserves about 20 trees; two barrels of oil; 7,000 gallons of water; and 4,100 kilowatt hours of electricity.

Communities recycle in different ways. Some have curbside pickup. The recyclables may be separated into bottles, cans, and newspapers, or picked up together. Charitable organizations might provide pickup service. They might collect aluminum cans, newspapers, or cardboard. People collect these products to help charities earn money. Some communities have buy-back centers. These are private companies that pay for recyclable products. Some communities have reverse vending machines. Beverage containers can be returned for a refund as cash or a voucher.

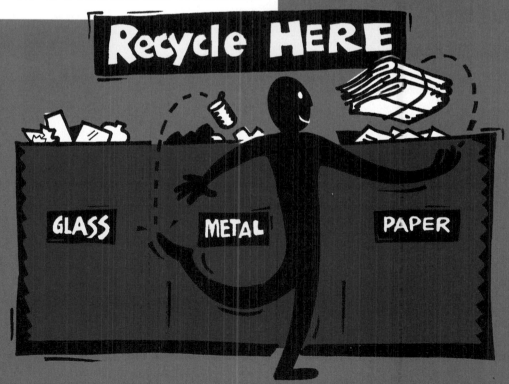

Recycling takes effort. You and others must be willing to handle your trash in special ways. Find out how your community program works. The usual categories for recycling are:

Glass

Glass bottles might be cleaned and reused. Glass products might be crushed and used to make new glass.

Metals

Metal cans, including aluminum cans, can be recycled. Other products, such as aluminum foil and frozen food trays, also can be recycled.

Plastic

Many kinds of plastic can be recycled, including the plastic bottles used for soft drinks.

Paper

Paper is the most common product to be recycled. Save newspapers, magazines, school papers, and cardboard containers. These products can be processed to make other paper products.

Composting

Composting is becoming more important as a method of recycling. **Composting** is the breakdown of plant remains and once-living materials into simpler substances. Mowed grass, dead leaves, leftover food, and vegetable peels are mixed in with straw. This mixture is stirred every few days. Bacteria help to decompose the organic material. It turns into a rich soil. Composting helps reduce the amount of garbage sent to landfills for disposal.

Swap Shop

Life Skill

I will precycle, recycle, and dispose of waste properly.

Materials: Items no longer used as explained in directions

Directions: One person's trash is another person's treasure. Organize a Swap Shop to recycle and reduce trash.

1. **Look through your possessions.** Choose items you no longer need or use that you might consider throwing away. The items should be in fair to good condition. Examples are old magazines or sports equipment you no longer use.

2. **Decide on a day for all students to bring in their items.** Arrange the items on a table in your classroom.

3. **Have students choose items they would like to have.** Students can take the items home.

4. **Suggest to your principal that the school have a Swap Shop.** Get your school involved in recycling.

Lesson 45

Review

Vocabulary

Write a separate sentence using each of the vocabulary words listed on page 480.

Health Content

Write responses to the following:

1. What are 14 ways to conserve energy? **page 482**
2. What are nine ways to conserve water? **page 483**
3. What are four actions that promote land conservation? **page 484**
4. What are ten ways to precycle? **page 486**
5. What are products that can be sorted and recycled? **page 488**

Appreciating the Environment

Vocabulary

pleasant sounds

visual environment

visual pollution

validation

visual validation

support network

social-emotional environment

Life Skills

- **I will protect the natural environment.**
- **I will take actions to improve my visual environment.**
- **I will take actions to improve my social-emotional environment.**

Your environment is everything that is around you. It includes sounds, your visual surroundings, and the family and friends who care about you. All of these parts of the environment can affect your health.

The Lesson Objectives

- Identify ways pleasant sounds promote your health.
- State ways a pleasant visual environment promotes your health.
- Explain how having a support network can promote your health.

Creating Pleasant Sounds

To what would you rather wake up? The jarring sounds of a jackhammer? The soft chirps of songbirds? Or maybe your favorite music? Your environment includes what you hear regularly. Loud noises harm health and cause hearing loss. **Pleasant sounds** are sounds that promote health.

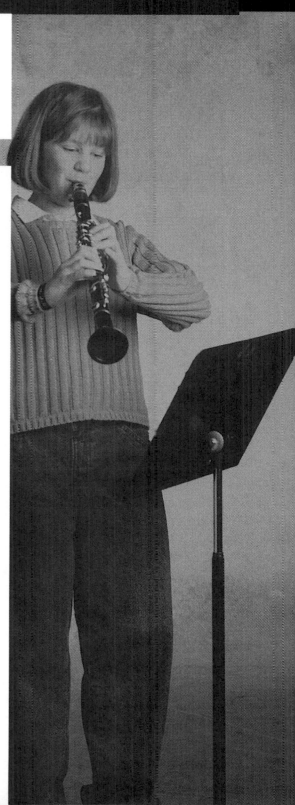

- **Pleasant sounds can motivate and energize you.** Your heart rate speeds up to music with a fast beat and slows down to music with a slower beat. Music can change electrical rhythms in your brain. When the school band plays the fight song, you feel motivated to cheer for your team. When you play upbeat music, you want to get up and dance. Try exercising to pleasant, upbeat music. You will get in the mood to exercise and feel less tired while exercising.

- **Pleasant sounds can improve mood and reduce depression.** If you feel depressed, try playing a favorite compact disc. You will feel pleasure in listening to sounds you enjoy. Learning to play a musical instrument can help lift your depression. When you focus on playing a musical instrument, you listen to sounds you enjoy. You get the added benefits of tuning out your problems and worries. You also get a sense of accomplishment. Music is not the only pleasant sound. You might improve your mood by listening to laughter or waves breaking on the shore.

- **Pleasant sounds can reduce the effects of body changes caused by the alarm stage of the general adaptation syndrome.** When you are stressed, your heart rate increases and your blood pressure can rise. You feel tense and anxious. Calm music with a slow beat can slow your heart rate. It can lower blood pressure and decrease anxiety. Relaxing, soothing sounds in nature also can reduce stress. Listen to the songs of birds, the wind in the trees, or soft steady rainfall.

Make a point to have pleasant sounds part of your environment. Visit a waterfall. Play uplifting music. Attend a symphony. Get up early to listen to the birds.

Creating a Pleasant View

If you are like most people, sight is your dominant sense. Most of what you learn from your environment comes from seeing. **Visual environment** is everything a person sees regularly. It includes what you see in your outdoor environment and in your indoor surroundings. A pleasant visual environment can affect your health in five ways.

A Pleasant Visual Environment:

- **Improves your mood.** When you look at beautiful scenes, you feel uplifted. The sight of a sunset or attractive painting causes you to feel more positive. If you are feeling depressed, a pleasant view can reduce your feelings of sadness.

- **Improves your concentration.** When you are working at a clean desk in a neat room, you concentrate better. **Visual pollution** is sights that are unattractive. Clutter and trash are visual pollution in an indoor environment. They can distract you when you are trying to work.

- **Helps relieve stress.** When you are stressed, looking at scenes of nature helps you to relax. Your heart rate slows. Your blood pressure returns to normal. You feel less anxious. You have less muscle tension.

- **Contributes to quality of life.** A neighborhood that has a pleasant visual environment is linked to a decrease in crime and violence. If you live in a neighborhood where people take care of their homes and yards, you enjoy living there. You feel proud to live there. You feel a sense of community.

- **Improves social health.** You are part of the visual environment. You show that you have respect for yourself when you have a clean and neat appearance. Others find you attractive.

Ways You Can Improve Your Visual Environment

- **Give yourself visual validations.** A **validation** is a statement that is true. A **visual validation** is something placed in the environment that reminds a person of his or her successes. You can put things in your visual environment that show what you have accomplished. You are not bragging or showing off when you do this. You are reminding yourself that you are capable and that you can reach your goals. Examples are a paper on which you received an "A" or a trophy. Visual validations can remind you that you are loved. You can arrange cards that people who love you have sent you. Perhaps you have a favorite saying or quote. You can write it on an index card and tape it to a mirror.

- **Change the colors in your visual environment.** Researchers have found that colors play a part in health and well-being. More than one vivid color in a room, such as red or yellow, is distracting. Dull colors, such as gray and beige, have a calming effect and reduce tension. However, adding one vivid color to a room with dull colors can energize and motivate you. Use your favorite color often. If you like blue, paint your room blue or get a blue bedspread. If you like green, get some plants.

- **Visit an art museum.** Look at paintings, sculpture, and three-dimensional art works. Great works of art can lift your spirits. Art can challenge you to look at the world in new ways. It gives you a break from your usual way of looking at things. You can face the world with renewed energy.

- **Clean up your visual environment.** Keep your room neat and clean. Organize your belongings. Throw litter in the trash.

Developing a Support Network

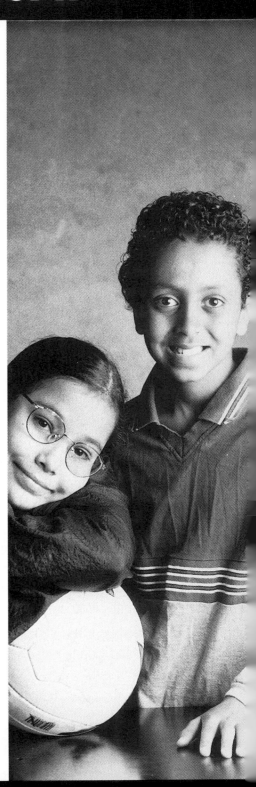

Do you have friends you can go to when you need to talk? Friends you can count on when you need help? If you answered yes, then you already know the value of a support network. A **support network** is a group of people who help and encourage a person. It is part of a person's social-emotional environment. The **social-emotional environment** is the quality of the contacts one has with the people with whom one interacts. A positive social-emotional environment promotes health in several ways. A positive social environment:

- **Improves self-respect.** Suppose your friends appreciate that you are special. They accept you as you are. They encourage you to choose responsible behavior. When your actions are worthy, you respect yourself.

- **Helps you to be resilient.** People in your support network encourage you to take healthful risks. If you do not succeed in something, your support network will make you feel cared about. You will still feel you are worthwhile. Suppose you compete in a contest at school and do not win. Your support network will praise you for trying and encourage you to keep trying.

- **Reduces your risk of illness.** Research shows that people who have a support network reduce their level of stress. High levels of stress can lead to illness. When you share your problems with caring friends and family, you feel less anxious. You experience less depression.

A support network involves give and take. Do not expect your family and friends to do all of the giving. You must do your part to support others. Keep confidences. Show genuine interest in and concern for others. Listen and encourage others. Try doing things others like to do, even if you think you might not like them. Make time for your support network. Even small gestures mean a lot. Send a card. Draw a funny cartoon for a friend who needs cheering. Call a friend just to say "I'm thinking about you." The old saying "to have a friend is to be one" is still true.

Friendly Web

Life Skill I will take actions to improve my social-emotional environment.

Materials: Ball of yarn

Directions: Complete this activity to make a support network or web.

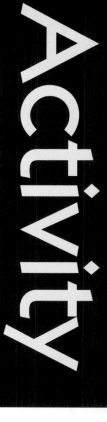

1. Your teacher will arrange your class in a circle with desks or with seated students on the floor.

2. One student takes the ball of yarn and holds the free end.

3. The student throws the yarn to another student. The student who throws the yarn says, "(Name of other student) is in my support network. I can be a friend to (name) by listening without criticizing."

4. The student to whom the yarn was thrown performs step 3 but states a different way to be supportive. The student must hold onto a piece of the yarn so that a web or network is formed.

5. Continue throwing the ball of yarn until all students have had a turn.

Lesson 46

Review

Vocabulary

Write a separate sentence using each of the vocabulary words listed on page 490.

Health Content

Write responses to the following:

1. What are three ways pleasant sounds promote your health? **page 491**

2. What are five ways a pleasant visual environment promotes your health? **page 492**

3. What are four ways you can improve your visual environment? **page 493**

4. What are three ways a support network promotes your health? **page 494**

5. What are ways you can support others? **page 494**

Unit 9 Review

Health Content

Review your answers for each Lesson Review in this unit. Then write answers to each of the following questions.

1. How can an ecosystem be destroyed? **Lesson 43 page 459**

2. How can you protect yourself from the thinning of the ozone layer? **Lesson 43 page 460**

3. How can teens living in poverty improve their environment? **Lesson 43 page 464**

4. How can you keep the air clean? **Lesson 44 page 470**

5. Why is it risky to breathe radon? **Lesson 44 page 472**

6. Why is it dangerous for PCBs and dioxins to get into a water supply? **Lesson 44 page 476**

7. How can you conserve land? **Lesson 45 page 484**

8. What are ways you can precycle? **Lesson 45 page 486**

9. How do pleasant sounds promote health? **Lesson 46 page 491**

10. How does a support network promote health? **Lesson 46 page 494**

Vocabulary

Number a sheet of paper from 1–10. Select the correct vocabulary word. Write it next to the corresponding number. DO NOT WRITE IN THIS BOOK.

cataract	sick building syndrome
ozone layer	support network
particulates	teratogen
precycling	toxic waste
radwaste	validation

1. _____ is the process of reducing waste by buying recycled products. **Lesson 45**

2. _____ is an illness that results from indoor air pollution. **Lesson 44**

3. _____ are tiny particles in the air. **Lesson 44**

4. A(n) _____ is an environmental agent that crosses the placenta of a pregnant female and causes miscarriage or birth defects. **Lesson 43**

5. A(n) _____ is a statement that is true. **Lesson 46**

6. The _____ is a layer in the upper atmosphere where ozone traps dangerous ultraviolet radiation from the sun. **Lesson 43**

7. A(n) _____ is a loss of transparency of the lens of the eye. **Lesson 43**

8. _____ is radioactive waste material. **Lesson 45**

9. _____ is waste that is poisonous. **Lesson 45**

10. A(n) _____ is a group of people who help and encourage you. **Lesson 46**

The Responsible Decision-Making Model™

You are feeling very stressed. You feel you just want to be left alone. You isolate yourself from your friends. Answer the following questions on a separate sheet of paper. Write "Does not apply" if a question does not apply to this situation.

1. Is it healthful to isolate yourself from your friends when you are stressed? Why or why not?

2. Is it safe to isolate yourself from your friends when you are stressed? Why or why not?

3. Is it legal to isolate yourself from your friends when you are stressed? Why or why not?

4. Will you show respect for yourself and others if you isolate yourself from your friends when you are stressed? Why or why not?

5. Will your parents or guardian approve if you isolate yourself from your friends when you are stressed? Why or why not?

6. Will you demonstrate good character if you isolate yourself from your friends when you are stressed? Why or why not?

What is the responsible decision to make in this situation?

Health Literacy

Effective Communication

Interview five people to learn whether they precycle and how they precycle. Summarize your findings to share with classmates.

Self-Directed Learning

Search the Internet for the Environmental Protection Agency site. Write down five facts about protecting the environment.

Critical Thinking

Consider where you live. What are three changes in your lifestyle you might have to make if the average temperature increases? Decreases?

Responsible Citizenship

Have your class plan a "Keep Our School Beautiful" day. Discuss and take actions to improve your visual environment in your school.

Multicultural Health

Rank the importance of these issues in a country different from your own: pollution; changes in climate; depletion of natural resources; and overcrowded conditions. Rank the importance of these issues in your country and compare the two countries.

Family Involvement

Share with your family ways you have learned to conserve water. Ask your parents or guardian for additional suggestions. Make a list of actions all family members can take to conserve water.

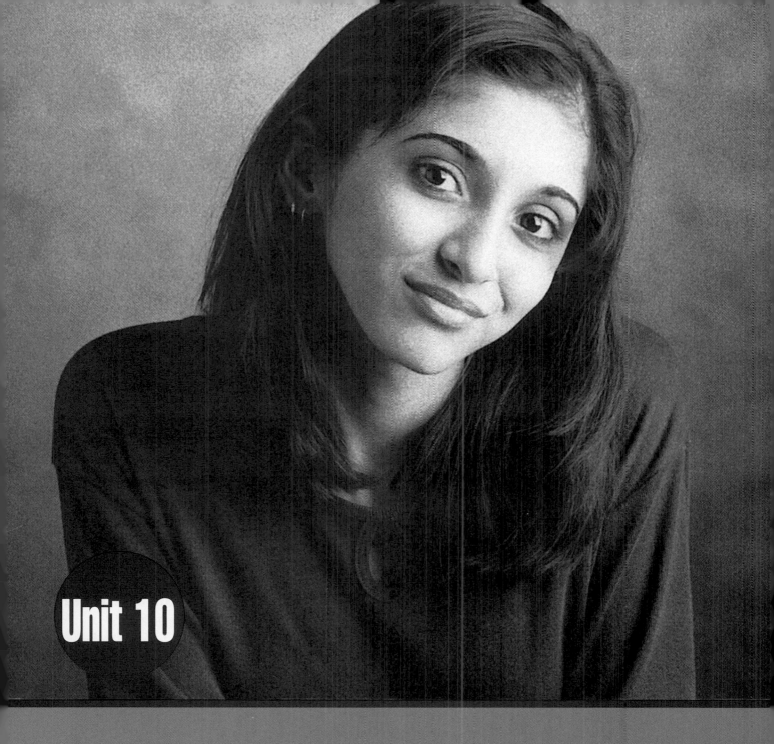

Unit 10

Injury Prevention and Safety

The Violence Prevention Guide

Vocabulary*

violence

violent behavior

victim of violence

protective factors

*A complete listing of vocabulary words appears at the end of the lesson.

- **I will practice protective factors to reduce the risk of violence.**
- **I will practice self-protection strategies.**
- **I will stay away from gangs.**
- **I will respect authority and obey laws.**
- **I will not carry a weapon.**
- **I will participate in victim recovery if I am harmed by violence.**

Violence is the use of physical force to injure, damage, or destroy oneself, others, or property. **Violent behavior** is behavior that threatens or uses force to injure, damage, or destroy a person or property. A **victim of violence** is a person who is harmed or killed by violence. In this lesson, you will learn ways to protect yourself from violence. You will learn what to do if you are a victim of violence.

The Lesson Objectives

- Describe how to recognize violence.
- List protective factors that help reduce your risk of violence.
- Explain the steps in victim recovery.

Protecting Yourself from Violence

How can you protect yourself from violence? **Protective factors** are ways that a person might behave and characteristics of the environment in which a person lives that promote health, safety, and well-being.

You are going to learn about 20 protective factors for violence. Some protective factors describe your behavior. You have some protection from violence when you choose these behaviors. Some protective factors describe the environment. You have some protection from violence when you live in a protective environment.

Think about your lifestyle. How many of the protective factors describe your behavior? How many of the protective factors describe the environment in which you live? Total the number. The closer the number is to 20, the greater protection you have from violence. Review the protective factors that do not describe your behavior or environment. Can you make changes in your lifestyle so that you will have greater protection from violence?

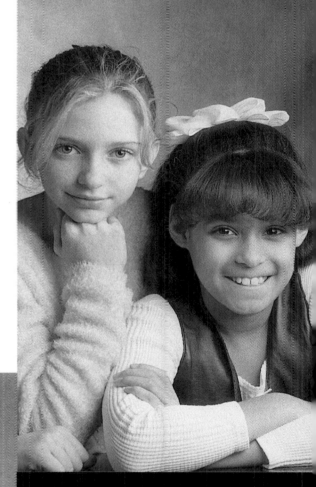

Say No!
Say No!
Say No!
Say No!

Protective Factors
That Help Reduce Your Risk of Violence

1.
Recognizing violent behavior

2.
Having self-respect

3.
Being raised in a healthful family

4.
Living in a nurturing environment

5.
Having social skills

6.
Being able to manage anger

7.
Being able to manage stress

8.
Participating in physical and recreational activities

9.
Practicing suicide prevention strategies

10. Being able to resolve conflict

11. Avoiding discriminatory behavior

12. Making responsible decisions

13. Being able to resist negative peer pressure

14. Avoiding the use of alcohol and other harmful drugs

15. Staying away from weapons

16. Staying away from gangs

17. Showing respect for authority and obeying laws

18. Practicing self-protection strategies

19. Participating in recovery if you have been a victim of violence

20. Changing your behavior if you have been a juvenile offender

Protective Factors
That Help Reduce Your Risk of Violence

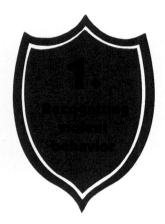

1. **Recognizing violent behavior** You have learned different types of violent behavior. You pay attention when you or someone you know behaves in these ways. Tell a trusted adult if someone around you behaves in violent ways. Ask an adult for help if you behave in violent ways. Never take a lazy attitude about violence or think violent behavior has no effect. Do not watch television programs, videotapes, and movies that show acts of violence. Choose music carefully to avoid listening to lyrics about violent behavior. Recognizing violent behavior helps protect you from violence.

Bullying

Bullying is an attempt by a person to hurt or frighten people who are weaker or smaller. A **bully** is a person who hurts or frightens people who are weaker or smaller. A bully might act in different ways. A bully might place a hand in the face of someone in order to threaten that person. A bully might call someone names or make cruel remarks to them. A bully tries to control others.

Fighting

Fighting is taking part in a physical struggle. Teens might have fistfights. They might push, punch, kick, or pull hair. Fighting is risky behavior. Many teens are injured because of fighting.

Homicide

Homicide (HAHM·uh·syd) is the accidental or purposeful killing of another person. **Murder** is killing someone on purpose. Most homicides follow arguments and fights between people who know each other. One way to protect yourself from murder is to avoid fighting.

Suicide

Suicide is the intentional taking of one's own life. Teens who commit suicide usually are depressed. They might have family difficulties. They might be troubled about a relationship with a friend. Often, they are using alcohol or other drugs. Keeping yourself and others alive should be a priority. In Lesson 5, there are suggestions for what to do if you or someone else is depressed.

Sexual Harassment

Sexual harassment is unwanted sexual behavior that ranges from making unwanted sexual comments to forcing another person into unwanted sex acts. Sexual harassment sometimes occurs in schools. Title IX, a federal law, makes it clear that sexual harassment should never occur in schools.

Rape

Rape is the threatened or actual use of physical force to get someone to have sex without giving consent. Laws help to define what it means to have sex "without giving consent." A person who does not willingly say yes has not given consent. Having sex with this person is considered rape. A person who is a minor (under the age of adulthood as defined by state law) cannot give consent. If an adult has sex with a minor, it is considered rape. A person who does not have certain mental abilities is protected by the law. Having sex with this person can be considered rape.

Abuse

Abuse (uh·BYOOS) is the harmful treatment of another person. Abuse can be physical, emotional, sexual, or due to neglect. **Physical abuse** is harmful treatment that results in physical injury to the victim. Results of physical abuse include broken bones, bruises, and cuts. **Emotional abuse** is "putting down" another person and making the person feel worthless. Emotional abuse includes name-calling, threats, and put-downs. Emotional abuse can have lasting effects. Victims might feel depressed, or have low self-esteem. **Sexual abuse** is sexual contact that is forced on a person. The victim of sexual abuse might or might not know the person who has abused them. Sexual abuse sometimes occurs between family members. **Incest** is sexual abuse between family members. **Neglect** is failure to provide proper care and guidance. Neglect includes failure to provide food or safe shelter for children or the elderly.

Domestic Violence

Domestic violence is violence that occurs within a family. **Child abuse** is the harmful treatment of a minor. Child abuse is one example of abuse within a family, but there are others. A husband or wife might be abused by a spouse. Someone might be harmed by a former spouse. The abuse might involve brothers, sisters, stepbrothers, or stepsisters. Sometimes children abuse their parents. **Parent abuse** is the harmful treatment of a parent.

Now you know different types of violent behavior. Each of these behaviors is wrong. It is wrong for you to behave in violent ways. It is wrong for others to behave in violent ways.

Signs of Abuse

A person who has been a victim of abuse might:

- have poor grades;
- have little interest in schoolwork;
- be poorly dressed or have poor hygiene;
- be depressed or show suicidal tendencies;
- run away from home;
- be shy or afraid of others;
- miss school frequently;
- show aggressive behavior toward others.

I will practice self-protection strategies.

Protective Factors
That Help Reduce Your Risk of Violence

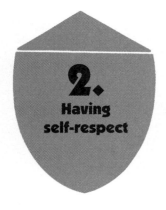

2. **Having self-respect** You feel good about yourself if you have self-respect. You do not want to harm yourself. You stay away from others who might harm you. Other people are more likely to respect you when you have self-respect. They are less likely to harm you. There are ways to get this important layer of protection from violence. Having self-respect helps protect you from violence.

Ways to Develop Self-Respect

- Use self-control to act on responsible values.
- Change behavior that is not reponsible.
- Spend time with teens in your support network.
- Treat others the way you want to be treated.
- Get regular physical exercise to generate feelings of well-being.
- Present a neat and clean appearance.

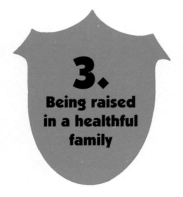

3. **Being raised in a healthful family** You have another layer of protection from violence when you are close to your family. Being close to family members helps you feel valued and loved. Adults in healthful families teach you to behave in responsible ways. They teach you how to respect others by showing respect for you. You are less likely to hang out with friends who make wrong decisions when you have the support of your family. You stay away from gangs. Being raised in a healthful family helps protect you from violence.

Protective Factors
That Help Reduce Your Risk of Violence

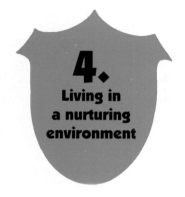

4. **Living in a nurturing environment** A nurturing **environment** is surroundings that help a person grow, develop, and succeed. The saying "Life is not fair" is true to some extent. Some teens are able to succeed more easily than others. For example, some teens live in safe neighborhoods. Their families might have enough money to buy the things they need. As a result, they are filled with hope. They might work hard when they do not get the things they need at first. Teens living in a nurturing environment have some protection from violence.

Other teens live in difficult environments. They might live in unsafe neighborhoods. Their families might be poor. People living in their neighborhood might steal or harm others to get what they need. There is much violence around them.

Teens who live in difficult environments can still make choices to protect themselves from violence. These teens can obey the law, although their situations are difficult. They can make wise choices, attend school, and prepare for their futures. If drugs are sold in their neighborhoods, they can stay away from people who sell them. They can stay away from gangs and weapons, too. These teens can try their best, although they know life is not always fair.

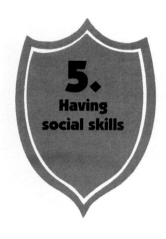

5. **Having social skills** Social skills are skills a person can use to relate well with others. They make it easier for other teens to like you. Other teens include you in enjoyable activities. You do not hang out with the wrong crowd, because you feel liked and accepted. You do not give in to negative peer pressure to choose harmful actions. Having social skills helps protect you from violence.

Protective Factors
That Help Reduce Your Risk of Violence

6.
Being able to manage anger

6. **Being able to manage anger** Anger is the feeling of being irritated or annoyed. Feeling angry is OK. But, you know that you must express your anger in appropriate ways. **Anger management skills** are ways of expressing anger without doing something harmful. Practicing anger management skills protects you from violence. When you feel angry, you use these skills rather than blowing up or acting out.

You also might have hidden anger. Hidden anger is anger that is not recognized and is expressed in an inappropriate way. If you have hidden anger, you might feel angry much of the time. You might make sarcastic or cruel remarks. You might blow up suddenly. These behaviors might provoke another person to behave violently toward you. Hidden anger also can cause you to release your anger on someone or something other than the cause of the anger. For example, you might destroy school property when you are really angry about a family situation. Anger management skills can help you deal with hidden anger.

Anger Management Skills

- Use self-statements to control your anger.
- Get involved in physical activity.
- Use I-messages to express angry feelings.
- Use active listening techniques.
- Do something creative.
- Talk with your parents, guardian, or mentor.
- Write a letter to express your angry feelings.
- Plan ahead and recognize your anger triggers.

Refer to Lesson 4 for more information about anger management skills.

Protective Factors
That Help Reduce Your Risk of Violence

7.

Being able to manage stress

7. **Being able to manage stress** Stress management skills are techniques to cope with the body changes produced by stress. They help you reduce anxiety and tension. You use these skills in difficult situations. Difficult situations do not cause you to "snap." You think clearly and respond in healthful ways Practicing stress management skills helps protect you from violence.

Stress Management Skills

- Use responsible decision-making skills.
- Get enough rest and sleep.
- Participate in physical activities.
- Use time management skills.
- Write in a journal.
- Spend time with close friends.
- Talk with parents and other trusted adults.
- Help others.
- Express affection in appropriate ways.
- Care for pets.
- Change your outlook.
- Keep a sense of humor.

Refer to Lesson 5 for more information about stress management skills.

Protective Factors
That Help Reduce Your Risk of Violence

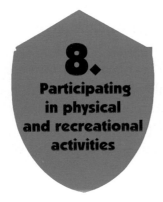

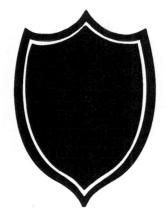

8. Participating in physical and recreational activities
Physical activities are activities that require the use of muscles and energy. Playing baseball, basketball, hockey, and soccer are physical activities. Taking a walk and jogging are physical activities. **Recreational activities** are activities that involve play, amusement, and relaxation. Playing chess and other board games are recreational activities. Going to an amusement park is a recreational activity. Attending a dance and going to camp are recreational activities. There are many benefits to participating in these activities. They provide an outlet for physical energy. This is one way they help protect you from violence. Suppose you are very angry or upset. When you have an outlet for physical energy, you are less likely to blow up. After getting involved in these activities, you are calmer. You have a better atttitude. This is because these activities release beta-endorphins. Remember, these are substances that make you feel good. There are other ways these activities help protect you from violence. They take up your free time. Then you are not idle and wondering what to do. Contests and games also teach you to follow rules and respect authority. When you participate, you see the need for rules and authority. You know it keeps order and is best. You learn what to do when you lose and somebody else wins.

9. Practicing suicide prevention strategies **Depression** is the feeling of being sad, unhappy, or discouraged. Everyone feels sad at times. But prolonged depression is not normal. Suppose you feel down in the dumps. Suppose you do not look forward to anything. Suppose you cannot sleep and do not feel like eating. These are signs that you need help. Talk to your parents or guardian. If needed, they can arrange for professional help. Teens who have depression that lasts are at risk for making a suicide attempt. Did you know that suicide is considered violence? It is violence because it involves self-harm. Practicing suicide prevention strategies helps protect you from violence.

Protective Factors
That Help Reduce Your Risk of Violence

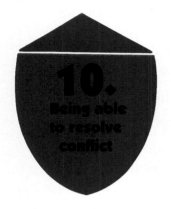

10. Being able to resolve conflict Conflict resolution **skills** are steps that can be used to resolve a disagreement in a healthful, safe, legal, respectful, and nonviolent way. When conflict arises, you use these steps rather than fighting or destroying property. You get help if you cannot reach a solution to the conflict. You approach a trusted adult.

Conflict Resolution Skills

- Remain calm.
- Set the tone.
- Define the conflict.
- Take responsibility for personal actions.
- Use I-messages to express feelings.
- Listen to the needs and feelings of others.
- List and discuss possible solutions. Evaluate each solution.
- Agree on a solution.
- Keep your word and follow the solution upon which you agreed.
- Ask for the assistance of a trusted adult or obtain mediation if the conflict cannot be resolved.

Refer to Lesson 6 for more information about conflict resolution skills.

Steps in the Mediation Process

- Keep a neutral position.
- Set ground rules.
- Define the conflict.
- Identify solutions to the conflict.
- Evaluate suggested solutions.
- Agree to try a solution.
- Schedule a follow-up meeting.

You might participate in mediation. **Mediation** is a process in which a third person helps people in conflict reach a solution. Lesson 6 outlined both conflict resolution and mediation skills. Practicing conflict resolution and mediation skills helps protect you from violence.

Protective Factors
That Help Reduce Your Risk of Violence

11.
Avoiding discriminatory behavior

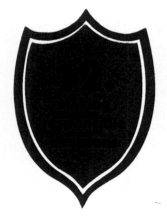

11. Avoiding discriminatory behavior To discriminate (dis·KRIM·uh·nayt) is to treat some people or groups of people differently from others. To prevent violence, you treat others with respect.

- You do not tease others or put others down.
- You do not laugh at jokes about other people.

Avoiding discriminatory behavior helps protect you from violence. You can take three actions to avoid discriminatory behavior.

- Share in another person's emotions or feelings. Put yourself in the other person's situation. This is what is meant by walking a mile in someone else's shoes.
- Ask others to stop discriminatory behavior. Do not remain silent when others make discriminatory remarks. Speak up and state your disapproval.
- Learn about people who are different from you. You will find that you have much in common. You will gain a better understanding of their emotions and feelings.

12. Making responsible decisions You evaluate the possible consequences before you make a decision. You make decisions that are healthful, safe, and legal. Your decisions show respect for yourself and others, follow family guidelines, and demonstrate good character. Making responsible decisions helps protect you from violence.

Suppose you decide to take a short cut through an area where gangs hang out. You use *The Responsible Decision-Making Model*™ to evaluate the consequences of your decision. You realize that you will place yourself in a situation that might lead to violence. This is an example of how making responsible decisions helps protect you from violence.

Protective Factors
That Help Reduce Your Risk of Violence

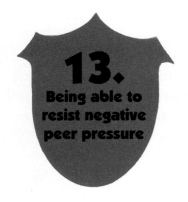

13.
Being able to resist negative peer pressure

13. Being able to resist negative peer pressure

Resistance skills are skills that are used when a person wants to say NO to an action or to leave a situation. You use resistance skills when peers want you to do something that is wrong. You say NO if they tell you not to worry because you will not get caught. You know that you might get away with wrong behavior once, but you still say NO. Eventually, you would pay a price and that price is often one you would regret later. You do not want anyone to get hurt. You do not want to break something and have to pay for it. You do not want someone to get angry and try to get even with you. You know if you do something illegal, you will be in trouble with the law. Being able to resist negative peer pressure helps protect you from violence.

Using Resistance Skills

- No, I will not use illegal drugs. I do not want to break the law.
- No, I will not carry a weapon. I do not want to risk being injured or killed.
- No, I will not shoplift. I do not want to be a juvenile offender.
- No, I will not get into fights. I will not risk being injured or injuring someone else.
- No, I will not join a gang. I do not want to have enemies in other gangs.
- No, I will not drink alcohol. I want to think clearly and be able to make responsible decisions.
- No, I will not skip school. I want to obey my family rules.
- No, I will not hitchhike. I do not want to risk being a victim of violence.
- No, I will not make fun of other people. I will not discriminate.
- No, I will not write graffiti on the wall. I will not destroy property.
- No, I will not go out alone at night with a person I do not know well. I will not risk being a victim of acquaintance rape.

Protective Factors
That Help Reduce Your Risk of Violence

Guidelines to Preventing Violence Involving Alcohol and Other Drugs

- Do not associate with people who use, make, or sell drugs.
- Stay away from gangs.
- Stay away from areas in which there is drinking or drug trafficking.
- Stay away from people who carry weapons.

14. Avoiding the use of alcohol and other harmful drugs When you are drug-free, you are able to think clearly. You consider the consequences of your behavior. You stay away from others who use alcohol and other harmful drugs. Avoiding the use of alcohol and other harmful drugs helps protect you from fights. You are less likely to be a victim of sexual assault, rape, and murder. Avoiding the use of alcohol and other harmful drugs helps protect you from violence.

Alcohol and other harmful drugs increase the risk of violence in the following ways.

- **Alcohol** Alcohol depresses the nervous system and changes mood and behavior. People who are angry or aggressive might act on these feelings. Most fights, assaults, and murders are associated with alcohol use.

- **Stimulants** Stimulants might cause a person to become impulsive and believe other people are going to harm him or her. The person might begin fights.

- **Marijuana and hallucinogens** People who use these drugs have a distorted view of reality. They might have hallucinations and resort to violent actions.

- **PCP** People who use PCP can become very angry, aggressive, and irritable. They might get out of control. They might harm people who try to control their actions.

- **Anabolic steroids** People who use anabolic steroids have mood swings and outbursts of anger called roid rages. They might harm others during these outbursts.

- **Sedative-hypnotics** People who take high doses of sedative-hypnotics can become angry and aggressive. They might resort to violent actions.

Protective Factors
That Help Reduce Your Risk of Violence

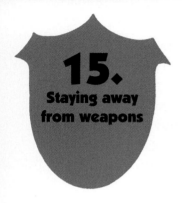

15.
Staying away from weapons

15. Staying away from weapons A **weapon** is an instrument or device used for violence. A weapon might be a handgun. It might be a kitchen knife. It might be a brick that is thrown at someone. Any instrument or device used to harm someone is a weapon. A **concealed weapon** is a weapon that is hidden from view. It is against the law for someone to have a concealed weapon. Take seriously someone who says he or she has a weapon or will use a weapon. Recently, some teens said ahead of time they were going to use weapons at school. The next day they did use weapons. They killed four classmates. Tell a responsible adult if another teen brags that he or she is going to hurt someone. Follow guidelines to prevent violence involving a weapon. Staying away from weapons helps protect you from violence.

Guidelines to Prevent Violence Involving a Weapon

- Do not purchase a weapon illegally.
- Do not carry a concealed weapon.
- Do not carry a weapon to school.
- Encourage other teens to avoid buying, carrying, or concealing a weapon.
- Do not pretend you are going to use a weapon.
- Avoid being around people who buy, carry, conceal, or use weapons.
- Do not argue with someone who has a weapon.
- Avoid being in situations in which there might be a weapon.
- Leave a weapon where you found it.
- Tell a responsible adult if you find a weapon.

Protective Factors
That Help Reduce Your Risk of Violence

16.
Staying away from gangs

16. **Staying away from gangs** **Gangs** are groups of young people who band together and participate in violent or criminal behavior. Belonging to a gang often means being with young people who have enemies. Rivalry exists among gangs. Gang rivalry and hatred result in fighting and other acts of violence. Gang members often have criminal records. Then it is difficult to get jobs.

You do not belong to a gang and you stay away from gang members. When gang members tell you to join and that they will protect you, you say NO. Gang membership is risky. You do not want money that comes from criminal activity or drug trafficking. Staying away from gangs helps protect you from violence.

Ways to Resist Belonging to a Gang

- Avoid being around gang members.
- Avoid being in locations that are gang turf.
- Avoid wearing colors or clothes that are gang-related.
- Do not participate in writing graffiti.
- Attend school and participate in school activities.
- Avoid staying out late at night.

Protective Factors
That Help Reduce Your Risk of Violence

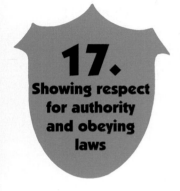

17.
Showing respect for authority and obeying laws

17. Showing respect for authority and obeying laws

A **law** is a rule of conduct or action that represents the beliefs of a majority of people in a community, state, or nation. Laws protect your rights and safety. Laws are regulated by people with authority. **Authority** is the power and right to govern and to apply laws. You show respect for authority and obey laws. You are responsible for your actions. You do not blame others or circumstances for what you do. Showing respect for authority and obeying laws helps protect you from violence.

When you show respect for authority and obey laws, you do not act in violent ways. You do not fight. You do not bully others. You do not hurt others. You settle disagreements peacefully. You do not get involved with people who believe violence is acceptable. You choose peers who show respect for authority and obey laws.

Your peers have tremendous influence over your actions. Suppose members of your peer group get into trouble or belong to a gang. You might be pressured to behave as your peers are behaving. You might start committing crimes such as stealing or destroying property. You might be pressured to harm another person. If you are arrested, you could face being placed on probation. You might be placed in a correctional facility, such as a group home or detention center.

You do not face these consequences if you show respect for authority and obey laws. When you show respect for authority and obey laws, you do not get into situations where you might harm others or others might harm you. You choose friends who obey laws. You protect yourself against violence.

Protective Factors
That Help Reduce Your Risk of Violence

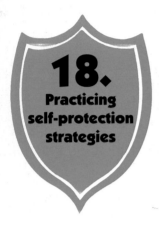

18. **Practicing self-protection strategies** Self-protection **strategies** are strategies that can be practiced to protect oneself and decrease the risk of becoming a victim. There are four keys to self-protection:

- Always trust your feelings about people and situations. You might have a gut feeling about someone or something. When you do, trust yourself. Avoid the person or situation.

- Always be alert. Pay close attention to the people around you. Be aware of what they are doing.

- Do not take your safety for granted. Learn ways to protect yourself in different situations. Do not let your guard down.

- Get help. Call the police or 9-1-1 if you feel threatened.

You need a plan to protect yourself when you are at home. Follow the guidelines for protecting yourself when at home.

Self-Protection Strategies for the Home

- Never let a stranger into your home.
- Always give the impression that someone else is at home besides you.
- Do not hide extra keys outside.
- Be cautious about giving out information.
- Keep doors and windows locked.

Protective Factors
That Help Reduce Your Risk of Violence

Whenever you are in public, there is a risk that others might harm you. Follow the guidelines for ways to protect yourself in public places.

Self-Protection Strategies for Public Places

- Avoid walking alone at night or in high-risk areas.
- Stay on well-lighted streets.
- Keep your distance if someone in a car asks for directions.
- Never accept a ride from a stranger or person you do not trust.
- Never hitchhike.
- Do not talk with strangers.
- Carry a whistle or buzzer to get attention if you need it.
- Use pay phones only when they are in well-lighted places and when others are around.

One type of violence that occurs is acquaintance rape. Acquaintance rape is rape that is committed by someone known to the victim. Follow the guidelines for ways to protect yourself when in social situations.

Self-Protection Strategies When in Social Situations

- Stay away from places where you will be alone with a person whom you do not know well or whom you do not trust.
- Do not go anywhere with a stranger, even if you are supposed to meet other people.
- Trust your gut feelings about other people.
- Choose to be with other people when you socialize with someone the first few times.
- Do not use alcohol or other harmful drugs.
- Pay attention to warning signs that indicate a person might harm you. A person might:

  show no respect for you;

  have a dominating attitude;

  be extremely jealous;

  be physically rough;

  have a history of violent or abusive behavior.

Protective Factors
That Help Reduce Your Risk of Violence

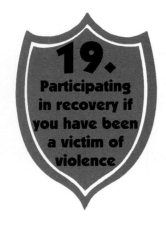

19. Participating in recovery if you have been a victim of violence A **victim of violence** is a person who is harmed or killed by violence. Some teens become victims of violence. Victims of violence might sustain physical as well as emotional injuries. Some injuries heal. But, some injuries can last a lifetime. It is important for victims of violence to get medical help for any physical injuries. They also need help to recover from the emotional effects of violence. There is an important reason why. Many adults who behave in violent ways were victims of violence as children or teens. Victims of violence need help so they do not behave in violent ways. If you have been a victim of violence, get help. You want to recover and gain self-confidence. Participating in recovery if you have been a victim of violence helps protect you from violence. Later in this lesson, you will learn more about victim recovery.

20. Changing your behavior if you have been a juvenile offender A **juvenile offender** is a legal minor who commits a criminal act. Juveniles are responsible for many violent crimes. **Rehabilitation** is the process of helping people change negative behavior to positive behavior. Juvenile courts usually attempt to rehabilitate juveniles rather than punish them. Juvenile offenders might be placed on probation. **Probation** is a sentence in which an offender remains in the community under the supervision of a probation officer for a specific period of time. Juvenile offenders who are on probation have to meet certain conditions and restrictions. They might have to perform community service. Teens who have been juvenile offenders must change their behavior.

Victim Recovery

Victims of violence can experience many different emotions. They might feel depressed and cry often. They might not want to talk with others about what happened. They might have difficulty paying attention in school. Victims of violence often are afraid. They might be fearful around others.

Some victims develop a severe stress disorder. **Post traumatic stress disorder (PTSD)** is a condition in which a person relives a stressful experience again and again. Symptoms include difficulty sleeping and concentrating.

Victims of violence find it difficult to ask for help. They might be embarrassed or afraid of what others will think or say. They might believe they did something to deserve harm. They might begin to act in violent ways themselves.

Victims of violence might have concerns about their health status. They might have become infected with a sexually transmitted disease (STD). They might have become infected with HIV, the virus that causes AIDS. Female victims of rape might have become pregnant.

Victims of all types of violence can continue to suffer for many years. **Victim recovery** is a person's return to physical and emotional health after being harmed by violence. Victim recovery often involves four steps:

1. **getting medical care for physical injuries;**
2. **getting counseling for emotional pain;**
3. **asking for support from family members and friends;**
4. **learning self-protection strategies to avoid becoming a victim again.**

Survivor of Violence

A victim of violence is a person who is harmed or killed by violence. Most people know this term and definition. But a newer term is being used for people who have been harmed by violence. Survivor of violence is the new term. This term is more empowering. It focuses on the actions a person who has been harmed can take. It focuses on right now and the future instead of the past. A survivor of violence is a person who has been harmed by violence and is taking steps toward recovery.

Activity

Shielded from Violence

Life Skill I will practice protective factors to reduce the risk of violence.

Materials: Notebook paper, pen or pencil, scissors, poster paper, markers, glitter, other art supplies as needed

Directions: Your classmates will share ideas about ways to protect themselves from violence. Then you will design your own shield.

1. **On a sheet of notebook paper, copy each of the protective factors from pages 502–503.** Skip a line between each factor. Cut and fold each protective factor into a separate slip. Your teacher will collect the slips and mix them up.

2. **Your teacher will form your class into a circle.** Students can sit on the floor or in desks arranged in a circle.

3. **One student starts by drawing a protective factor.** The student must name one way (s)he can practice that factor. For example, if the protective factor is, "resisting gang membership," the student might say, "I will not wear colors that are gang related." The student then writes what he or she said on the back of the slip and keeps it.

4. **Each student takes several turns until every student has drawn at least five different factors.**

5. **Draw an outline of a shield on a piece of poster paper.** Copy the actions you have written on your slips of paper on to the shield.

6. **Decorate your shield and display in your classroom or in a hallway where all students can see it.**

Lesson 47

Review

Vocabulary

Write a separate sentence using each of the vocabulary words listed below.

violence
violent behavior
victim of violence
protective factors
bullying
bully
fighting
homicide
murder
suicide
sexual harassment
rape
abuse
physical abuse
emotional abuse
sexual abuse
incest
neglect
domestic violence
child abuse
parent abuse
nurturing environment
social skills
anger management skills

stress management skills
physical activities
recreational activities
depression
conflict resolution skills
mediation
discriminate
resistance skills
weapon
concealed weapon
gangs
law
authority
self-protection strategies
juvenile offender
rehabilitation
probation
post traumatic stress disorder (PTSD)
victim recovery

Health Content

Write responses to the following:

1. What are 20 protective factors that help reduce the risk of violence? **pages 502–503**
2. Why is it important to recognize violent behavior? **page 504**
3. Describe kinds of violent behavior. **pages 504–506**
4. What are five kinds of abuse? **page 505**
5. What choices must be made by teens living in a difficult environment ? **page 509**
6. What are eight anger management skills? **page 510**
7. How does participating in physical and recreational activities reduce violence? **page 512**
8. What are ten conflict resolution skills? **page 513**
9. What are seven steps in the mediation process? **page 513**
10. What are two ways to treat others with respect and avoid discriminatory behavior? **page 514**
11. What are ten guidelines to prevent violence involving a weapon? **page 517**
12. What are six ways to resist belonging to a gang? **page 518**
13. Why is it important to show respect for authority and obey laws? **page 519**
14. What are four keys to self-protection? **page 520**
15. What are five self-protection strategies to follow at home? **page 520**
16. What are eight self-protection strategies to follow in public places? **page 521**
17. What are six self-protection strategies to follow that reduce the risk of acquaintance rape? **page 521**
18. Why do victims of violence need to participate in recovery? **page 522**
19. Why might victims of violence have difficulty asking for help? **page 523**
20. What are four steps in victim recovery? **page 523**

Preventing Unintentional Injuries

Vocabulary

accident

unintentional injury

smoke detector

heat detector

firearm

suffocation

electricity

poisoning

carbon monoxide (CO)

carbon monoxide detector

pedestrian

safety belt

child safety restraint

air bags

all-terrain vehicle (ATV)

Life Skills

- **I will follow safety guidelines to reduce the risk of unintentional injuries.**
- **I will follow guidelines for motor vehicle safety.**

Many teens are injured in accidents in the home and in the community. An **accident** is an event that is not planned to happen. An **unintentional injury** is an injury caused by an accident. Unintentional injuries are a leading cause of death among teens. This lesson contains safety guidelines you can follow to stay safe at home and in your community.

The Lesson Objectives

- Identify steps to prevent these unintentional injuries: falls, suffocation, electric shock, poisoning, and farm injuries.
- Give steps for the family fire escape plan.
- Explain ways to be safe around firearms.
- Describe safety guidelines for: pedestrians, riding in a motor vehicle, riding a bicycle, riding an ATV, and protecting against animal bites.

Falls

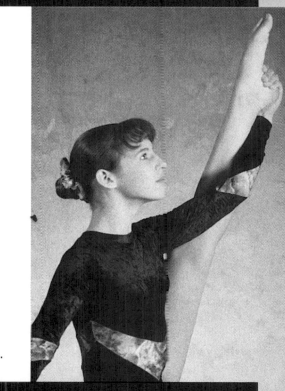

Falls cause more deaths than any other type of home accident. In addition, many people are seriously injured.

There are steps you can take to prevent falls in your home.

- Place rubber mats in the bathtub and shower to avoid slipping.
- Place a nonskid backing on floor rugs.
- Keep objects off walkways and stairways.
- Keep stairway areas well-lighted.
- Clear ice and snow from steps and sidewalks.
- Use a stepladder with handrails to reach high shelves.
- Make certain that ladders are in good condition. When standing on a ladder, keep your body in the center of the step to avoid tipping to the side.
- Do not run in your home, especially up and down the stairs.

Fires

Most home fires could be prevented, as they are caused by carelessness. Some ways in which people are careless and cause home fires include:

- falling asleep in bed or on a couch with a lighted cigarette;
- overloading electrical outlets;
- running electrical cords under rugs;
- playing with matches or cigarette lighters;
- leaving food cooking on the stove;
- having oil-soaked rags or other flammable objects in the home.

Your home should be equipped with both a smoke detector and a heat detector. A **smoke detector** is a device that sounds an alarm when smoke is detected. A **heat detector** is a device that sounds an alarm when the room temperature rises above a certain level. A fire can spread before a heat detector will send warning signals. Smoke detectors are more effective than heat detectors in detecting fires. An earlier alarm is given because smoke rises above fire.

Your family should prepare for a fire emergency.

- Test your heat detector and smoke detector so that you will be familiar with the warning sound.

- Know different ways to escape from your home should you hear the warning sound.

- Decide on a place to meet outside the home. Should there be a fire, your family will want to know if all members have escaped.

Family Fire Escape Plan

1. **Pay attention if you hear the warning sound.**

2. **Alert everyone in your home if a fire begins.**

3. **Crawl on your hands and knees to stay below the smoke line when escaping from a fire.**

4. **Feel the door for heat. Only when the door is cool should a door be opened. Even then, it should be opened slowly. Keep the door shut if it is hot.**

5. **Stuff rugs, blankets, or clothes around a door if smoke enters through the cracks.**

6. **Call the fire department or 9-1-1 after you have escaped.**

7. **Meet family members at the designated meeting place.**

8. **Do not go back into a burning building. Tell the fire officials if people or animals are inside the building.**

Electric Space Heaters and Kerosene Heaters

Fires can be caused by electric space heaters or kerosene heaters. Choose an electric space heater that shuts off automatically if tipped over. Follow these safety tips for using a kerosene heater.

- Keep the heater away from area walkways.

- Refuel a heater only with adult supervision.

- Do not refuel a heater while it is lit.

- Do not fill the tank to the top with cold kerosene. When heated, the kerosene will expand and spill over the top.

- Use the kind of kerosene recommended by the manufacturer. Never use gasoline in a kerosene heater. It can explode.

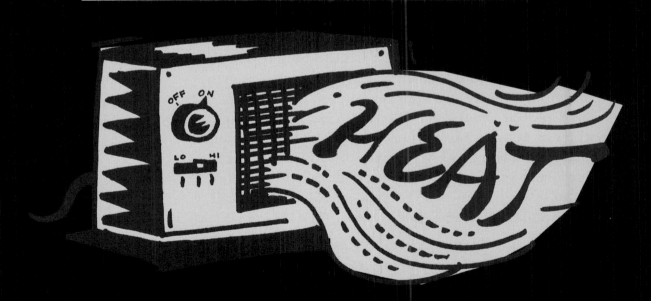

Firearms

A **firearm** is a weapon from which shot is ejected when gunpowder explodes. Many firearm accidents occur in the home. Young people often are curious about firearms and might handle them without knowing how. Firearms should be kept in a secure place and stored unloaded. Ammunition should be locked away and stored separately from the firearm.

The handling of firearms should be done only under the close supervision of a responsible adult. Teens who plan to go hunting should have the permission of their parents or guardian and the appropriate hunting license. They should be taught how to properly use and carry firearms. Firearms should be treated as if they were loaded at all times. They should never be pointed at another person or at oneself. Most firearm accidents can be avoided if simple safety precautions are observed.

Suffocation Injuries

Suffocation (su·fuh·KAY·shun) is a condition in which a person lacks oxygen due to an obstruction to the passage of air into the lungs. Most suffocation injuries occur in young children. Young children might put objects, such as marbles or buttons, in their mouths. These objects might block the airway passage and cause suffocation. Young children also suffocate when they choke on food, such as hard candy or grapes. The Teen's Guide to First Aid will tell you what to do if someone chokes. (See Lesson 50.)

Plastic bags, pillows, and blankets also can cause suffocation in small children. You might have a younger sibling or you might baby-sit. Here are things you can do to prevent suffocation injuries:

- Keep small objects, such as marbles, out of the reach of young children.
- Cut food into small pieces to make it easier to swallow.
- Keep plastic bags, such as garbage bags, away from young children.
- Never let a child put a plastic bag over his or her head.
- Check sleeping children often to be certain a pillow or blanket is not blocking their breathing.

Electric Shock

Electricity is a current that provides a source of energy. Electricity can run motors and produce light and heat. It is needed to make televisions, hair dryers, and telephones work. Electricity runs through wires. You can be shocked if you have direct contact with electric wires. Electric shock can cause injury and death.

Here are ways to prevent electric shock:

- Read the directions before using an electrical product.
- Do not use an electrical product when the wires are cracked or worn.
- Place only the recommended number of plugs in an electrical outlet.
- Pull on the plug, not the wire, when unplugging an electrical product.
- Keep electrical products away from water and other liquids.
- Do not use electrical products when you are wet, standing in water, or taking a bath or shower.

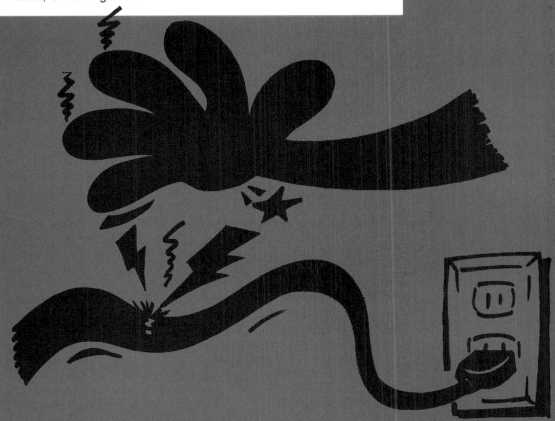

Follow a...

Health Behavior Contract

Copy the health behavior contract on a separate sheet of paper.

DO NOT WRITE IN THIS BOOK.

Name: _____ **Date:** _____

Life Skill: I will follow safety guidelines to reduce the risk of unintentional injuries.

Effect On My Health: Poisoning is a harmful chemical reaction that can occur when a drug or other substance enters the body. Poisoning can cause sickness or death. Breathing toxic gases and vapors can harm the central nervous system. I can avoid breathing toxic gases and vapors if I wear a protective mask or respirator.

My Plan: I will make a plan to avoid poisoning in my home.

I will list five household cleaners my family uses. I will wear a protective mask or respirator if I use these products.

1.

2.

3.

4.

5.

I will talk to my parents or guardian. We will decide where to keep medicines to keep our home child-proof for poisoning. The place we will keep medicines is:_____.

I will talk to my parents or guardian about installing a CO detector. A place we might put a CO detector is _____.

How My Plan Worked: (Complete after making your home safe.) I will write a paragraph to say why I want to protect myself from breathing poisons.

Poisoning

Poisoning is a harmful chemical reaction that can occur when a drug or other substance enters the body. Poisoning can cause sickness or death. Many cases of poisoning involve young children. Young children might swallow household products or take medications that were not intended for them. There are ways to prevent poisoning in young children.

- Household products and medicines should be kept out of the reach of young children.
- Household products and medicines should be purchased in childproof containers.

There are other causes of poisoning that can affect adults as well as children. Overdoses of medicine, mixing medicines, or taking the wrong medicine can cause poisoning. Breathing gases or vapors from gas leaks or faulty heating equipment also can cause poisoning.

Of particular concern is carbon monoxide poisoning. **Carbon monoxide** (KAR·buhn muh·NAHK·syd) **(CO)** is an odorless, tasteless, colorless, poisonous gas. When a person breathes CO, CO replaces oxygen in the red blood cells. As a result, some red blood cells transport CO instead of oxygen. Body cells do not get enough oxygen and a person suffocates. The signs of CO poisoning include dizziness, fatigue, headache, confusion, nausea, irregular breathing, and vomiting.

There are many potential sources of CO in the home. Heaters, stoves, and appliances fueled by gas, kerosene, or oil might produce CO if they are not installed and maintained properly. Cars, motorcycles, and lawnmowers also can produce CO. Blocked chimneys and flues can cause CO buildup. The use of a charcoal grill inside the home can release CO into the air.

Actions to Take to Prevent CO Poisoning:

- Install a CO detector in your home. A **carbon monoxide detector** is a device that sounds an alarm when there is a dangerous level of CO in the air.
- Know the signs of CO poisoning.
- Get fresh air and medical help if signs of CO poisoning occur.
- Never keep a car, motorcycle, or lawnmower running in a closed or attached garage.
- Have a qualified service technician check your home's central and room heating appliances.
- Open doors and windows when using unvented kerosene and gas space heaters.
- Have your chimney and flue checked for blockages.
- Never use a range or oven to heat a room.

Farm Injuries

Many people are injured working on farms, or being near farm equipment or animals. One out of every five fatal farm accidents involves a person under the age of 16. Most farm accidents can be prevented if the following safety guidelines are followed.

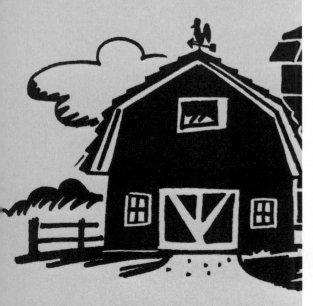

Be careful around farm equipment. Many accidents occur because people do not keep a safe distance from farm equipment. They get their hands caught in moving rollers, knives, sickles, chains, or other moving parts. They fall into storage areas and suffocate.

Be careful around farm animals. Do not approach animals without the consent of a responsible adult. Treat all animals kindly. Do not try to surprise an animal or take food from an animal that is eating. If you are going to handle an animal, ask for instructions. A responsible adult, such as an agricultural teacher or county extension agent, can give you instructions.

Protect your hearing. Farm equipment is noisy. Whenever possible, stay away from noisy equipment. Wear ear plugs to shield your ears from noise.

Protect yourself from chemicals. Chemicals might be used to spray farm plants. These chemicals can be dangerous if inhaled into the lungs. Whenever possible, avoid areas that are being sprayed. If necessary, wear a mask that protects the respiratory passages. Wear clothing to keep chemicals from getting on the body.

Follow guidelines to prevent fires. A large number of farm fires are caused by carelessness. Many are caused by lightning. They can be prevented by the use of lightning rods on buildings and roofs. Some fires are caused by cigarettes or matches that have been thrown near hay or other substances that ignite easily. Other fires occur when hay and grain are stored without being thoroughly dried. Fire extinguishers should be placed in several locations.

Have an emergency plan. Be prepared for emergencies. Someone on the farm should be trained in basic first aid. A first aid kit should be readily available. Everyone should know where the first aid kit is kept and what to do if an emergency occurs.

Follow the Road to Safety

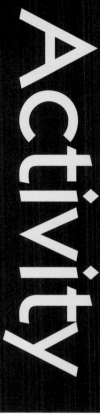

Life Skill

I will follow safety guidelines to reduce the risk of unintentional injuries.

Materials: Poster paper, markers, chips, one die

Directions: Use safety guidelines you have learned in this lesson to create and play a board game.

1. **Get into groups of four or five as instructed by your teacher.**

2. **Create a board game using poster paper and markers.** Design a path with spaces. Write a safety guideline in each space and assign points. Include actions that would NOT be safety guidelines. Examples include: "Never use a range or oven to heat a room +2 points"; and "Place household cleaner in a cabinet near the floor -2 points." Use different colored chips for markers. Make a start and finish line.

3. **Play Follow the Road to Safety.** Each player rolls the die and moves his or her marker the number of steps indicated on the die. The first person to reach the finish line wins the game.

Pedestrian Safety

A **pedestrian** is a person who is walking. Walking is the safest form of transportation. However, many pedestrians are injured or killed each year. There are ways you can stay safe when you are walking. First, *do not use alcohol or other harmful drugs, because they interfere with judgment and might cause you to be injured.* Second, follow safety guidelines for pedestrians. Do not take foolish chances.

Safety Guidelines for Pedestrians

- Never enter a street between two parked motor vehicles.
- Never attempt to cross a street as a traffic signal is changing.
- Never use headphones while walking or jogging in traffic areas.
- Never hitchhike.
- Always use sidewalks and crosswalks.
- Always walk along the side of a road against the traffic.
- Always wear light-colored clothing when you are walking at dusk or when it is dark.

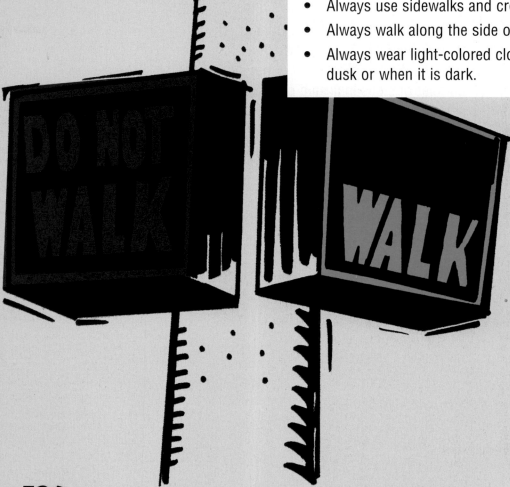

Motor Vehicle Safety

The leading cause of accidental deaths in teens is motor vehicle accidents. The reason for most of these accidents is an error by the driver. *Carefully select the people with whom you ride in a motor vehicle.* Follow safety guidelines for riding in a motor vehicle.

Safety Guidelines for Riding in a Motor Vehicle

- Never ride in a motor vehicle driven by someone who has been drinking alcohol or using other harmful drugs. Remember, alcohol and other harmful drugs interfere with reaction time and judgment.

- Never ride in a motor vehicle driven by someone who exceeds the speed limit. It is difficult to control a motor vehicle when speeding, especially in weather conditions such as rain or ice.

- Never ride in a motor vehicle with someone who is driving dangerously or showing off. Skidding, "doing doughnuts," or fishtailing can lead to accidents.

- Never ride in a motor vehicle driven by someone who argues or challenges other drivers. This can lead to accidents and fights that cause injuries.

- *Always wear a safety belt and place small children in a child safety restraint.* A **safety belt** is a seat belt and shoulder strap. A **child safety restraint** is a seat designed for a small child that is to be secured in the back seat of a motor vehicle. Some motor vehicles might also have air bags. **Air bags** are cushions in motor vehicles that inflate within a fraction of a second after a collision.

The use of safety belts and child safety restraints is now required by law in many states. Although required to by law, many teens do not "buckle up." Some teens believe safety belts are inconvenient and uncomfortable. They might think they would be better off unrestrained, even if they might be thrown from a motor vehicle. They might fear that they might be trapped underwater or in a fire. However, a person's chance of being killed is 25 times greater when thrown from a motor vehicle than when remaining in the motor vehicle. Very few accidents involve a car plunging into water or catching on fire.

Follow a...
Health Behavior Contract

Name:_____ **Date:**_____

Life Skill: I will follow guidelines for motor vehicle safety.

Effect On My Health: A safety belt is a seat belt and a shoulder strap. Laws require people to wear a safety belt when riding in a motor vehicle. Wearing a safety belt helps protect me from injury. If the motor vehicle stops suddenly, I will not hit the windshield or the seat in front of me. This protects my teeth and mouth from injury. If I am in a motor vehicle crash, I am less likely to be injured if I am wearing a safety belt.

My Plan: I will obey laws and wear a safety belt at all times. On an index card, I will write the life skill *I will follow guidelines for motor vehicle safety.* I will put the index card in the motor vehicle in which I ride most often. Each time I get into the motor vehicle for the next two weeks I will make a note on the index card. I will write the date and time. I will put initials next to the date and time to indicate that I used a safety belt.

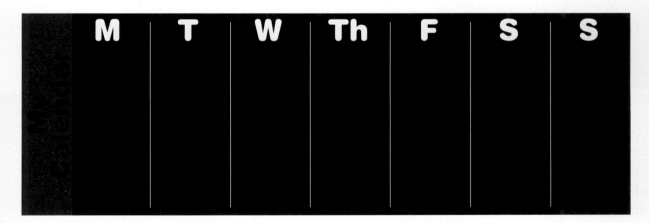

M	T	W	Th	F	S	S

How My Plan Worked: (Complete after two weeks.) I will check my index card. I will say how I felt about sticking to my promise to use a safety belt. I will write a few sentences to say how my behavior influenced the behavior of other people riding in the motor vehicle.

Bicycle Safety

Bicycle riding is gaining in popularity. Besides being a means of transportation, it is a way to exercise. However, bicycle riding can be dangerous when safety rules are not followed. The most dangerous bicycle accidents are those that involve motor vehicles. About one-half of these accidents occur at intersections. Usually, the person riding the bicycle did not obey a traffic law. Most serious injuries and deaths occur when no bicycle helmet is worn. You can reduce the risk of being injured while riding a bicycle by following safety guidelines.

Safety Guidelines for Riding a Bicycle

- Wear a bicycle helmet.
- Obey traffic rules.
- Ride single file with the traffic.
- Do not ride double.
- Use a hand signal and look back before turning left.
- Watch for the sudden opening of a car door when approaching a parked car.
- Watch for cars and trucks backing out of driveways.
- Keep your bicycle in good working order.
- Wear clothing that will not get caught in the chain or spokes of the bicycle.
- Use lights and reflectors at night.
- Wear light-colored clothing at night.
- Wear shoes at all times.
- Use crosswalks to walk a bicycle across a busy intersection.

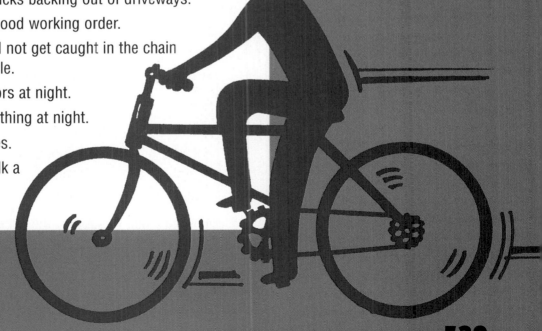

All-Terrain Vehicles

An **all-terrain vehicle (ATV)** is a vehicle that is built to travel easily over rough ground. An ATV is built to travel where other vehicles cannot go. At first, ATVs were used by people who worked in areas that they could not get to with other kinds of transportation. Now ATVs are produced for recreation. People use them for camping, exploring, trail riding, and racing. Knowing more about ATVs can prevent injury.

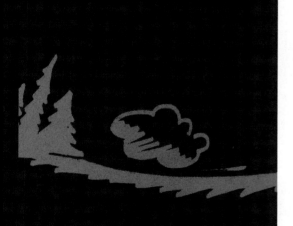

What to Know About All-Terrain Vehicles

1. **Learn how to operate an ATV safely.** The ATV Safety Institute (ASI) provides courses that teach people how to operate an ATV. Instructors teach skills such as braking, turning, and shifting. They explain clutch and throttle control and how to position the body.

2. **Follow state laws for operating ATVs.** Know your state laws regarding ATV use.

3. **Wear protective clothing.** The following protective clothing is recommended for teens:
   - A full-faced helmet
   - Eye goggles
   - A long-sleeved jersey with elbow pads
   - Riding pants with hip and thigh pads
   - Boots
   - Gloves with finger and knuckle guards
   - Chest protector and shoulder pads with elbow and full back protection
   - Knee protectors
   - Kidney belt to support the back and stomach firmly

4. **Select the appropriate size ATV for your age.** Many injuries occur when teens under the age of 16 ride ATVs designed for adults.

5. **Inspect the ATV before riding.** Be certain that all parts of the ATV are in good working condition.

6. **Follow safety guidelines.** Always keep the following set of riding rules in mind:

   - Do not operate an ATV without first having instruction.
   - Obtain a copy of the rules for riding ATVs from your local police department, and follow these rules at all times.
   - Practice riding your ATV on a level surface before riding on a tougher terrain.
   - Study a trail map before riding your ATV.
   - Keep both hands on the handlebars or steering wheel.
   - Never ride double on a one-passenger machine.
   - Do not follow another rider closely. It is difficult to see ahead and to stop quickly.
   - Always ride on the far right side of a trail.
   - Watch the grade carefully when a trail starts downhill.
   - Always yield to other vehicles.
   - Be cautious and look for pedestrians.
   - Use hand signals for stops and turns.
   - Keep a repair kit and first aid kit with you at all times.
   - Never ride by yourself in a secluded area.

Safety Around Animals

Most states now have laws that require owners to keep their pets on a leash when they are not on their own property. These laws were designed to prevent animals from harming people. Still, many people are bitten by animals. Dogs are the animals most likely to bite people. There are safety guidelines that protect you and others from animal bites.

Safety Guidelines for Protection from Animal Bites

- Keep your pet on a leash on your property.
- Do not approach strange animals.
- Do not feed strange animals.
- Do not provoke an animal by yelling or throwing something at it.
- Do not leave small children unattended near animals.
- Get medical help when bitten by an animal.

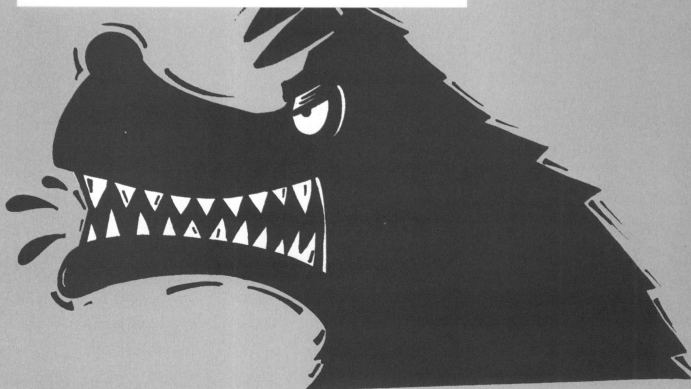

Apply...

The Responsible Decision-Making Model™

A classmate was in a fight at school yesterday. Today (s)he shows you a gun (s)he brought to school to protect himself or herself. Your friend wants you to keep the gun in your locker. (S)he says no one will suspect you.

Answer the following questions on a separate sheet of paper. Write "Does not apply" if a question does not apply to this situation.

1. Is it healthful to keep a gun in your locker? Why or why not?
2. Is it safe to keep a gun in your locker? Why or why not?
3. Is it legal to keep a gun in your locker? Why or why not?
4. Will you show respect for yourself and others if you keep a gun in your locker? Why or why not?
5. Will your parents or guardian approve if you keep a gun in your locker? Why or why not?
6. Will you demonstrate good character if you keep a gun in your locker? Why or why not?

What is the responsible decision to make in this situation?

Lesson 48

Review

Vocabulary

Write a separate sentence using each of the vocabulary words listed on page 526.

Health Content

Write responses to the following:

1. What are eight steps to prevent falls in the home? **page 527**
2. What are eight steps for the family fire escape plan? **page 528**
3. How can you stay safe around firearms? **page 530**
4. What are five ways to prevent suffocation injuries in young children? **page 530**
5. What are six ways to prevent electric shock? Two ways to prevent poisoning in young children? **pages 531–533**
6. What are six safety guidelines to prevent farm injuries? **page 534**
7. What are seven safety guidelines for pedestrians? Five safety guidelines for riding in a motor vehicle? **pages 536–537**
8. What are 13 safety guidelines for riding a bicycle? **page 539**
9. What are 14 safety guidelines for riding an ATV? **page 541**
10. What are six safety guidelines to protect against animal bites? **page 542**

Staying Safe During Extreme Weather Conditions and Natural Disasters

Vocabulary

weather

natural disaster

heat cramps

heat exhaustion

heatstroke

wind-chill factor

hypothermia

frostbite

electrical storm

lightning

hurricane

tornado

tornado watch

tornado warning

earthquake

flood

Life Skill • **I will follow safety guidelines for severe weather and natural disasters.**

Newspaper headlines often report extreme weather conditions and natural disasters. The **weather** is the condition of the atmosphere at a particular time or place. A **natural disaster** is an event caused by nature that results in damage or loss. To stay safe, you can follow safety guidelines for extreme weather conditions and natural disasters.

The Lesson Objectives

- Identify health conditions that might occur during hot and cold weather.
- State ways to stay safe during hot and cold weather.
- Explain safety guidelines to follow during: an electrical storm; a hurricane warning; a tornado watch or warning; an earthquake; a flood.

Safety During Hot Weather

Imagine that it is a hot day and the temperature is climbing. You must protect yourself from heat cramps, heat exhaustion, and heatstroke. **Heat cramps** are painful muscle spasms that occur most often in the legs and arms due to excessive fluid loss through sweating. **Heat exhaustion** is extreme tiredness due to the inability of the body temperature to be regulated. **Heatstroke** is a sudden attack of illness from exposure to high temperatures. Heatstroke can be life-threatening.

Four Ways to Stay Cool When the Temperature Is Hot

1. **Drink plenty of fluids.**
2. **Avoid becoming too exhausted.**
3. **Wear lightweight, loose-fitting clothing.**
4. **Stay in the shade or in the coolest area of an apartment, house, or building.**

Safety During Cold Weather

Imagine it is a cold day and the temperature is dropping. You can see your breath when you exhale outdoors. The radio announcer warns of the low wind-chill factor. The **wind-chill factor** is a measure of the air temperature which takes into account the chilling effect of the wind.

Continued exposure to cold temperatures can produce serious health conditions. **Hypothermia** (hy·poh·THUHR·mee·uh) is a reduction of the body temperature so that it is lower than normal. It can cause death if the body is not warmed up. Another serious condition due to cold temperatures is frostbite. **Frostbite** is the freezing of body parts, often the tissues of the extremities.

How to Stay Warm When the Temperature Is Cold

- **Wear layers of clothing.**
- **Keep clothing as dry as possible.**
- **Wear boots and gloves that are loose enough to allow circulation of blood.**
- **Stay inside when the wind-chill factor is very low.**

Safety During an Electrical Storm

An **electrical storm** is a storm in which there are bolts of lightning. **Lightning** is the flashing of light caused by electricity in the air. If you are struck by lightning, serious injury and death can occur.

Safety Guidelines to Follow During an Electrical Storm

- Do not stand under a tree or in the open. Try to find a ravine or low spot for shelter if you are caught out in the open.
- Do not swim or stay near water. Do not take a bath or shower. Electricity travels through water.
- Stay away from metal objects.
- Do not use the telephone because electricity can travel through the wires.
- Unplug electrical appliances.
- Stay away from the fireplace.

Safety During a Hurricane

A **hurricane** is a tropical storm with heavy rains and winds in excess of 74 miles per hour. In the United States, the southern Atlantic states are most at risk for hurricanes. Most hurricanes occur during August, September, and October.

Safety Guidelines to Follow During a Hurricane Warning

- Follow the warnings issued by the National Hurricane Service. These warnings are on the television and radio.
- Leave the area if advised to do so.
- Contact your local hurricane emergency office or American Red Cross chapter and ask for the community hurricane preparedness plan. This plan includes information on nearby shelters.
- Keep a safety kit containing bottled water, a radio, a flashlight, candles, and matches.

Safety During a Tornado

A **tornado** is a violent, rapidly spinning windstorm that has a funnel-shaped cloud. In the United States, tornadoes are most common in the midwestern and southern states. Most tornadoes occur in the spring and early summer months.

A **tornado watch** is a caution issued by the National Weather Service that the weather conditions are such that a tornado is possible. People in the area should be alert and prepared for possible danger. A **tornado warning** is a caution that a tornado has been sighted. These are broadcast over radio and television stations.

Safety Guidelines to Follow During a Tornado Watch or Tornado Warning

- Seek shelter in a basement or underground cellar if possible.
- Stay in the center of the ground floor, in a room with no windows, or in a closet, if there is no basement.
- Crawl under something solid, such as a heavy piece of furniture.
- Seek shelter in a low area, such as a ravine, gully, or ditch, if you are outside.

Safety During an Earthquake

An **earthquake** is a violent shaking of Earth's surface caused by the shifting of plates that make up Earth's crust. Most areas of the United States are at risk for earthquakes. To date, most earthquakes in the United States have been in western states. An earthquake in Los Angeles caused much damage.

When an earthquake occurs, the greatest number of injuries occurs from falling objects. This is why you are safest when you stay clear of objects that can fall. If you are riding in a car, it is recommended that you stop and get out. If you are on a bridge, you want to get off quickly. The bridge might collapse. Then you might become injured.

During an earthquake, there might be broken power lines. Remember, the broken power lines are hot. You cannot touch these power lines. If you do, you risk electrocution.

Suppose you are inside your home when an earthquake occurs. Suppose you are at school or inside another building. Get under a table or desk. Then if objects fall they will not strike you in the head.

Safety Guidelines to Follow During an Earthquake

- Stay calm and do not panic.
- Stay clear of any objects that can fall.
- Stay away from broken power lines.
- Get under a table or desk if you are inside a building.
- Stop and get out if riding in a car.
- Get off a bridge as quickly as possible.

Safety During a Flood

A **flood** is a rising and overflowing of a body of water onto normally dry land. You might turn on the news and hear of flash flood warnings. A flash flood is a flood that occurs suddenly. Warnings of a flash flood might occur when there is heavy rainfall. Areas near a body of water that receive heavy rainfall are at risk for floods.

Suppose your family lives near a body of water. Suppose your family lives in an area that gets heavy rainfall. Your family should prepare for floods. You should have a supply of batteries, flashlights, and a radio. The electricity might be out if flooding occurs. You should have a supply of fresh water. Your family might keep some bottled water. It is not safe to drink water from a flood. Your family should also keep a first aid kit. Family members should know the safest and quickest route to take away from your home.

Safety Guidelines to Prepare for and Follow During a Flood

- Leave your home and community if warned to do so by officials.
- Keep a supply of batteries, flashlights, and a radio available.
- Learn the safest and quickest route to take from your home to shelter.
- Keep supplies of fresh water and food that do not need refrigeration or heat.
- Turn off all electrical circuits in the home if a flood occurs.
- Close all gas lines that lead into the home.
- Move all valuables to the top floors in a home to help prevent their destruction.
- Keep the family car in good working order and keep the gas tank filled so that you can leave the area quickly.
- Have a first aid kit available.
- Do not drive where water is over the road.

Eye Out for the Storm

Life Skill

I will follow safety guidelines for severe weather and natural disasters.

Materials: Newspaper, paper, pen or pencil

Directions: Combine your imagination with your knowledge of how to stay safe during natural disasters to create a story.

1. **Look through a newspaper or visit the Internet to find an article about a natural disaster.**

2. **Write a two-page story based on the article.** Include safety guidelines for the disaster throughout your story.

Lesson 49

Review

Vocabulary

Write a separate sentence using each of the vocabulary words listed on page 544.

Health Content

Write responses to the following:

1. What are three health conditions that might occur during hot weather? **page 545**

2. What are four ways to stay cool when the temperature rises? **page 545**

3. What are two serious health conditions that can result from continued exposure to cold temperatures? **page 546**

4. What are four ways to stay warm when the temperature is cold? **page 546**

5. What are six safety guidelines to follow during an electrical storm? **page 547**

6. What are four safety guidelines to follow during a hurricane warning? **page 547**

7. What is the difference between a tornado watch and a tornado warning? **page 548**

8. What are four safety guidelines to follow during a tornado watch or tornado warning? **page 548**

9. What are six safety guidelines to follow during an earthquake? **page 549**

10. What are ten safety guidelines to prepare for and follow during a flood? **page 550**

The Teen's Guide to First Aid

Vocabulary*

first aid

emergency

universal precautions

Medic Alert tag

emergency dispatcher

actual consent

implied consent

Good Samaritan laws

***A complete listing
of vocabulary words
appears on page 553.**

Life Skill

• **I will be skilled in first aid procedures.**

First aid is the immediate and temporary care given to a person who has been injured or suddenly becomes ill. It is important for you to learn first aid skills. An **emergency** is a serious situation that occurs without warning and calls for quick action. You will know what to do when someone needs help. You will not panic. You will be safer in your own activities.

The Lesson Objectives

- Discuss what items should be kept in a first aid kit.

- Discuss universal precautions.

- Explain how to: be prepared for emergencies at home; be alert to emergencies; respond to an emergency; make an emergency telephone call; get consent to give first aid; and check a victim.

- Explain first aid procedures for: choking; rescue breathing; CPR; heart attack; stroke; bleeding; shock; poisoning; marine animal stings; tick bites; burns; injuries to muscles, bones, and joints; sudden illness; heat-related illnesses; and cold-temperature related illnesses.

Aid Me If I'm Wrong

Activity

 Life Skill I will be skilled in first aid procedures.

Materials: Index cards, pen or pencil

Directions: Play Aid Me If I'm Wrong to help you learn the meanings of terms used in first aid.

1. **Your teacher will pass out index cards and assign each student two to three words from the vocabulary list below.**

2. **Find the definitions of your words in this lesson.** Write the definitions on one side of your index card. Skip a line between each definition you write. Underline the vocabulary words.

3. **Find vocabulary words you have not been assigned.** Write the vocabulary words without their definitions on the line above the assigned vocabulary words. For example your card might look like this:

burn

A <u>strain</u> is an overstretching of muscles and/or tendons.

bruise

A <u>fracture</u> is a break or a crack in a bone.

4. **Your teacher will collect the cards and divide your class into two teams.**

5. **Your teacher will read each definition out loud but insert the vocabulary word you were not assigned.** (S)he will call on students on each team to give the correct vocabulary word.

first aid
emergency
universal precautions
Medic Alert tag
emergency dispatcher
actual consent
implied consent
Good Samaritan laws
victim assessment
choking
universal distress signal
abdominal thrusts
rescue breathing
cardiopulmonary
  resuscitation (CPR)

heart attack
cardiac arrest
stroke
wound
closed wound
open wound
bruise
incision
laceration
abrasion
avulsion
puncture
infection
tetanus

lockjaw
nosebleed
knocked-out tooth
shock
poison
Lyme disease
burn
first-degree burn
second-degree burn
third-degree burn
electrical burn
chemical burn
splint
fracture
open fracture

closed fracture
dislocation
sprain
strain
sudden illness
heat-related illnesses
heat cramps
heat exhaustion
heatstroke
cold-temperature related
  illnesses
frostbite
hypothermia

The First Aid Kit

It is important to keep first aid kits where they might be needed. Keep a first aid kit at home and in the family car. Carry a first aid kit when you participate in outdoor activities, such as camping and hiking. Ask where first aid kits are kept when you are away from home. You can purchase a first aid kit from a drugstore or the local chapter of the American Red Cross. You also can purchase items and put together a first aid kit yourself. Keep items needed to follow universal precautions in your first aid kit. Universal precautions are discussed later. Add special medicines you or family members need. Check the first aid kit often. Some of the items have expiration dates and will need to be replaced. Be certain flashlight batteries work.

activated charcoal

syrup of ipecac

plastic bags

triangular bandage

gauze pads and roller gauze

cold pack

disposable gloves

adhesive tape

hand cleaner

adhesive bandages

small flashlight and extra batteries

scissors and tweezers

blanket

antiseptic ointment

Follow a...

Health Behavior Contract

Name:_____ **Date:**_____

Copy the health behavior contract on a separate sheet of paper.

DO NOT WRITE IN THIS BOOK.

Life Skill: I will be skilled in first aid procedures.

Effect On My Health: First aid is the immediate and temporary care given to a person who has been injured or suddenly becomes ill. My family needs to have a first aid kit. I need to know the location of the first aid kit. Then I will be able to get the first aid kit quickly if I need it. I also need to know the emergency telephone numbers for the fire department, police, poison control center, my physician, and my dentist. Then I will be able to get help quickly. I will be less likely to panic. I will make better decisions in an emergency situation. The victim for whom I provide first aid will get better care.

My Plan: I will make a list of items that need to be in a first aid kit. I will ask my parents or guardian where we will keep our first aid kit. I will write the emergency telephone numbers on a notepad and place them by our telephone.

Items in first aid kit	Location of first aid kit	Emergency phone numbers
		Fire Department:
		Police:
		Poison Control Center:
		Physician:
		Dentist:

How My Plan Worked: I will notify all family members of the first aid kit and where it will be kept. I will go over with them the emergency telephone numbers that are on the notepad.

Universal Precautions: Protect Your Health

You must protect your health when giving first aid to another person. A victim's body fluids might contain harmful pathogens. For example, blood and other body fluids might contain HIV or HBV. HIV is found in blood, semen, vaginal secretions, and urine. A person who is infected with HIV will develop AIDS. HBV also is found in blood. A person who is infected with HBV can develop hepatitis B. You can help a victim and reduce your risk of infection with these pathogens.

Universal precautions are steps taken to prevent the spread of disease by treating all human blood and body fluids as if they contained HIV, HBV, and other pathogens. Follow universal precautions in any situation in which you might have contact with blood and other body fluids.

FOLLOW UNIVERSAL PRECAUTIONS
- Wear Disposable Latex Gloves
- Always Use a Face Mask

Universal Precautions

1. Wear disposable latex or vinyl gloves. Your hands and fingers might have tiny cuts or openings you cannot see. Pathogens in a victim's blood or other body fluids might enter your bloodstream through these tiny cuts or openings. Wearing latex or vinyl gloves helps protect you from contact with the victim's blood. Do not wear the same gloves more than once. Do not wear the same gloves to give first aid to another victim.

2. Wash your hands with soap and water after removing gloves. This provides extra protection.

3. Use a face mask with a one-way valve when performing first aid for breathing emergencies. You might have tiny cuts or openings in your lips or mouth. There might be blood in the saliva or vomit in the victim's mouth. The victim might be bleeding from the mouth or nose. The face mask helps protect you from the victim's blood. Follow the instructions provided with the face mask. Do not use the face mask to give first aid to more than one victim without sterilizing it.

4. Take other precautions to avoid contact with the victim's blood. Cover any cuts, scrapes, or rashes on your body with a plastic wrap or sterile dressing. Avoid touching objects that have had contact with the victim's blood.

5. Do not eat or drink anything while giving first aid. Wash hands after giving first aid and before eating or drinking. This will help prevent pathogens from entering your body.

6. Do not touch your mouth, eyes, or nose while caring for a victim.

Plan Ahead If You Play Sports

Suppose you are on a sports team. Plan ahead to know what to do if an emergency occurs. Ask your coach what to do if you or a teammate is injured and begins to bleed. Find out who will give first aid. Find out where the first aid kit will be. Discuss what you learn with your parents or guardian.

Emergencies at Home: Be Prepared

Your family should be prepared for an emergency.

1. Keep the local emergency telephone number by your telephone.

2. Keep a list of other important telephone numbers by your telephone, such as the telephone number for the:

   • **fire department;**
   • **police;**
   • **poison control center;**
   • **your physician;**
   • **your dentist.**

3. Keep the names and telephone numbers of neighbors who would help, too. Be certain that your family's address is easy to read from the street. This allows emergency helpers to locate your residence quickly.

4. Keep family medical records where you can get them quickly. Know where insurance cards are. These records provide valuable information when medical help is needed.

5. Wear a Medic Alert tag if you have a health condition. A **Medic Alert tag** is a medical identification tag that provides medical information about the person wearing it. It is usually worn as a necklace or bracelet.

6. Keep first aid kits where they might be needed.

7. Keep available items needed to follow universal precautions.

Emergencies Around You: Be on the Lookout

You can recognize and report emergencies that happen around you. Your senses of hearing, sight, and smell can help you recognize an emergency. Pay attention to what you hear, see, and smell.

Unusual noises can alert you to an emergency. You might hear someone scream, cry, moan, or call for help. You might notice the sound of screeching tires, a gun being fired, two automobiles crashing into one another, or glass breaking. These sounds alert you that something is wrong.

Unusual sights can alert you to an emergency. You might see smoke or fire coming from a building. You might see someone carrying a weapon and running from a store. An automobile might be on the side of the road with its lights flashing. Electrical wires might be down during a storm. These sights warn you an emergency might exist. The way a person looks and behaves also might catch your attention. An empty medicine container might be next to a person who is lying down and not moving. A person might have slurred speech and stagger while walking. A person might be choking and turning a pale blue color.

Unusual or strong odors can alert you to an emergency. You might wake up to the smell of smoke. There might be the odor of gas. There might be the odor of a strong-smelling chemical in the air. These odors warn of possible danger. They might alert you to a fire.

How to Respond to an Emergency

You must make responsible decisions when an emergency exists. Evaluate the situation carefully. Consider your safety first. Do not put your life in danger to save someone else. Instead, obtain emergency help. Suppose you hear the sound of a gun being fired. Someone might be wounded and need help. The responsible decision might be to call the police. Police officers can protect themselves from harm. If you go outside to see what happened, you risk being shot. Suppose a house is on fire and you know there is a small child inside. Flames are soaring from the house. It is not safe to enter the house. You would risk being injured, too. If you are injured, you will not be able to help the child, either. The responsible decision might be to get a firefighter to enter the house. Firefighters wear protective clothing and are trained to rescue victims.

Consider the impact of the emergency situation. How many people are involved? The number of victims will affect the resources needed for help. Suppose several teens are injured in an automobile accident. The extent of their injuries will vary. What kind of care will each victim need? You will need this information when you call for help.

The emergency situation might pose a threat to others in the community. Suppose a building is on fire. The fire might spread to another building. More people might be injured. How might the people in the other building be alerted to the fire? Suppose there is a victim of violence. The person or people who harmed the victim are still at large. How can other people stay safe until the police arrive?

You might be with other people during an emergency. How can you work together to respond to the emergency? If an adult is present, the adult should be in charge. If there is more than one person available, one person should call for help. The other person or people should stay with the victim(s).

How to Make an Emergency Telephone Call

Be prepared to make an emergency telephone call. Learn the telephone numbers to call in your community. Check out the telephone numbers to call when you travel to another community. In many communities, calling 9-1-1 will reach assistance for fire, police, and medical emergencies. The local phone book will tell whether a community has a 9-1-1 emergency assistance telephone number. Dial the operator (the number 0) if you do not know the correct number to call.

An emergency dispatcher will answer the telephone when you call 9-1-1. An **emergency dispatcher** is a person who decides who to contact when there is a call for help. The call may be directed to the police, fire station, poison control center, rescue squad, or emergency medical team.

Guidelines to Follow When Making an Emergency Telephone Call:

1. Remain calm and speak clearly.

2. Describe the exact location of the emergency. Give the address and ways for emergency personnel to find the location. Naming the closest intersection or a landmark is helpful.

3. Give your name, what happened, the number of people involved, the condition of the injured people, and the help that has been given.

4. Give the telephone number of the telephone you are using. This makes it possible for someone to call you back if you get disconnected or if more information is needed.

5. Listen carefully if you are told how to care for the victim. Write down directions if necessary. Give directions to other people who are caring for the victim.

6. Do not hang up the telephone until you are told to do so.

7. Return to the victim. Provide care if appropriate. Stay with the victim until help arrives.

No Prank Calls

Never make prank calls to your local emergency telephone number.

More than 35 percent of all calls made to 9-1-1 are for nonemergencies.

The emergency dispatcher must take time to answer the telephone and evaluate each call. Unnecessary calls and prank calls can take time away from real emergency calls. These calls might slow down help to people who really need it.

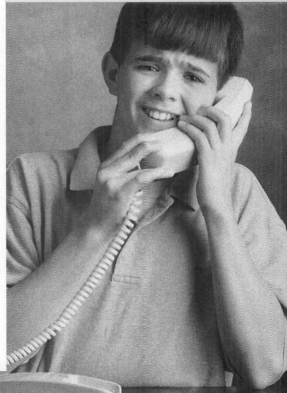

How to Obtain Consent to Give First Aid

You must have consent to give first aid. Consent means permission. There are two types of consent.

Actual Consent

Actual consent is oral or written permission from a mentally competent adult to give first aid. Tell the victim who you are, what you plan to do, and the first aid training that you have had. If the person gives you permission, this is actual consent. Do not give first aid to a conscious adult who does not give you permission.

A parent or guardian must give actual consent if the victim is a child or is not mentally competent. A supervising adult with legal permission from parents to care for an infant or child also can give actual consent. Do not give first aid to a conscious infant or child when a parent or guardian says NO. Do not give first aid to a conscious infant or child when a supervising adult with legal permission to care for an infant or child says NO.

Implied Consent

Implied consent is unspoken understanding that first aid may be given if no one who can give actual consent is conscious or present. You have implied consent to give first aid to:

- a mentally competent adult victim who is unconscious;
- an adult victim who is not mentally competent, when no adult who can grant actual consent is present;
- an infant or child when no adult who can grant actual consent is present.

Good Samaritan Laws

Good Samaritan laws are laws that protect people who give first aid in good faith and without gross negligence or misconduct. Many states have Good Samaritan laws to protect people who give first aid. Lawsuits usually do not occur if a person giving first aid has the skills to do so. Lawsuits do occur when a minor injury is made worse because of the first aid given. Good Samaritan laws cannot provide complete legal protection. Anyone giving first aid should be properly trained and apply the correct procedures and skills.

Perform only the first aid skills you have been trained to give. Do not perform skills beyond your knowledge such as those you might see on a television show.

How to Check the Victim

A **victim assessment** is a check of the injured or medically ill person to determine if:

- the victim has an open airway;
- the victim is breathing;
- the victim's heart is beating;
- the victim is severely bleeding;
- the victim has other injuries.

FOLLOW UNIVERSAL PRECAUTIONS

Wear Disposable Latex Gloves and Always Use a Face Mask

1.

Call the local emergency number and obtain medical care immediately.

Ask the victim what happened. A victim who is able to speak to you is breathing and has a pulse.

2.

Tap the victim and shout loudly to see if the victim responds.

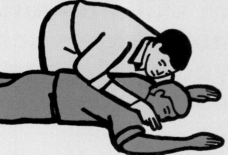

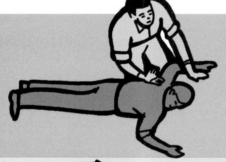

3.

Check for breathing if the victim does not respond.

a) Place your finger under the nose or near the mouth to feel for air being exhaled.

b) Listen for signs of breathing.

4.

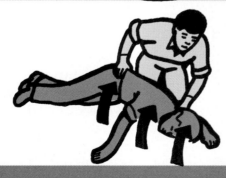

If there are no signs of breathing...

Support the head and neck and position the victim on the back.

5. Tilt the head back and lift the chin of the victim. The victim's mouth should be open.

6. Make a five-second recheck for signs of breathing. (Repeat step 3.)

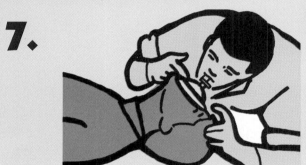

7. **If there are still no signs of breathing...**

Wear a face mask or shield for protection. Follow instructions provided with the mask. Blow two slow breaths of air into the victim's mouth.

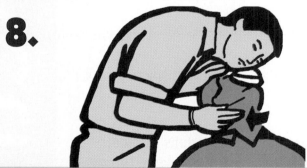

8. Check to see if the victim has a pulse for five to ten seconds. Use your index and third finger and check the carotid artery in the victim's neck.

9.

10. Check the victim's body for severe bleeding. Be certain to follow universal precautions to avoid contact with the victim's blood.

Check for other injuries.

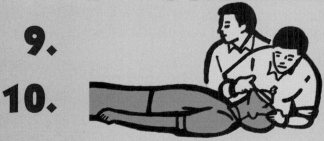

First Aid for Choking

Choking is an emergency in which the airway is blocked. A piece of food or other small object might block the airway. A conscious victim will cough to try to dislodge it. If a victim can talk, the victim is getting enough air. Encourage the victim to continue trying to cough up the object. Call for help if the victim cannot cough up the object.

A victim might not get enough air to talk or cough. Or the cough might be very weak. This tells you that the airway is completely blocked. The victim might indicate that (s)he is not breathing. The **universal distress signal** is a warning that a person has difficulty breathing and is shown by clutching at the throat with one or both hands.

The airway must be opened quickly when someone is choking. **Abdominal thrusts** are a series of thrusts to the abdomen that force air from the lungs to dislodge an object. The method of giving abdominal thrusts is different for adults, children, and infants.

Practice Abdominal Thrusts

Life Skill

I will be skilled in first aid procedures.

Materials: A one gallon plastic milk container, black marker

Directions: Complete the following activity to practice giving abdominal thrusts.

1. **Outline the front "chest" area on a one-gallon milk container.** Use a marker to make the lungs and the rib cage.

2. **Place a cork in the milk container to represent something upon which a person is choking.**

3. **Practice abdominal thrusts for adults or older children who are conscious and choking.** Wrap your hands around the milk carton. Make a fist with one hand. Place the thumb side of the fist into the part of the milk carton just below the rib cage. Grab your fist with the other hand. Give five quick abdominal thrusts to dislodge the cork from the milk carton. Apply pressure inward and push up in one smooth movement.

Activity

When an Adult or Older Child Is Conscious and Is Choking

1. FOLLOW UNIVERSAL PRECAUTIONS
- Wear Disposable Latex Gloves
- Always Use a Face Mask

Call the local emergency number and obtain medical care immediately.

> Ask the victim if (s)he is choking. Do not do anything if the victim can speak or cough easily. Encourage the victim to continue coughing to dislodge the object.

2.

If the victim cannot speak, breathe, or cough...

> Stand behind the victim and wrap your hand around the victim's waist. Make a fist with one hand. Place the thumb side of the fist into the victim's abdomen above the navel and below the rib cage. Grab your fist with the other hand.

3.

> Give five quick abdominal thrusts. Apply pressure inward and push up toward the victim's diaphragm in one smooth movement. Repeat the cycle of five abdominal thrusts until the object is dislodged.

The victim might need rescue breathing after the object is dislodged. Stay with the victim and watch for breathing difficulties.

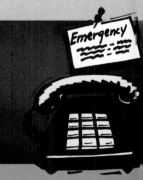

Call the local emergency number and obtain medical care immediately.

When an Adult or Older Child Is Not Conscious and Is Choking

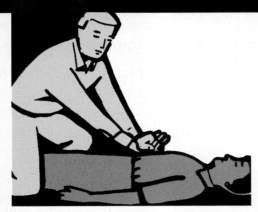

1.

Call the local emergency number and obtain medical care immediately.

Roll the victim on his or her back. Place the heel of your hand just above the navel. Point your fingers toward the victim's head and give five quick abdominal thrusts.

The victim might need rescue breathing if the object is not dislodged.

When an Infant or Young Child Is Choking

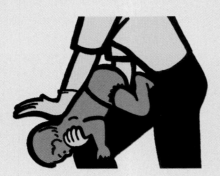

1.

If the victim cannot cough, cry, or breathe...

Place the victim face down on your forearm or upper leg. Support the victim's head by placing your hand around the lower jaw and chest. Use the heel of your other hand and give five quick blows to the victim's back between the shoulder blades.

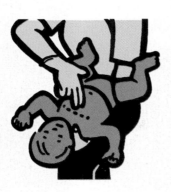

2.

Place the victim face up on your upper leg. Make certain that the victim's head is lower than the trunk. Press two or three fingers in the center of the breastbone (just below an imaginary line between the nipples). Give five quick chest thrusts. Repeat back blows and chest thrusts until the object is dislodged.

The victim might need rescue breathing after the object is dislodged. Stay with the victim and watch for breathing difficulties.

When You Are Choking

Call the local emergency number and obtain medical care immediately.

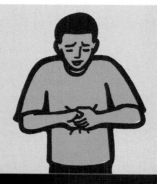

1. Get the attention of someone around you. Use the universal distress signal if you are unable to speak.

2. Give yourself abdominal thrusts if no one can help you. Make a fist with one hand and grab the fist with your other hand. Give yourself five quick abdominal thrusts. Apply pressure inward and push up toward your diaphragm in one smooth movement. Repeat until the object is dislodged.

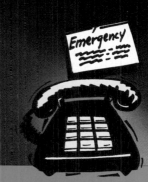

Call the local emergency number and obtain medical care immediately.

FOLLOW UNIVERSAL PRECAUTIONS
- Wear Disposable Latex Gloves
- Always Use a Face Mask

Rescue Breathing

Suppose a person is swimming and begins to drown. Suppose someone has a heart attack and stops breathing. A victim will become unconscious without oxygen after a period of time. When the heart muscle does not get oxygen, the heart stops beating. Blood carrying oxygen stops circulating to body organs.

A person can live without oxygen for a few minutes. However, the longer a person is without oxygen the more damage there will be to body organs. For example, suppose a person has been without oxygen for a period of time. The brain cells did not receive oxygen during this time. This person can have brain damage. This person can have damage to other body organs that did not get oxygen.

Without quick first aid, a victim who is not breathing will have damage to body organs. The victim can die. **Rescue breathing** is a way of breathing air into an unconscious victim who is not breathing, but has a pulse. Rescue breathing gives a victim the oxygen needed to stay alive. For rescue breathing to help, it must be given quickly. You must know the proper technique.

When you give rescue breathing, you need to follow universal precautions. Always wear a face mask for rescue breathing. If you do not, you will have contact with the body fluids in the victim's mouth. Try out a face mask in a nonemergency situation. Read the directions for wearing it. Then you will be prepared when you need to put it on quickly.

Wear disposable latex gloves, too. You might have to clear out vomit or an object from the victim's mouth. The victim might have other injuries and there might be blood.

Follow Universal Precautions

A face mask or shield should be worn for rescue breathing. Place it between your mouth and nose and the victim's mouth and nose. This helps prevent you from having contact with the victim's body fluids.

FOLLOW UNIVERSAL PRECAUTIONS
• Wear Disposable Latex Gloves
• Always Use a Face Mask

Using a Face Mask
Adults and Children

Follow the instructions provided with the face mask. The folllowing instructions might be included with a face mask:

1. Apply rim of mask between the victim's lower lip and chin, thus pulling back the lower lip to keep the mouth open under the mask. Position the end marked "nose" over the victim's nose.

2. Seal mask. Open airway and blow slowly.

3. Remove your mouth. Allow the victim to exhale. Continue until the chest rises (If the victim vomits, remove the mask and clear the victim's airway. Reapply mask.)

For Infants

Follow procedures except reverse the mask so the end marked "nose" is under the chin.

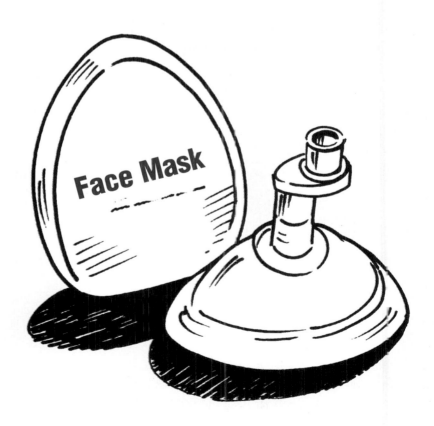

Face Mask

Rescue Breathing for Adults and Older Children

FOLLOW UNIVERSAL PRECAUTIONS
• Wear Disposable Latex Gloves
• Always Use a Face Mask

1.

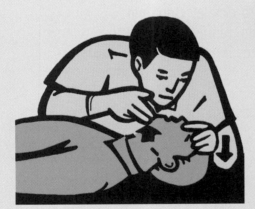

Call the local emergency number and obtain medical care immediately.

Roll the victim on his or her back. Tilt the victim's head back in the following way. Place one hand under the victim's chin and lift up while pressing down on the victim's forehead with your other hand. Pinch the victim's nostrils shut.

2.

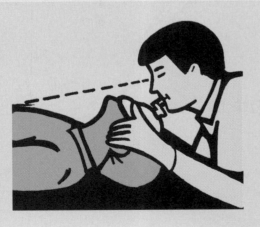

Wear a face mask or shield for protection. Follow instructions provided with mask. Apply mask. Open airway. Give two slow breaths. Watch to see if the victim's chest slowly rises.

3.

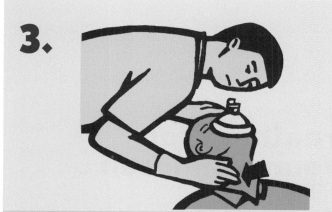

Check to see if the victim has a pulse. Use your index and third finger and find the carotid artery in the neck. The carotid artery is the large artery where the pulse can be felt.

4.

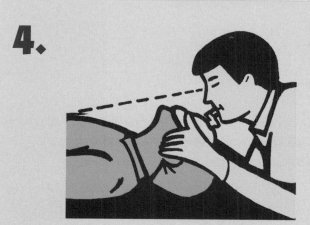

If the pulse is present, but the victim is still not breathing...

Give one slow breath about every five seconds. Remove your mouth after each breath so the victim can exhale.

5.

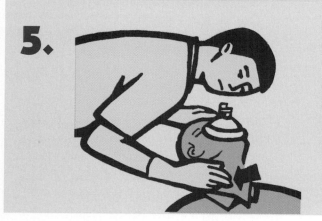

Recheck pulse and breathing every minute. Continue rescue breathing as long as the victim is not breathing, but has a pulse.

If the victim does not have a pulse, the heart is not beating. CPR is needed. CPR is illustrated in the next section.

CPR should be used only if you are trained to use it.

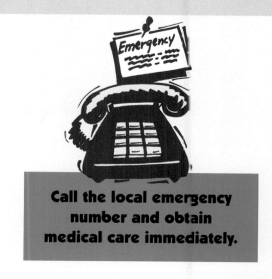

Call the local emergency number and obtain medical care immediately.

Rescue Breathing for Infants and Young Children

FOLLOW UNIVERSAL PRECAUTIONS
- Wear Disposable Latex Gloves
- Always Use a Face Mask

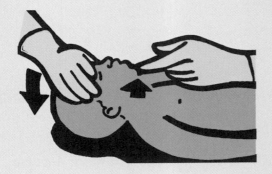

1.

Call the local emergency number and obtain medical care immediately.

Roll the victim on his or her back. Tilt the victim's head back slightly.

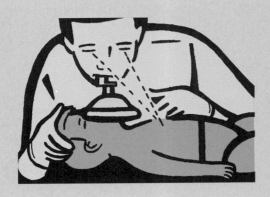

2.

Wear a face mask or shield for protection. Follow instructions provided with mask. Apply mask. Open airway. Give two slow breaths. Watch to see if the victim's chest slowly rises. Remove your mouth to allow the victim to exhale.

3.

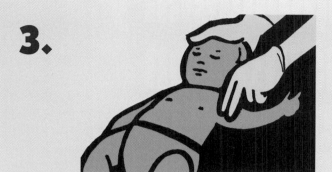

Check to see if the victim has a pulse. Use your index and third finger and check the brachial artery on the inside of the upper arm.

4.

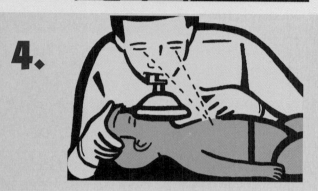

If the pulse is present, but the victim is still not breathing...

Give one slow breath about every three seconds. Remove your mouth after each breath so the victim can exhale. Recheck pulse and breathing every minute.

5.

Continue rescue breathing as long as the victim is not breathing, but has a pulse.

If the victim does not have a pulse, the heart is not beating. CPR is needed. CPR is illustrated in the next section.

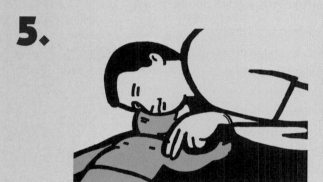

CPR should be used only if you are trained to use it.

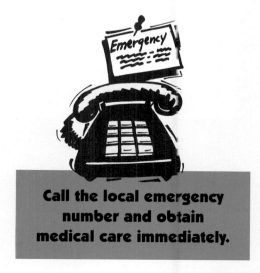

Call the local emergency number and obtain medical care immediately.

Cardiopulmonary Resuscitation

Cardiopulmonary resuscitation (CPR) is a first aid technique that is used to restore heartbeat and breathing. Think about the letters CPR to remember the name of this first aid skill. C stands for cardio or heart. P stands for pulmonary or the lungs. R stands for resuscitation. In this first aid technique, the heart (cardio) and lungs (pulmonary) are helped to work (resuscitation).

CPR is an advanced first aid skill. For this reason, people who give CPR require training. You should not give CPR if you are not trained to do so. The American Red Cross offers training in CPR. They have special instructors who provide the training. These instructors are certified as first aid instructors. They keep their certification current.

You can call the American Red Cross to learn where courses are offered. Perhaps your teacher is certified to teach CPR. Perhaps someone else in your school is certified to teach CPR. Talk with your parents or guardian. Find out if they or other family members are trained to give CPR. This is a first aid technique that adults should learn. You do not know when a family member or other close person might need to have CPR.

People who give CPR should follow universal precautions. A face mask should be worn. If a face mask is not worn, there can be contact with fluids in the victim's mouth. The victim also might be bleeding from the nose. Wear disposable latex gloves. The victim's airway might have to be cleared. The victim might have other injuries. The victim might have been bleeding.

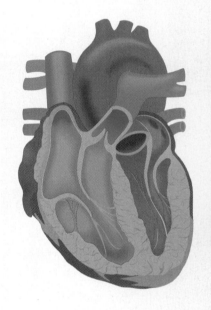

FOLLOW UNIVERSAL PRECAUTIONS
• Wear Disposable Latex Gloves
• Always Use a Face Mask

CPR should be used only if you are trained to use it.

CPR should be used only if you are trained to use it.

CPR

The ABCs of CPR help you determine the need for CPR.

A-Airway — Open the victim's airway.

B-Breathing — Perform rescue breathing if breathing has stopped.

C-Circulation — Perform CPR if pulse is absent.

Cardiopulmonary Resuscitation for Adults and Older Children

FOLLOW UNIVERSAL PRECAUTIONS
With Disposable Latex Gloves
Always Use a Face Mask

CPR should be used only if you are trained to use it.

1.

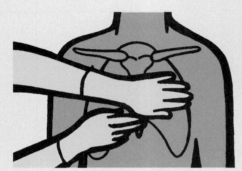

Make a victim assessment.

Call the local emergency number and obtain medical care immediately.

A person who is trained in CPR should:

Roll the victim on his or her back. Find the lower part of the breastbone and measure up the width of two fingers from that point. Place the heel of your other hand on the sternum next to the fingers. Place the other hand on top of the first hand.

2.

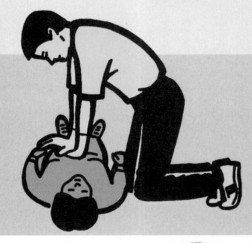

Position shoulders over hands to exert pressure straight down. Compress the chest 15 times (at a rate of 80 compressions per minute). Exert enough pressure to depress the breastbone one and one-half to two inches. Each compression forces blood from the heart to other parts of the body.

3.

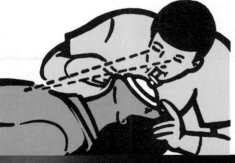

Wear a face mask or shield for protection. Follow instructions provided with mask. Apply the mask. Open the airway. Give two slow breaths. Watch to see if the victim's chest slowly rises. Remove the mouth to allow the victim to exhale.

4.

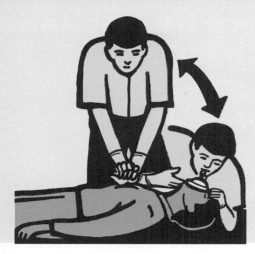

Do three more sets of 15 compressions and two slow breaths.

5.

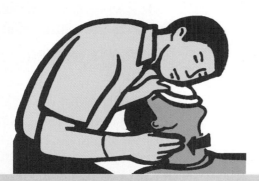

Make a five-second check to see if the victim has a pulse and is breathing.

6.

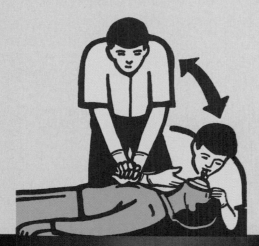

If the victim does not have a pulse...

Continue sets of 15 compressions and two slow breaths.

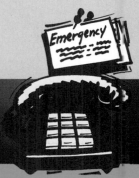

Call the local emergency number and obtain medical care immediately.

Cardiopulmonary Resuscitation for Children

FOLLOW UNIVERSAL PRECAUTIONS
• Wear Disposable Latex Gloves
• Always Use a Face Mask

CPR should be used only if you are trained to use it.

1.

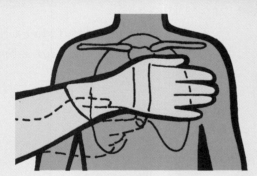

Make a victim assessment.

Call the local emergency number and obtain medical care immediately.

A person who is trained in CPR should:

Roll the victim on his or her back. Place the heel of your hand on the center of the breastbone.

2.

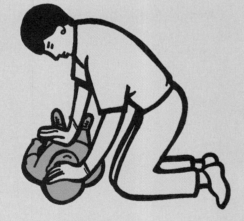

Position shoulders over the hand to exert pressure straight down. Compress the chest five times (at a rate of 60 compressions per minute).

3.

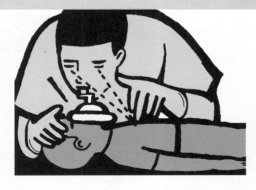

Wear a face mask or shield for protection. Follow instructions provided with mask. Apply the mask. Open the airway. Give one slow breath. Watch to see if the victim's chest slowly rises. Remove the mouth to allow the victim to exhale.

4.

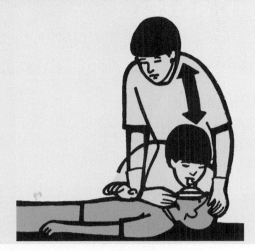

Repeat sets of five compressions and one slow breath for about one minute (12 sets).

5.

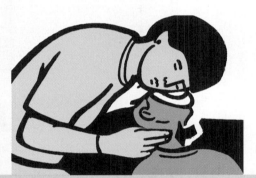

Make a five-second check to see if the victim has a pulse and is breathing.

6.

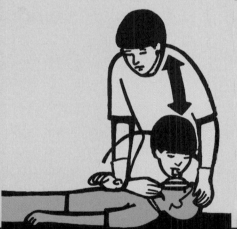

If the victim does not have a pulse...

Continue sets of five compressions and one slow breath. Recheck pulse and breathing every few minutes.

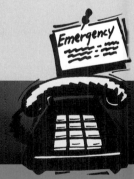

Call the local emergency number and obtain medical care immediately.

Cardiopulmonary Resuscitation for Infants

FOLLOW UNIVERSAL PRECAUTIONS
- Wear Disposable Latex Gloves
- Always Use a Face Mask

CPR should be used only if you are trained to use it.

1.

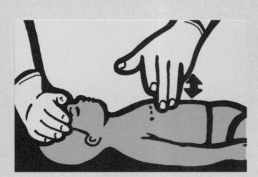

Make a victim assessment.

Call the local emergency number and obtain medical care immediately.

A person who is trained in CPR should:

Roll the victim on his or her back. Place the third and fourth finger on the center of the breastbone. Compress the chest five times.

2.

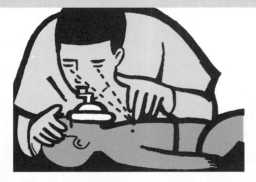

Wear a face mask or shield for protection. Follow instructions provided with mask. Apply mask. Open airway. Give one slow breath. Watch to see if the victim's chest slowly rises. Remove the mouth to allow the victim to exhale.

3.

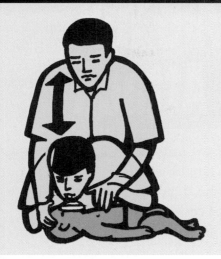

Repeat sets of five compressions and one slow breath for about one minute (12 sets).

4.

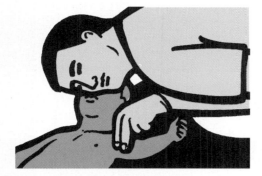

Check to see if the victim has a pulse and is breathing.

5.

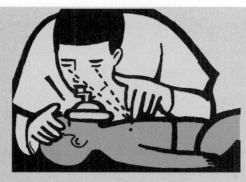

If the victim does not have a pulse...

Continue sets of five compressions and one slow breath. Recheck for pulse and breathing every few minutes.

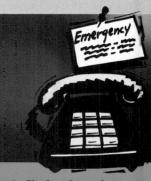

Call the local emergency number and obtain medical care immediately.

First Aid for Heart Attack

A **heart attack** is the death of part of the heart muscle caused by a lack of blood flow to the heart. The blocked blood vessel prevents blood from getting to the heart tissue. Without blood, the heart tissue does not receive oxygen. This usually causes pain in the center of the chest, beneath the breastbone. **Cardiac arrest** is the death of the heart muscle. Prompt action must be taken for warning signs of heart attack to prevent cardiac arrest.

The Warnings Signs of Heart Attack

- **Persistent pain or pressure in the center of the chest that is not relieved by resting or changing position**
- **Pain that spreads from the center of the chest to the shoulder, arm, neck, jaw, or back**
- **Dizziness**
- **Sweating**
- **Fainting**
- **Difficulty breathing**
- **Shortness of breath**
- **Pale or bluish skin color**
- **Moist face**
- **Irregular pulse**

First aid for heart attack involves these steps:

Call the local emergency number and obtain medical care immediately.

1. Have the victim stop activity and rest in a comfortable position.

2. Ask the victim about his or her condition. Does the victim have a history of heart disease? Is the victim taking any medication?

3. Comfort the victim until help arrives.

4. Observe the victim for changes in condition.

If cardiac arrest occurs, the victim is not breathing and has no pulse...

A person who is trained in CPR should:

5. Perform CPR and rescue breathing.

CPR should be used only if you are trained to use it.

FOLLOW UNIVERSAL PRECAUTIONS
- Wear Disposable Latex Gloves
- Always Use a Face Mask

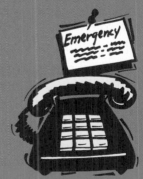

Call the local emergency number and obtain medical care immediately.

First Aid for Stroke

A **stroke** is a condition caused by a blocked or broken blood vessel in the brain. A stroke can occur when a clot moves through the bloodstream and lodges in the brain. A clot can form inside one of the arteries in the brain, or a blood vessel in the brain can burst. A head injury or tumor can cause an artery to burst. Blood cannot get to all parts of the brain and some tissue dies.

The damage that occurs depends on the part of the brain that is affected. A victim might suffer a loss of vision or slurred speech. Body parts can become paralyzed. Sometimes blood cannot flow to parts of the brain that control heart rate or breathing and death results. Prompt action must be taken for signs of stroke to prevent disability or death.

The Warning Signs of Stroke

- **Conscious or unconscious victim**
- **Slow breathing rate**
- **Unequal pupil size**
- **Slurred speech**
- **Paralysis on one side of the body**
- **Blurred vision**
- **Severe headache**

First aid for stroke involves these steps:

Call the local emergency number and obtain medical care immediately.

1. Keep the victim lying down with the head and shoulders raised to relieve the force of blood on the brain.
2. Check the airway. Keep the victim's air passage open.
3. Position the victim on his or her side if there is fluid or vomit in the mouth.
4. Do not give the victim anything to drink.
5. Comfort the victim until help arrives.

FOLLOW UNIVERSAL PRECAUTIONS

- Wear Disposable Latex Gloves
- Always Use a Face Mask

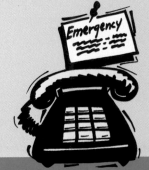

Call the local emergency number and obtain medical care immediately.

First Aid Puzzle

Life Skill

I will be skilled in first aid procedures.

Materials: Paper, pen or pencil.

Directions: Design and complete a crossword puzzle using the clues given. Work alone or in a group.

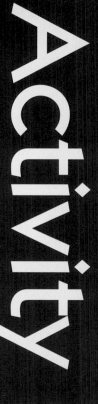

Activity

1. _____ **disease:** a bacterial disease transmitted through a tick

2. Immediate and temporary care

3. An emergency in which the airway is blocked

4. _____ **consent:** unspoken understanding that first aid may be given if no one who can give actual consent is conscious or present

5. A dangerous reduction in blood flow to the body tissues

6. A cut that causes a jagged or irregular tearing of the skin

7. An overstretching of muscles and/or tendons

8. _____ **burn:** a burn that occurs when chemicals in a laboratory or in products get on the skin or into the eyes or body

9. A wound caused by rubbing or scraping away of the skin

10. _____ **laws:** laws that protect people who give first aid

11. A break or crack in a bone

12. **Cardiac** _____: the death of the heart muscle

13. An injury in which the skin's surface is broken

14. An injury caused by heat, electricity, chemicals, or radiation

15. _____ **breathing:** a way of breathing air into an unconscious victim

16. **Universal** _____: a warning that a person has difficulty breathing

17. **First-**_____ **burn:** a burn which affects the top layer of skin

18. Medical identification tag that provides information about the person wearing it

19. _____ **resuscitation:** a first aid technique that is used to restore heartbeat and breathing

20. _____ **burn:** a burn that occurs when electricity travels through the body

21. A cut caused by a sharp-edged object

22. A condition caused by a blocked or broken blood vessel in the brain

23. The movement of a bone from its joint

24. The freezing of body parts

25. _____**-degree burn:** a burn that involves all layers of the skin and some underlying tissues

26. A wound produced when a pointed instrument pierces the skin

27. **Actual** _____: oral or written permission from a mentally competent adult to give first aid

28. _____ **tooth:** a tooth that has been knocked out of its socket

29. An injury to the ligaments, tendons, and soft tissue around a joint caused by undue stretching

30. _____ **precautions:** steps taken to prevent the spread of disease

31. A wound in which damage to soft tissues and blood vessels causes bleeding under the skin

32. An injury to the body's soft tissues

First Aid for Bleeding

A **wound** is an injury to the body's soft tissues. A **closed wound** is an injury to the soft tissues under the skin. An **open wound** is an injury in which the skin's surface is broken. There are many types of wounds.

Types of Wounds

Bruise

A **bruise** is a wound in which damage to soft tissues and blood vessels causes bleeding under the skin. The tissues change color and swell. A bruise might appear red and change to blue or purple. Large bruises might indicate serious damage to deeper body tissues.

Incision

An **incision** is a cut caused by a sharp-edged object, such as a knife, razor, scissors, or broken glass. Bleeding from an incision can be heavy. There might be damage to large blood vessels, nerves, and deep soft body tissues if the cut is deep.

Laceration

A **laceration** is a cut that causes a jagged or irregular tearing of the skin. Bleeding can be heavy. There is the risk of infection because foreign matter is forced through the skin.

Abrasion

An **abrasion,** or scrape, is a wound caused by rubbing or scraping away of the skin. There is the risk of infection as dirt and other matter can become ground into the wound. An abrasion can be painful if the scraping away of the skin exposes nerve endings.

Avulsion

An **avulsion** is a wound in which the skin or other body tissue is separated or completely torn away. This injury can result in a piece of skin hanging as a flap. It might result in a body part, such as a finger, being completely torn from the body. Bleeding is heavy if deeper tissues are damaged.

Puncture

A **puncture** is a wound produced when a pointed instrument pierces the skin. A needle, nail, piece of glass, knife, or gunshot can cause a puncture wound. Puncture wounds do not usually bleed much unless a major blood vessel is damaged. The risk of infection from a puncture wound is high. A tetanus shot might be given if the victim has not had one recently.

Preventing Infection

A wound must be kept clean to prevent infection. An **infection** is a condition in which pathogens enter the body and multiply. Wash minor wounds with soap and water. Do not wash more serious wounds that require medical care. Closely watch the wounded area for signs of infection. There might be swelling and redness. The wounded area might become warm, throb with pain, or discharge pus. Red streaks might develop by the wound and move toward the heart.

There are steps to take when signs of infection occur.

1. **Keep the area clean and soak it with warm water.**
2. **Apply an antibiotic ointment.**
3. **Elevate the infected area.**
4. **Seek medical attention.**

An Ounce of Prevention— Have You Had Your Tetanus Shot?

If you have ever stepped on a nail or been bitten by an animal, your doctor might have given you a tetanus shot. Some wounds, especially puncture wounds, put you at risk for infection with tetanus. **Tetanus,** or **lockjaw,** is a bacteria that grows in the body and produces a strong poison that affects the nervous system and muscles. A DPT is an immunization given in childhood to protect against tetanus, diphtheria, and pertussis (whooping cough). A booster shot is needed every five to ten years after the childhood series. A booster shot is also needed when a wound is caused by a dirty object, such as a rusty nail.

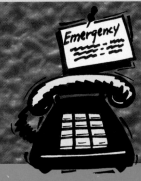

Call the local emergency number and obtain medical care immediately.

How to Control Bleeding

1.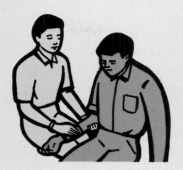

The first priority in any wound is to stop severe bleeding and prevent germs from entering the wound. A person with a wound can bleed to death in a matter of minutes.

Call the local emergency number and obtain medical care immediately.

Cover the wound with a clean cloth or sterile dressing and apply direct pressure with your hand. Add more cloth if the blood soaks through, but do not remove the first piece of cloth. Do not remove any foreign objects that are lodged deep in the wound.

2.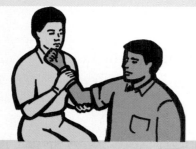

Elevate the wounded body part above the level of the heart. This helps reduce blood flow to the area.

3.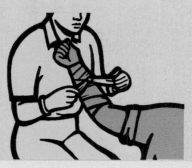

Cover the cloth or sterile dressing with a roller bandage.

4.

If bleeding does not stop...

Continue to apply direct pressure to the wound. Locate the closest pressure point. The pressure point technique compresses the main artery that supplies blood to the affected body part. This technique stops circulation within the limb. It is important to remember that if the use of pressure points is necessary, it should be used with direct pressure and elevation. Using pressure points to stop bleeding is not a substitute for direct pressure.

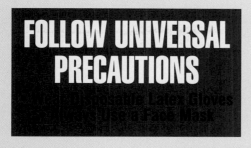

FOLLOW UNIVERSAL PRECAUTIONS

Wear Disposable Latex Gloves and Use a Face Mask

Nosebleeds

A **nosebleed** is a loss of blood from the mucous membranes that line the nose. Many teens have nosebleeds. Most nosebleeds are caused by a blow to the nose or cracked mucous membranes in the nose. Nosebleeds are usually easy to control.

1. Have the victim sit with his or her head slightly forward and pinch the nostrils firmly together. Sitting slightly forward helps the blood flow toward the external opening of the nose instead of backward down the throat.

2. The nostrils should be pinched firmly together for about five minutes before releasing. The victim should breathe through the mouth and spit out any blood in the mouth.

3. An ice pack may be applied to the bridge of the nose.

4. Repeat this procedure for another ten minutes if the bleeding does not stop.

5. Get prompt medical help if bleeding continues or if you suspect serious injury.

FOLLOW UNIVERSAL PRECAUTIONS
- Wear Disposable Latex Gloves
- Always Use a Face Mask

Knocked-Out Tooth

A **knocked-out tooth** is a tooth that has been knocked out of its socket. There are various recommendations on how to respond to this emergency.

1. Place a sterile dressing in the space left by the missing tooth. Have the victim bite down to hold the dressing in place.

2. Place the tooth in a cup of cold milk, or in water if milk is not available. Do not touch the root of the tooth.

3. The victim should see a dentist immediately. The sooner the tooth is placed back inside the socket, the better the chance it can be saved.

Mouth Protectors Aren't Just for Football

Two million teeth a year get knocked out, mostly from sports-related injuries. Most of those injuries could have been prevented by wearing a mouth protector. A mouth protector is a device that helps prevent injury to the mouth. It also cushions blows that might cause jaw fractures and head injuries.

The American Dental Association recommends that any person involved in an activity that might injure the mouth should wear a mouth protector. These activities include organized sports and other recreational activities. Mouth protectors should be worn when bicycling and in-line skating.

Mouth protectors are available in sporting goods stores. Custom-fitted mouthguards are designed and constructed by dentists.

Sports Requiring Mouth Protection

Acrobatics

Basketball

Boxing

Discus throwing

Field hockey

Football

Gymnastics

Handball

Ice hockey

Lacrosse

Martial arts

Racquetball

Rugby

Shotputting

Skateboarding

Skiing

Skydiving

Soccer

Squash

Surfing

Volleyball

Water polo

Weightlifting

Wrestling

Source: American Dental Association

FOLLOW UNIVERSAL PRECAUTIONS

First Aid for Shock

Any serious injury or illness can lead to shock. **Shock** is a dangerous reduction in blood flow to the body tissues. The body organs fail to function properly when they do not receive oxygen. Shock can lead to collapse, coma, and death if untreated. Signs of shock include rapid, shallow breathing; cold, clammy skin; rapid, weak pulse; dizziness; weakness; and fainting. First aid for shock involves the following steps:

Call the local emergency number and obtain medical care immediately.

1. Have the victim lie down. Elevate the legs about 8 to 12 inches above the level of the heart unless you suspect head, neck, or back injuries or broken bones in the hips or legs. Leave the victim lying flat if you are unsure of the victim's injuries.

2. Improve the victim's circulation.

   A Airway Keep the victim's airway open.

   B Breathing Perform rescue breathing if necessary. Remember to use a face mask or shield.

   C Circulation If you have completed CPR training, perform CPR if the victim has no pulse.

3. Control for external bleeding. Wear latex gloves.

4. Help the victim maintain normal body temperature. Cover the victim with a blanket if (s)he is cold.

5. Do not give the victim anything to eat or drink.

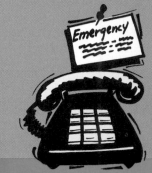

Call the local emergency number and obtain medical care immediately.

FOLLOW UNIVERSAL PRECAUTIONS

- Wear Disposable Latex Gloves
- Always Use a Face Mask

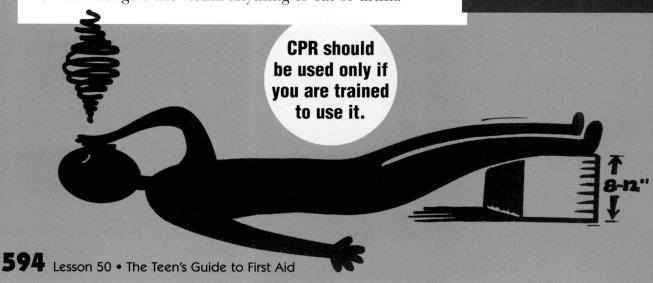

CPR should be used only if you are trained to use it.

8–12"

Work Safe!

Millions of teens age 14 to 17 work. According to The National Institute for Occupational Safety and Health or NIOSH, many teens are injured on the job every year. Some common injuries are sprains, strains, cuts and lacerations, heat burns, fractures, and dislocations. Some causes of the injuries are falls (tripping or slipping on something), being overtired, contact with hot objects or substances, and being hit by falling objects.

You might not have a job now. But if you do get a job, you need to know safety and health guidelines. Teens are protected by safety and health standards set by the Occupational Safety and Health Administration or OSHA.

Your employer will show you how to perform your job safely. You must follow safety and health rules where you work. Ask if you do not understand how to do something. Wear protective equipment if it is required. Be aware of safety hazards, such as clutter by a fire escape exit. Know your company's fire escape plan. Learn what to do if you run into a potentially violent customer. Know who to call if you or someone else gets injured.

Here is a list of jobs or job duties that you are not permitted to perform if you are under eighteen.

1. Manufacturing or storing explosives
2. Coal mining
3. Logging and sawmilling
4. Exposure to radioactive substances
5. Meat packing or processing
6. Power-driven bakery machines
7. Manufacturing brick, tile, and related products
8. Wrecking, demolition, and ship-breaking operations

First Aid for Poisoning

A **poison** is a substance that causes injury, illness, or death if it enters the body. Poisoning can occur when a person:

- **swallows a poison;**
- **breathes a poison;**
- **has poison on the skin that is absorbed into the body.**

Most cases of poisoning occur when small children swallow medicines or products, such as cleaning solutions or pesticides. Some people are poisoned by certain foods, such as shellfish or mushrooms. Some substances cause poisoning in larger amounts. For example, a person can be poisoned by taking too many pills or by drinking too much alcohol too quickly. Combinations of drugs, such as alcohol and sleeping pills, can cause poisoning.

Poisoning also can occur from breathing the fumes of household products, such as glue, paints, and cleaners. Certain gases cause poisoning. For example, a well-known tennis athlete died from carbon monoxide poisoning. Chlorine that is added to swimming pools is dangerous to breathe. Fumes from certain drugs, such as crack cocaine, also can cause poisoning.

Some poisons get on the skin and are absorbed into the body. Products, such as pesticides and fertilizers, can cause poisoning if they get on the skin. People using these products should wear gloves and clothing to prevent poisoning. They also should wear a mask to keep from breathing in fumes from these products. Poisons from plants, such as poison ivy and poison oak, can get on the skin. They are absorbed into the body and cause a reaction.

Poisoning can occur when a needle is used to inject drugs into the body. Bites or stings from insects, spiders, bees, snakes, and marine life can cause poisoning.

The signs of poisoning include difficulty breathing, nausea, vomiting, chest and abdominal pain, sweating, and seizures. Skin rashes and burns on the lips or tongue also might indicate poisoning.

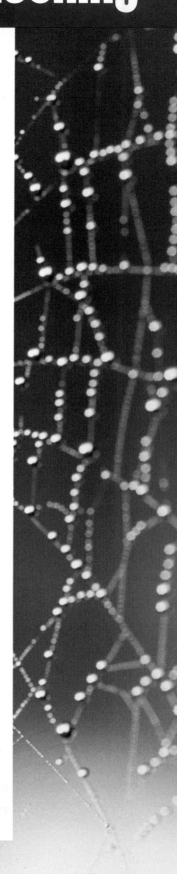

Steps to be taken when you suspect someone has been poisoned:

Call the local emergency number and obtain medical care immediately.

1. Be cautious. Protect your health and safety. Do not risk injury.

2. Move the victim to a safe location if necessary.

3. Treat the victim for life-threatening emergencies.

A	**Airway**	Keep the victim's airway open.
B	**Breathing**	Perform rescue breathing if necessary. Remember to use a face mask or shield.
C	**Circulation**	If you have completed CPR training, perform CPR if the victim has no pulse.

4. Gather information about the cause of poisoning. Determine the type of poison. Ask the victim what the type of poison might be. Be on the lookout for empty bottles and containers or needles. Recognize fumes and odors that might be the cause. Be alert to the environment. Are there bees, snakes, or poisonous plants in the area? Try to determine how much poison has been taken and when.

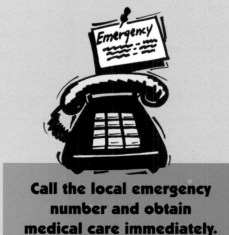

Call the local emergency number and obtain medical care immediately.

CPR should be used only if you are trained to use it.

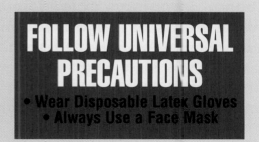

FOLLOW UNIVERSAL PRECAUTIONS
• Wear Disposable Latex Gloves
• Always Use a Face Mask

The Poison Control Center will tell you whether or not to induce vomiting in the victim. Victims who have swallowed acid substances, bleach or gasoline products should not vomit. These substances can burn the esophagus, mouth, and throat if the victim vomits. A victim with seizures or who is unconscious or semiconscious might be advised not to vomit. You might be advised to dilute the poison by having the victim drink water or milk.

Syrup of ipecac is a liquid used to induce vomiting in victims who have swallowed certain poisons. It can be bought at local drug stores. Victims between the ages of 1 to 12 are given one tablespoon of the syrup followed by two glasses of water. Victims over age 12 are given two tablespoons of the syrup followed by two glasses of water. The victim usually vomits within 20 minutes after taking the syrup.

The victim might be advised to take activated charcoal after vomiting. Activated charcoal is a product used to absorb poisons that have been swallowed. It is sold in both liquid and powder forms at drug stores. It counteracts the effects of the poison that remains after a person has vomited.

Lead Poisoning

Children sometimes get lead poisoning by eating paint chips that contain lead. However, teens and adults can get lead poisoning, too. You can be exposed to lead if you eat food that is stored and served in dishes that contain lead. You can breathe in fumes from burning lead-painted wood in your home fireplace. You can breathe in fumes from paint that has lead.

Lead attaches to red blood cells. It accumulates in bone. Symptoms of lead poisoning develop over several weeks or longer. You might have headaches, poor appetite, vomiting, and stomach cramps. You also might have a metallic taste in your mouth. See a physician if you have symptoms that might be from lead poisoning.

Use syrup of ipecac only if told to do so by a poison control center or physician.

Poisonous Plants

Touching poisonous plants, such as poison ivy, poison sumac, or poison oak, can result in skin redness, swelling, and itching. If you touch a poisonous plant:

1. Wash the affected body parts with soap and water immediately.

2. Remove any clothing that might have some of the poison on it.

3. Use over-the-counter drugs to relieve the reactions that result.

4. Call a physician if the reactions are severe.

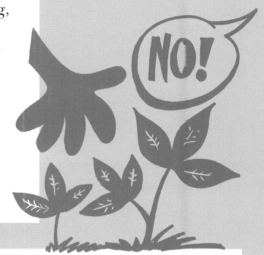

FOLLOW UNIVERSAL PRECAUTIONS
• Wear Disposable Latex Gloves
• Always Use a Face Mask

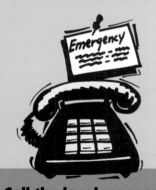

Call the local emergency number and obtain medical care immediately.

Snakebites

Poisoning can occur from being bitten by a poisonous snake, such as a coral snake or a pit viper. Examples of pit vipers are rattlesnakes, copperheads, and water moccasins. Symptoms of a bite from a poisonous snake include pain at the site of the wound, rapid pulse, dimmed vision, vomiting, and shortness of breath. The victim might experience shock and become unconscious.

Call the local emergency number and obtain medical care immediately.

1. Treat for shock.

2. Keep the victim still. This will reduce the speed with which the poison can travel through the body.

3. Keep the bitten area below the level of the heart.

4. Get the victim of a snakebite prompt medical care.

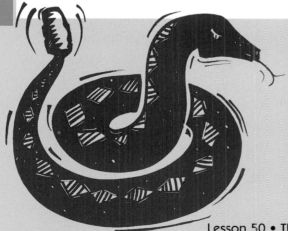

Bee Stings

Stings from bees are one of the most common insect-related problems. Bee stings can create a serious health problem for people who are allergic. These people should carry medication to prevent a serious allergic reaction. They also should wear a Medic Alert tag.

Most people do not have an allergic response to bee stings. The bee will leave its stinger in the skin when it stings.

Call the local emergency number and obtain medical care immediately.

1. Remove the stinger. Do not try to remove the stinger with a tweezer. The tweezer will force the bee's venom into the body. Flick the stinger away with a nail file, fingernail, credit card, or a similar object. Hornets, wasps, and yellow jackets do not leave stingers in the skin.

2. Place something cold over the area to relieve the pain.

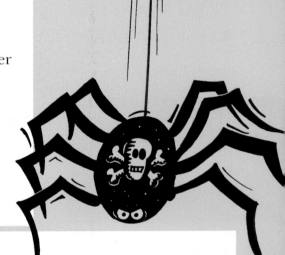

FOLLOW UNIVERSAL PRECAUTIONS

Spider Bites

Being bitten by a black widow spider can be deadly. A bite from this spider will produce a dull, numbing pain. Headache, muscular weakness, vomiting, and sweating might occur.

Call the local emergency number and obtain medical care immediately.

1. Wash the bitten area with soap and water.

2. Apply ice to relieve the pain.

3. Get prompt medical help. An antivenum might be given. An antivenum is a medicine that reduces the effects of the poison.

A bite from the brown recluse spider also is dangerous. A bite from this spider produces an open ulcer. Chills, nausea, and vomiting might follow.

1. Wash the affected part with soap and water.

2. Get prompt medical help.

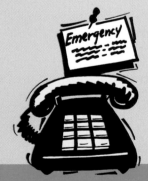

Call the local emergency number and obtain medical care immediately.

Marine Animal Stings

Stings from marine animals, such as the sting ray, man-of-war, sea anemone, jellyfish, sea urchin, or spiny fish, can cause serious allergic reactions. Breathing difficulties, heart problems, and paralysis can result. A victim should be removed from the water as soon as possible.

Call the local emergency number and obtain medical care immediately.

For stings from a sting ray, sea urchin, or spiny fish:

1. Remove the sting ray, sea urchin, or spiny fish.
2. Flush the area where the sting is located with water.
3. Do not move the injured part.
4. Soak the injured area with hot water for 30 minutes to relieve pain.
5. Clean the wounded area and apply a bandage.
6. Seek medical attention. A tetanus shot might be required.

For stings from a jellyfish, sea anemone, or man-of-war:

1. Remove the victim from the water as soon as possible.
2. Soak the area with vinegar as soon as possible. Vinegar offsets the effects of the toxin from the sting. Rubbing alcohol or baking soda can be used if vinegar is not available.
3. Do not rub the wound. Rubbing spreads the toxin and increases pain.

FOLLOW UNIVERSAL PRECAUTIONS

- Wear Disposable Latex Gloves
- Always Use a Face Mask

Prompt medical attention is needed for a victim who:

- does not know what stung him or her;
- has had a previous allergic reaction to a sting;
- has been stung on the face or neck;
- has difficulty breathing.

Tick Bites

A tick is an insect that attaches itself to any warm-blooded animal. It feeds on the blood of the animal. There is great concern about diseases spread by ticks. Two such diseases are Lyme disease and Rocky Mountain spotted fever. **Lyme disease** is a bacterial disease transmitted through a tick. The ticks that spread Lyme disease are those on field mice and deer. The ticks are very small. The bacteria that cause Lyme disease are transmitted through the bite of an infected tick. A rash starts and spreads to be about seven inches across. The center of the rash is light red and the outer ridges are darker red and raised. A victim might have fever, headaches, and weakness. Prompt medical attention is needed. Antibiotics are used for treatment.

Rocky Mountain spotted fever is a potentially life-threatening disease carried by a tick. Cases of this disease are not confined to the Rocky Mountain region. Symptoms include high fever, weakness, rash, leg pains, and coma. Prompt medical attention is needed. Antibiotics are used for treatment.

Do not put nail polish or petroleum jelly on a tick bite to suffocate the tick. Do not try to kill the tick by burning it with a match. These are not appropriate first aid procedures.

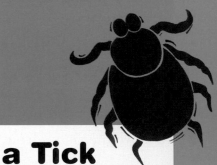

How to Remove a Tick

A tick should always be removed from the body.

1. Grasp the tick with tweezers as close to the skin as possible.

2. Use a glove or plastic wrap to protect your fingers if you do not have tweezers.

3. Pull the tick slowly away from the skin.

4. Wash the area with soap and water. Also, wash your hands with soap and water.

5. Apply an antibiotic ointment or antiseptic to the area to prevent infection.

6. Observe the area for signs of infection.

7. Obtain medical help if the tick cannot be removed or if part of it remains under the skin. Medical help also is needed if signs of Lyme disease or Rocky Mountain spotted fever develop.

First Aid for Burns

A **burn** is an injury caused by heat, electricity, chemicals, or radiation. The seriousness of a burn depends on:

- the cause of the burn;
- the length of time the victim was exposed to the source of the burn;
- the location of the burn on the body;
- the depth of the burn;
- the size of the burn;
- the victim's age and health condition.

Burns are usually described as first-degree burns, second-degree burns, or third-degree burns. These descriptions help explain the seriousness of the burn.

FOLLOW UNIVERSAL PRECAUTIONS

- Wear Disposable Latex Gloves
- Always Use a Face Mask

First-Degree Burns

A **first-degree burn** is a burn which affects the top layer of skin. Most sunburns are first-degree burns. The skin becomes red and dry and the area might swell. The area is painful to touch. First-degree burns usually heal in six days without permanent scarring.

First aid for a first-degree burn includes the following steps:

1. Stop the burning. Get the victim out of the sun. Put out flames that are burning clothes or skin.

2. Cool the burned area with water as soon as possible. Soak the area with water from a faucet or a garden hose, or have the victim get into the bath or shower. Use sheets or towels soaked in cold water to cool a burn on the face or other areas that cannot be soaked. Keep adding cool water.

3. Wear latex gloves. Loosely bandage the area with a dry, sterile, dressing.

4. Place cotton or gauze between burned fingers and toes.

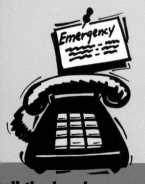

all the local emergency number and obtain edical care immediately.

Second-Degree Burns

A **second-degree burn** is a burn that involves the top layers of the skin. The skin becomes red. Blisters form and might open and discharge a clear fluid. The skin appears wet and mottled. Second-degree burns usually heal in two to four weeks. Slight scarring can occur.

First aid for a second-degree burn includes the following steps:

Call the local emergency number and obtain medical care immediately.

1. Stop the burning. Remove the victim from the source of the burn.

2. Cool the burned area with cool water or cold cloths.

3. Cover the area with a dry, sterile dressing or clean cloth. Keep the cover loose. This helps prevent infection and reduces pain. Do not break blisters or remove tissue.

4. Elevate the burned area.

5. Cover the victim with clean, dry sheets if burns cover large parts of the body. Treat for shock.

FOLLOW UNIVERSAL PRECAUTIONS
- Wear Disposable Latex Gloves
- Always Use a Face Mask

Third-Degree Burns

A **third-degree burn** is a burn that involves all layers of the skin and some underlying tissues. A third-degree burn might affect fat tissue, muscle tissue, bones, and nerves. The skin becomes darker and appears charred. The underlying tissues might appear white. A third-degree burn is painless if nerve endings are destroyed. Permanent scarring often occurs. Some victims require skin grafting and plastic surgery.

First aid for a third-degree burn includes the following steps:

Call the local emergency number and obtain medical care immediately.

1. Treat the victim for shock.

2. Check immediately if the victim is breathing. Give rescue breathing if necessary. Do not open blisters or remove pieces of tissue. Do not apply cold.

3. Cover the burned area with a dry, sterile dressing; clean cloth; or sheet.

Electrical Burns

An **electrical burn** is a burn that occurs when electricity travels through the body. The cause might be lightning or contact with faulty electrical equipment or with a power line. The seriousness of an electrical burn depends on the strength of the electrical current. It also depends on the path the current takes through the body. An electrical burn can be very deep. There might be a wound where the electrical current enters and where it leaves the body.

First aid for an electrical burn includes the following steps:

Call the local emergency number and obtain medical care immediately.

1. Do not go near the victim until the source of electricity is turned off.
2. Get prompt medical attention.
3. Treat the victim for shock.
4. Do not move the victim.
5. Cover the burn with a dry, sterile dressing. Do not use cool water or compresses as the victim might be in shock.

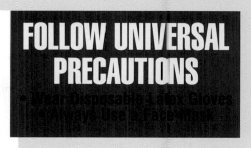

FOLLOW UNIVERSAL PRECAUTIONS
• Wear Disposable Latex Gloves
• Always Use a Face Mask

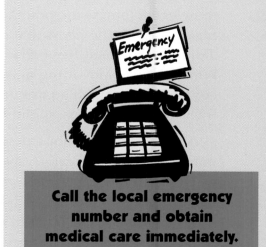

Call the local emergency number and obtain medical care immediately.

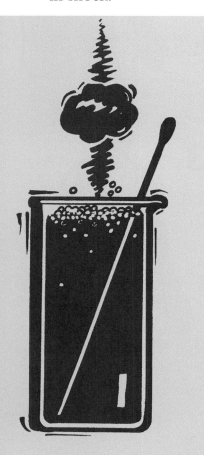

Chemical Burns

A **chemical burn** is a burn that occurs when chemicals in a laboratory or in products get on the skin or into the eyes or body. The burn continues as long as there is contact with the chemical.

First aid for a chemical burn includes the following steps:

Call the local emergency number and obtain medical care immediately.

1. Remove the source of the chemical. Have the victim remove any clothing with the chemical on it.
2. Flush the skin or eyes with cool, low-pressure, running water. If the chemical is dry or solid, brush it off with a cloth before flushing with water. Take special precautions if one eye is involved. Have the victim turn the head and run the water from the nose away from the eye. This keeps water with the chemical in it from running into the other eye.

First Aid for Injuries to Muscles, Bones, and Joints

There are 206 bones in the body and more than 600 muscles. A joint is the point at which two bones meet. Ligaments are the fibers that connect bones together. Tendons are tough tissue fibers that connect muscles to bones. Injuries involving muscles, bones, and joints are common in teens. The most common injuries are fractures, dislocations, sprains, and strains.

A **splint** is material or a device used to protect and immobilize a body part. A splint should only be used when you need to move a victim without emergency help and need to keep an injured body part still. A splint should only be used if it can be used without hurting the victim. A folded blanket, towel, sheet, or bandage might be used as a soft splint. Rolled-up newspapers or boards might be used as a rigid splint. Emergency medical personnel might use a board as a splint.

First aid when using a splint includes the following steps:

Call the local emergency number and obtain medical care immediately.

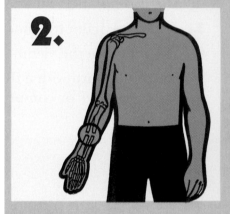

1. Attempt to splint the injury in the position you find it.

2. A splint for an injured bone must include the joints above and below the fracture.

3. A splint for an injured joint must include the bones above and below the injured joint.

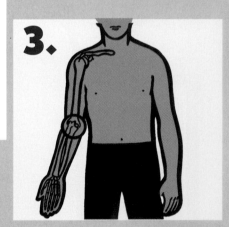

4. Check for circulation so that the splint is not too tight.

Fractures

A **fracture** is a break or a crack in a bone. An **open fracture** is a fracture in which there is a break in the skin. A **closed fracture** is a fracture in which there is no break in the skin. A fracture can be very serious if a break in a bone damages an artery or interferes with breathing. The signs of a fracture include pain, swelling, loss of movement, and deformity. Signs of a fracture of the skull include bleeding from the head or ears, drowsiness and headache.

First aid for fractures includes the following steps:

Call the local emergency number and obtain medical care immediately.

1. Treat for bleeding and shock.
2. Keep the injured part from moving. Use a splint when appropriate. Keep a victim with a head injury still.
3. Apply ice to the break or crack to prevent swelling.
4. Follow universal precautions. Control bleeding.
5. Get prompt medical help.

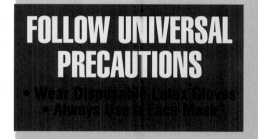

FOLLOW UNIVERSAL PRECAUTIONS
• Wear Disposable Latex Gloves
• Always Use a Face Mask

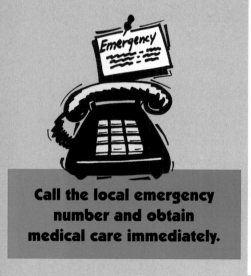

Call the local emergency number and obtain medical care immediately.

Dislocations

A **dislocation** is the movement of a bone from its joint. Dislocations often are accompanied by stretched ligaments. The signs of a dislocation are pain, swelling upon movement, loss of movement, and deformity.

First aid for a dislocation includes the following steps:

Call the local emergency number and obtain medical care immediately.

1. Splint above and below the dislocated joint.
2. Apply cold compresses.

Sprains

A **sprain** is an injury to the ligaments, tendons, and soft tissue around a joint caused by undue stretching. The signs of a sprain include pain that increases with movement or weight bearing, tenderness, and swelling.

First aid for sprains:

1. Follow the RICE treatment.
2. Get prompt medical help if a fracture is suspected.

Strains

A **strain** is an overstretching of muscles and/or tendons. One of the most common strains involves the muscles of the back. Signs of strain include pain, swelling, stiffness, and firmness to the area.

First aid for strains:

1. Follow the RICE treatment.
2. Get prompt medical help for a severe strain.

The RICE Treatment

The RICE treatment is a technique for treating injuries in which pain is lessened, swelling is limited, tissue damage is reduced, and faster healing is promoted.

Rest	Rest the injured part.
Ice	Apply cold, such as a cold compress, ice pack, or cold water.
Compression	Apply an elastic bandage to limit internal bleeding. Be careful not to apply the bandage too tightly. Check the body part for pain, numbness, change in color, or tingling. After 30 minutes, remove the bandage and the ice for 15 minutes. Then reapply the ice and bandage for 30 minutes. Repeat the procedure for three hours.
Elevation	Elevate the injured part above the level of the heart. This helps drain blood and fluid from the injured area.

First Aid for Sudden Illness

Sudden illness is an illness that occurs without warning signals of what is actually happening. It is difficult to determine if the situation is an emergency. Signs of sudden illness might include dizziness and confusion, weakness, changes in skin color, nausea, vomiting, and diarrhea. Seizures, paralysis, slurred speech, difficulty seeing, and severe pain might also indicate sudden illness.

FOLLOW UNIVERSAL PRECAUTIONS
- Wear Disposable Latex Gloves
- Always Use a Face Mask

First aid for sudden illness includes the following steps:

Call the local emergency number and obtain medical care immediately.

1. Give first aid for life-threatening conditions.
2. Keep the victim calm.
3. Cover the victim with a blanket if (s)he is chilled.
4. Do not give an unconscious victim anything to eat or drink.
5. Get prompt medical attention.

Fainting

6. If the victim has fainted: Put the victim on his or her back. Elevate the victim's legs eight to 12 inches above the level of the heart. (Do not elevate the legs if you suspect a head or back injury.) Loosen tight clothing. Do not splash water on the victim, slap the victim's face, or use smelling salts.

Vomiting

7. If the victim is vomiting: Turn the victim on his or her side.

Seizures

8. If the victim has a seizure: Place something under the victim's head to cushion the head from injury. Remove objects that might injure the victim. Loosen the clothing around the victim's neck. Do not restrain the victim. Do not place anything in the victim's mouth or between the teeth. Look for a Medic Alert tag.

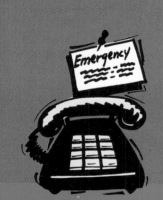

Call the local emergency number and obtain medical care immediately.

First Aid for Heat-Related Illnesses

Heat-related illnesses are physical conditions that can result when a person is exposed to higher than normal temperatures. Heat cramps, heat exhaustion, and heat stroke are the most common heat-related illnesses.

Heat Cramps

Heat cramps are painful muscle spasms that occur most often in the legs and arms due to excessive fluid loss through sweating.

First aid for heat cramps includes the following steps:

1. Have the victim rest in a cool, shaded area.
2. Give the victim cool water to drink.
3. Stretch the muscle gently.

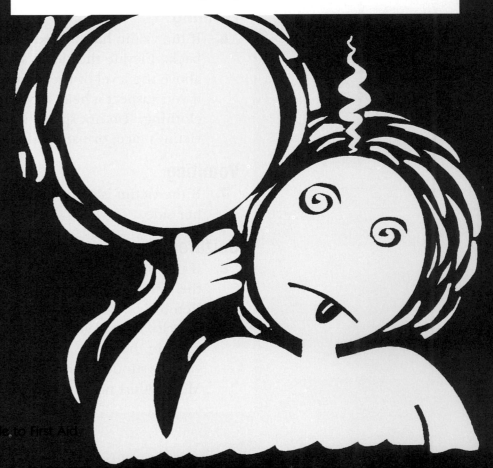

Heat Exhaustion

Heat exhaustion is extreme tiredness due to the inability of the body temperature to be regulated. Heat exhaustion can be life-threatening. A victim of heat exhaustion will have a body temperature that is below normal. Other signs of heat exhaustion include cool, moist, pale, or red skin; nausea; headache; dizziness; fast pulse; and weakness.

First aid for heat exhaustion includes the following steps:

Call the local emergency number and obtain medical care immediately.

1. Have the victim rest in a cool place.
2. Have the victim lie down and elevate the feet.
3. Give the victim cool water to drink.
4. Observe the victim for signs of heatstroke

FOLLOW UNIVERSAL PRECAUTIONS
- Wear Disposable Latex Gloves
- Always Use a Face Mask

Heatstroke (Sunstroke)

Heatstroke is a sudden attack of illness from exposure to high temperatures. Sweating ceases so that the body cannot regulate its temperature. The victim has a high body temperature and rapid pulse and respiration rate. The skin becomes hot and dry. A victim feels weak, dizzy, and has a headache. A victim might be unconscious.

First aid for heatstroke includes the following steps:

Call the local emergency number and obtain medical care immediately.

1. Have the victim rest in a cool place.
2. Remove heavy clothing.
3. Wrap the victim in cool, wet towels or sheets.
4. Place ice packs near the neck, armpits, and groin.
5. Continue cooling the victim until a body temperature of 102°F is reached.
6. Treat life-threatening emergencies.

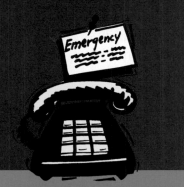

Call the local emergency number and obtain medical care immediately.

First Aid for Cold-Temperature Related Illnesses

Cold-temperature related illnesses are physical conditions that result from exposure to low temperatures, either below or above freezing. The most common cold-temperature related emergencies are frostbite and hypothermia.

Frostbite

Frostbite is the freezing of body parts, often the tissues of the extremities. Most cases of frostbite involve the fingers, toes, ears, and nose. A person who is exposed to subfreezing temperatures or snow is at risk for developing frostbite. Signs of frostbite include numbness in the affected area, waxy appearance of skin, and skin that is cold to touch and is discolored.

First aid for frostbite includes the following steps:

Call the local emergency number and obtain medical care immediately.

1. Do not attempt rewarming if a medical facility is nearby. Take the following steps if medical help is not available.

2. Remove any clothing or jewelry that interferes with circulation.

3. Handle the affected area gently.

4. Soak the affected body part in water that has a temperature between 100° and 105°F. Water that is too hot for the hand is too warm to use for the victim. Warming usually takes 25 to 40 minutes, until the tissues are soft.

5. Apply warm, moist cloths to the ears, nose, or face.

6. Do not rub the affected body part.

7. Do not allow a victim to walk on frostbitten toes or feet, even after rewarming.

8. Slightly elevate the affected part.

9. Place dry, sterile gauze between toes and fingers to absorb moisture and avoid having them stick together.

FOLLOW UNIVERSAL PRECAUTIONS
- Wear Disposable Latex Gloves
- Always Use a Face Mask

Hypothermia

Hypothermia (hy·poh·THUR·mee·uh) is a reduction of the body temperature so that it is lower than normal. Hypothermia results from overexposure to cool temperatures, cold water, moisture, and wind. The temperature can be as high as 50°F and a person can suffer from hypothermia.

Most cases of hypothermia are mild. The victim will shiver and feel cold. The pulse rate slows down and becomes irregular as the body temperature drops. Eventually, a victim can become unconscious. A victim can die if hypothermia is not treated.

First aid for hypothermia includes the following steps:

Call the local emergency number and obtain medical care immediately.

1. Get the victim into a warm environment.

2. Handle the victim gently.

3. Remove any wet clothing, and replace it with dry clothing.

4. Place something warm, such as blankets, above and below the victim.

5. Cover the victim's head.

For mild hypothermia (body temperature above 90°F):

6. Warm the victim. Use an electric blanket or tub of water with a temperature no greater than 105°F. Keep the victim's legs and arms out of the water. Do not have the victim's arms or legs covered by the electric blanket.

7. Place hot packs on the victim's head, neck, chest, and groin. Be careful not to burn the victim.

For profound hypothermia (body temperature below 90°F):

8. Do not rewarm a victim who can be transported to a medical facility within 12 hours.

9. Calm the victim.

10. Move the victim as little as possible.

11. Do not give CPR to the victim unless there is no pulse. Continue CPR until the victim is transported to a medical facility.

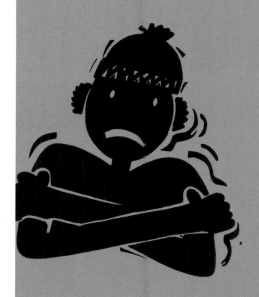

CPR should be used only if you are trained to use it.

FOLLOW UNIVERSAL PRECAUTIONS
- Wear Disposable Latex Gloves
- Always Use a Face Mask

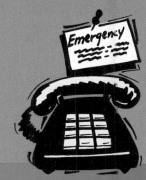

Call the local emergency number and obtain medical care immediately.

American Red Cross Courses

The American Red Cross offers courses to the public in first aid, taught by authorized American Red Cross personnel. According to the American Red Cross, after completing a standard first aid course, you will be able to:

- **Identify ways to prevent injury and illness**
- **Recognize when an emergency has occurred**
- **Provide basic care for injury and/or sudden illness until the victim can receive professional medical care**

People who successfully complete the standard first aid course receive a certificate from the American Red Cross. Contact your local chapter of the American Red Cross for further information on training courses available in your area.

Be a Better Baby-Sitter

Completing a caregiver's training or first aid course can help you gain the knowledge to care for infants and children safely. Some parents will ask potential caregivers if they have taken a first aid course, and recommend they do so. Your local chapter of the American Red Cross and other local health organizations might offer courses for the training of baby-sitters and caregivers.

These courses often include training in:

- ways to prevent injuries;
- basic first aid skills for emergencies;
- the needs and abilities of infants and children at different stages of development;
- signs of child abuse and steps to take when child abuse is suspected;
- communication skills.

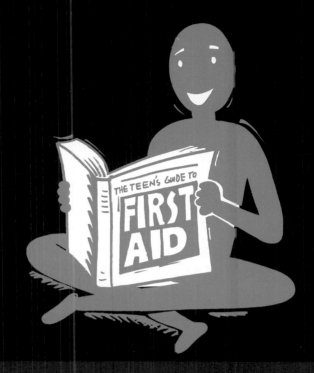

I will be skilled in first aid procedures.

Lesson 50

Review

Health Content

Write responses to the following:

1. What are items that are needed in a first aid kit? **page 554**

2. What are the universal precautions? **pages 556–557**

3. What are seven ways a family can prepare for a home emergency? **page 558**

4. What are seven guidelines for making an emergency telephone call? **page 561**

5. How do you obtain consent to give first aid? **page 562**

6. What are ten steps to follow when making a victim assessment? **pages 564–565**

7. What are six types of wounds in which bleeding might occur? **pages 588–589**

8. What are four steps to take when signs of infection occur? **page 590**

9. When should syrup of ipecac be used? **page 598**

10. What are first aid procedures for: choking; rescue breathing; CPR; heart attack; stroke; bleeding; shock; poisoning; marine animal stings; tick bites; burns; injuries to muscles, bones, and joints; sudden illness; heat-related illnesses; and cold-temperature related illnesses? **pages 566–613**

Unit 10 Review

Health Content

Review your answers for each Lesson Review in this unit. Then write answers to each of the following questions.

1. What are some types of violent behavior? **Lesson 47 pages 504–505**

2. How can you treat people with respect and avoid discriminatory behavior? **Lesson 47 page 514**

3. Why is it important for a victim of violence to participate in recovery? **Lesson 47 page 522**

4. What are actions you can take to prevent falls? **Lesson 48 page 527**

5. What safety guidelines should you follow if you are a pedestrian? **Lesson 48 page 536**

6. How can you stay warm when the temperature is cold? **Lesson 49 page 546**

7. How can you stay safe during an earthquake? **Lesson 49 page 549**

8. How can your family prepare for a home emergency? **Lesson 50 page 558**

9. What should you do when signs of infection in a wound occur? **Lesson 50 page 590**

10. What is the correct way to remove a tick? **Lesson 50 page 602**

Vocabulary

Number a sheet of paper from 1–10. Select the correct vocabulary word. Write it next to the corresponding number. DO NOT WRITE IN THIS BOOK.

air bags	laceration
avulsion	Lyme disease
bullying	probation
child abuse	suffocation
hypothermia	tornado warning

1. _____ is the harmful treatment of a minor. **Lesson 47**

2. _____ is a condition in which a person lacks oxygen due to an obstruction to the passage of air into the lungs. **Lesson 48**

3. _____ are cushions in motor vehicles that inflate within a fraction of a second after a collision. **Lesson 48**

4. _____ is a reduction of the body temperature so that it is lower than normal. **Lesson 49**

5. A(n) _____ is a caution that a tornado has been sighted. **Lesson 49**

6. _____ is an attempt by a person to hurt or frighten people who are weaker or smaller. **Lesson 47**

7. _____ is a sentence in which an offender remains in the community under the supervision of a probation officer. **Lesson 47**

8. _____ is a bacterial disease transmitted through a tick. **Lesson 50**

9. A(n) _____ is a wound in which the skin or other body tissue is separated or completely torn away. **Lesson 50**

10. A(n) _____ is a cut that causes a jagged or irregular tearing of the skin. **Lesson 50**

The Responsible Decision-Making Model™

Several days of hard rain have caused some flooding in your neighborhood. The street in front of your house is under five inches of water. The water is full of litter. Your friends come wading down the street and invite you to join them. Answer the following questions on a separate sheet of paper. Write "Does not apply" if a question does not apply to this situation.

1. Is it healthful to wade in the water? Why or why not?

2. Is it safe to wade in the water? Why or why not?

3. Is it legal to wade in the water? Why or why not?

4. Will you show respect for yourself if you wade in the water? Why or why not?

5. Will your parents or guardian approve if you wade in the water? Why or why not?

6. Will you demonstrate good character if you wade in the water? Why or why not?

What is the responsible decision to make in this situation?

Health Literacy

Effective Communication

Pretend you are a deejay who will announce and play the Top 40 Violence-Free Hits. Brainstorm titles with your classmates.

Self-Directed Learning

Search the Internet for the site of the National Safety Council. Copy or print out safety tips for extreme weather conditions and natural disasters.

Critical Thinking

Rank the twenty protective factors for violence in the order of their importance. Explain why you chose the first five as the most important.

Responsible Citizenship

Start a column in your school newspaper that reports positive happenings involving teens.

Multicultural Health

Research laws regarding motor vehicle safety in another country. Compare them to the laws in your country. For example, are the speed limits different? Is it mandatory to wear a seat belt? Relate the laws to the death rates from motor vehicle accidents in each country.

Family Involvement

Ask your parents or guardian whether your home has a first aid kit. If not, assist your parents or guardian in buying one or putting one together.

What Are 100 Life Skills I Should Practice?

Life skills are healthful actions that are learned and practiced for a lifetime. To take charge of your health, you need to practice life skills. There are ten units in this book. Ten life skills are recommended for each unit. A *Health Behavior Inventory* is a personal assessment tool that contains a list of life skills to which a person responds, "YES, I practice this life skill," or "NO, I do not practice this life skill." The *Health Behavior Inventory* on the following pages includes the 100 life skills that are in the ten units in this book. Use this *Health Behavior Inventory* to learn about your health behavior.

Health Behavior Inventory

Directions: Number from 1 to 100 on a separate sheet of paper. Read each life skill carefully. Write YES or NO next to the same number on your paper. Each YES response indicates a life skill you are working on right now. Each NO response indicates a life skill you are not working on right now. Leave a blank if you do not understand what the life skill involves. Some life skills might not relate to your life right now. Some might not apply to you. You will learn more about each life skill as you read this book. The listed life skills are not of equal value. You will learn that some life skills affect your health more than others.

Mental and Emotional Health

1. I will take responsibility for my health.
2. I will gain health knowledge.
3. I will practice life skills for health.
4. I will make responsible decisions.
5. I will use resistance skills when appropriate.
6. I will develop good character.
7. I will choose behaviors that promote a healthy mind.
8. I will communicate with others in healthful ways.
9. I will follow a plan to manage stress.
10. I will be resilient during difficult times.

Family and Social Health

11. I will use conflict resolution skills.
12. I will develop healthful family relationships.
13. I will make healthful adjustments to family changes.
14. I will work to improve difficult family relationships.
15. I will develop healthful relationships.
16. I will recognize harmful relationships.
17. I will develop skills to prepare for dating.
18. I will practice abstinence.
19. I will develop skills to prepare for marriage.
20. I will develop skills to prepare for parenthood.

Growth and Development

21. I will keep my body systems healthy.

22. I will recognize habits that protect female reproductive health.

23. I will recognize habits that protect male reproductive health.

24. I will learn about pregnancy and childbirth.

25. I will practice abstinence to avoid teen pregnancy and parenthood.

26. I will provide responsible care for infants and children.

27. I will achieve the developmental tasks of adolescence.

28. I will develop my learning style.

29. I will develop habits that promote healthful aging.

30. I will share with my family my feelings about dying and death.

Nutrition

31. I will select foods that contain nutrients.

32. I will eat the recommended number of servings from the Food Guide Pyramid.

33. I will follow the Dietary Guidelines.

34. I will plan a healthful diet that reduces the risk of disease.

35. I will evaluate food labels.

36. I will follow the Dietary Guidelines when I go out to eat.

37. I will protect myself from foodborne illnesses.

38. I will develop healthful eating habits.

39. I will maintain a desirable weight and body composition.

40. I will develop skills to prevent eating disorders.

Personal Health and Physical Activity

41. I will be well-groomed.

42. I will have regular examinations.

43. I will follow a dental health plan.

44. I will participate in regular physical activity.

45. I will get adequate rest and sleep.

46. I will develop and maintain health-related fitness.

47. I will develop and maintain skill-related fitness.

48. I will follow a physical fitness plan.

49. I will prevent physical activity-related injuries and illnesses.

50. I will be a responsible spectator and participant in sports.

Alcohol, Tobacco, and Other Drugs

51. I will not misuse or abuse drugs.

52. I will follow guidelines for the safe use of prescription and OTC drugs.

53. I will not drink alcohol.

54. I will avoid tobacco use and secondhand smoke.

55. I will not be involved in illegal drug use.

56. I will be aware of resources for the treatment of drug misuse and abuse.

57. I will practice protective factors that help me stay away from drugs.

58. I will use resistance skills if I am pressured to misuse or abuse drugs.

59. I will choose a drug-free lifestyle to reduce my risk of violence and accidents.

60. I will choose a drug-free lifestyle to reduce my risk of HIV, STDs, and unwanted pregnancy.

Communicable and Chronic Diseases

61. I will choose behaviors to prevent the spread of pathogens.

62. I will choose behaviors to reduce my risk of infection with communicable diseases.

63. I will choose behaviors to reduce my risk of infection with sexually transmitted diseases.

64. I will choose behaviors to reduce my risk of HIV infection.

65. I will choose behaviors to reduce my risk of cardiovascular diseases.

66. I will keep a personal health record.

67. I will choose behaviors to reduce my risk of cancer.

68. I will recognize ways to manage chronic health conditions.

69. I will recognize ways to manage asthma and allergies.

70. I will choose behaviors to reduce my risk of diabetes.

Consumer and Community Health

71. I will evaluate sources of health information.

72. I will recognize my rights as a consumer.

73. I will choose healthful entertainment.

74. I will develop media literacy.

75. I will take action if my consumer rights are violated.

76. I will make a plan to manage time and money.

77. I will make responsible choices about health care providers and facilities.

78. I will evaluate ways to pay for health care.

79. I will be a health advocate by being a volunteer.

80. I will investigate health careers.

Environmental Health

81. I will stay informed about environmental issues.

82. I will be a health advocate for the environment.

83. I will help keep the air clean.

84. I will help keep the water safe.

85. I will help keep noise at a safe level.

86. I will help conserve energy and natural resources.

87. I will precycle, recycle, and dispose of waste properly.

88. I will protect the natural environment.

89. I will take actions to improve my visual environment.

90. I will take actions to improve my social-emotional environment.

Injury Prevention and Safety

91. I will practice protective factors to reduce the risk of violence.

92. I will practice self-protection strategies.

93. I will stay away from gangs.

94. I will respect authority and obey laws.

95. I will not carry a weapon.

96. I will participate in victim recovery if I am harmed by violence.

97. I will follow safety guidelines to reduce the risk of unintentional injuries.

98. I will follow guidelines for motor vehicle safety.

99. I will follow safety guidelines for severe weather and natural disasters.

100. I will be skilled in first aid procedures.

Glossary

Sound	As in	Symbol	Example
ă	cat, tap	a	salivary (SA·luh·vehr·ee)
ā	may, same	ay	trachea (TRAY·kee·uh)
a	wear, dare	ehr	beta carotene (BAY·tuh KEHR·uh·teen)
ä	father, top	ah	amniotic (am·nee·AH·tik)
ar	car, park	ar	artery (AR·tuh·ree)
ch	chip, touch	ch	childbirth (CHYLD·berth)
ĕ	bet, test	e	melanin (MEL·uh·nuhn)
ē	pea, need	ee	emphysema (em·fuh·SEE·muh)
er	perk, hurt	er	hypothermia (HEYE·puh·THER·mee·uh)
g	go, big	g	malignant (muh·LIG·nuhnt)
ĭ	tip, live	i	cilia (SI·lee·uh)
ī	side, by	y, eye	angina (an·JY·nuh)
j	job, edge	j	cartilage (KAR·tuhl·ij)
k	cook, ache	k	quackery (KWA·kuh·ree)
ō	bone, know	oh	alveoli (al·vee·OH·ly)
ô	more, pour	or	beta-endorphins (BAY·tuh·en·DOR·fuhnz)
ȯ	saw, all	aw	audiologist (AW·dee·AH·luh·jist)
oi	coin, toy	oy	roid (ROYD) rage
ou	out, now	ow	power (POW·er)
s	see, less	s	cerebrum (suh·REE·bruhm)
sh	she, mission	sh	shadowing (SHA·doh·ing)
ŭ	cup, dug	uh	medulla (muh·DUH·luh)
u	wood, pull	u	pulmonary (PUL·muh·nehr·ee)
ü	rule, union	oo	nutrient (NOO·tree·uhnt)
w	we, away	w	water (WAH·ter)
y	you, yard	yu	urethra (yu·REE·thruh)
z	zone, raise	z	physician (fuh·ZI·shun)
zh	vision, measure	zh	malocclusion (MA·luh·KLOO·zhuhn)
ə	around, mug	uh	epididymis (ε·puh·DI·duh·muhs)

A

abdominal thrusts: a series of thrusts to the abdomen that force air from the lungs to dislodge an object.

abrasion: a wound caused by rubbing or scraping away of the skin.

abstinence: choosing not to be sexually active.

abuse (uh·BYOOS): the harmful treatment of another person.

accident: an event that is not planned to happen.

accident insurance: insurance that pays hospitalization, medical, and surgical expenses that result from accidents.

acid rain: rain and other precipitation (snow, sleet, hail) that has a high acid content resulting from air pollution.

acne: a skin disorder in which glands and hair follicles are inflamed.

acquaintance rape: rape that is committed by someone known to the victim.

Acquired Immune Deficiency Syndrome (AIDS): a condition that results when infection with HIV causes a breakdown of the body's ability to fight other infections.

active immunity: a resistance to disease due to the production of antibodies.

active listening: a type of listening in which a person lets others know that (s)he heard and understood what was said.

actual consent: oral or written permission from a mentally competent adult to give first aid.

addictive behavior: behavior that is repeated, is difficult to stop, and has harmful effects.

ADHD: a developmental disorder characterized by inattention and hyperactivity.

adipose (A·duh·pohs) **tissue:** the fat that accumulates around internal organs, within muscle, tissues and under the skin.

adolescence: a physical, emotional, and social transition from childhood to adulthood.

adoptive family: a family that consists of a parent(s) and a child or children who have become a permanent part of the family through the legal process.

adrenal glands: two glands that control the body's water balance, help in the digestive process, and secrete adrenaline.

adrenaline (uh·DREN·uhl·un): a hormone that prepares the body for quick action.

advertisement (ad): a paid announcement about a product or service.

advertising: a form of selling that provides information about products and services.

aerobic (uh·ROH·bik) **exercise:** an exercise that requires a continuous use of oxygen over an extended period of time.

affection: a warm feeling.

afterbirth: the placenta and other membranes that support the fetus.

Agent Orange: a substance containing dioxin that was sprayed on vegetation to kill it.

agility: the ability to move quickly and easily.

AIDS dementia complex: a loss of brain function caused by HIV infection.

air bags: cushions in motor vehicles that inflate within a fraction of a second after a collision.

air pollution: the contamination of air with undesirable gases, particles, dust, smoke, and chemicals.

Al-Anon: a support group for family members and friends of people with alcoholism and/or other addictions.

alarm stage: the first stage of the GAS in which adrenaline is secreted into the bloodstream.

Alateen: a support group for young people who have been affected by the behavior of someone with alcoholism and/or another addiction.

alcohol: a drug in certain beverages that slows down the central nervous system and harms body organs.

alcohol dementia (di·MEN·shuh): brain impairment with overall intellectual decline.

Alcoholics Anonymous (AA): a self-help treatment group in which people with alcoholism attend meetings and support each other to keep from drinking and to choose healthful behavior.

alcoholism: a disease in which there is physical and psychological dependence on alcohol.

allergen: a substance that causes an allergic reaction.

allergy: the reaction of the body to certain substances.

allied health professional: a trained practitioner who practices under some degree of supervision.

all-terrain vehicle (ATV): a vehicle that is built to travel easily over rough ground.

alveoli (al·vee·OH·ly): small air sacs at the ends of the bronchioles.

Alzheimer's Association: an organization that focuses on the prevention of Alzheimer's disease and the care and treatment of patients and families with Alzheimer's disease.

Alzheimer's disease: a disease characterized by a progressive loss of memory and mental function.

American Cancer Society: an organization that focuses on educating the public and health care professionals about cancer, provides cancer research, and offers services for patients and families dealing with cancer.

American Dental Association (ADA): an organization that sets standards for the education and conduct of dentists.

American Diabetes Association: an organization established to prevent and cure diabetes and to improve the life of people affected by diabetes.

American Heart Association: an organization devoted to reducing disability and death from cardiovascular diseases and stroke.

American Lung Association: an organization that focuses on the prevention and cure of lung disease.

American Medical Association (AMA): an organization that sets standards for the education and conduct of medical physicians.

American Public Health Association (APHA): an organization that establishes standards for scientific procedures in public health, conducts research, and makes policies in the public health field.

American Red Cross: an organization that provides relief to victims of disaster and helps people prevent, prepare for, and respond to emergencies.

amino acids: the building blocks that make up proteins.

amniotic sac: a thin membrane filled with fluid in which the developing baby floats.

Amount Per Serving: the number of calories in one serving and the number of Calories from Fat in one serving.

amphetamines (am·FE·tuh·meenz): chemically manufactured stimulant drugs that are highly addictive.

anabolic steroid (a·nuh·BAH·lik STIR·oyd): a synthetic drug that is used to increase muscle size and strength.

anaerobic (an·uh·ROH·bik) **exercise:** an exercise in which the body's demand for oxygen is greater than the supply.

anesthesiologist (a·nuhs·thee·zee·AH·loh·jist): a physician who specializes in the administration of drugs to prevent pain and induce unconsciousness during surgery.

anger: a feeling of being irritated and annoyed.

anger cues: body changes that occur when a person is angry.

anger management skills: ways of expressing anger without doing something harmful.

angina pectoris (an·JY·nuh PEK·tuhr·is): a chest pain that results from narrowed blood vessels in the heart.

anorexia nervosa: an eating disorder characterized by self-starvation and a weight of 15 percent or more below normal.

antibiotic (an·ti·by·AH·tik): a substance that kills bacteria or slows the growth of bacteria.

623

antibody: a protein that helps fight infection.

antioxidants (an·tee·AHK·suh·duhnts): substances that protect cells from being damaged by oxidation.

anti-perspirant: a product used to reduce the amount of perspiration.

aorta (ay·OR·tuh): the main artery in the body.

Apgar score: a scoring system to rate the health of a newborn baby.

appetite: the desire for food that is determined by environmental and psychological factors.

arrhythmia (ay·RITH·mee·uh): a heart condition in which the heartbeat is abnormal and irregular.

arteries (AR·tuh·reez): blood vessels that carry blood away from the heart.

arteriosclerosis (ahr·tee·ree·oh·skluh·ROH·sis): a general term used to describe several conditions that cause hardening and thickening of the arteries.

arthritis: the painful inflammation of joints in the body.

asbestos: a heat-resistant mineral that is found in building materials.

assertive behavior: the honest expression of thoughts and feelings without experiencing anxiety or threatening others.

Association for the Advancement of Health Education (AAHE): an organization for health educators that provides support, training, grants, and publications.

asthma (AZ·muh): a condition in which the bronchial tubes constrict, making breathing difficult.

Asthma and Allergy Foundation of America, The: an organization dedicated to finding a cure for and controlling asthma and allergic diseases through research, public education programs, and support groups.

astigmatism (uh·STIG·muh·ti·zuhm): a visual problem in which an irregular curvature of the lens or cornea causes blurred vision.

atherosclerosis (A·thuh·ROH·skluh·ROH·sis): a disease in which fat deposits on artery walls.

atrium (AY·tree·uhm): one of the upper two chambers of the heart.

Attention Deficit Hyperactive Disorder (ADHD): a developmental disorder characterized by inattention and hyperactivity.

audiologist (aw·dee·AH·luh·jist): an allied health professional who screens people for hearing problems and makes recommendations for hearing devices.

audiometer: a machine used to assess the range of sounds that a person can hear.

authority: the power and right to govern and to apply laws.

avulsion: a wound in which the skin or other body tissue is separated or completely torn away.

AZT: a drug that slows the multiplication of HIV.

B

B cells: cells that produce antibodies.

bacteria (bak·TIR·ee·uh): single-celled microorganisms.

bagging: inhaling chemicals from a paper bag.

balance: the ability to keep from falling.

balanced budget: a plan in which income is equal to expenses.

ball and socket joint: a joint that allows movement in a full circle.

bandwagon appeal: an advertising appeal that tries to convince a person that everybody is using a particular product or service and (s)he should, too.

barbiturates (bar·BI·chuh·ruhts): a type of sedative that was prescribed by physicians to help people sleep.

beryllium: a metal used to manufacture many products, including fluorescent light bulbs.

beta-blockers: drugs that slow the heartbeat rate and reduce the force of the heart's contractions.

beta-endorphins (BAY·tuh·en·DOR·fihnz): substances produced in the brain that help reduce pain and create a feeling of well-being.

biodegradable: having the ability to be broken down by living organisms.

biological age: a measure of how well a person's body parts are functioning.

biological therapy: treatment to improve the ability of immune cells to fight infection and disease.

biomechanics: the study of how the body functions during movement.

blackout: a period in which a person cannot remember what has happened.

blended family: a family that consists of two adults, one or both of whom has children from a previous relationship.

blister: a raised area containing liquid that is caused by an object rubbing against the skin.

blood alcohol concentration (BAC): the amount of alcohol in a person's blood.

blood pressure: the force of blood against the artery walls.

blood type: the kind of red blood cells a person has: A, B, AB, or O.

body composition: the percentage of fat tissue and lean tissue in the body.

body image: the perception a person has of his or her body's appearance.

body system: a group of organs that work together to perform a main body function.

botulism (BAH·chuh·li·zuhm): severe poisoning resulting from consuming foods with a preformed toxin.

braces: devices that are placed on the teeth and wired together to help straighten teeth.

brain stem: the lowest section of the brain.

brand loyalty appeal: an advertising appeal that tries to convince a person that one brand is better than the rest.

brand name: a product or service made by a certain company or manufacturer.

brand-name drug: a registered name or trademark given to a drug by a pharmaceutical company.

bronchi: two short tubes through which air enters the lungs.

bronchioles: small tubes that lead into the alveoli.

bruise: a wound in which damage to soft tissues and blood vessels causes bleeding under the skin.

budget: a plan for spending and saving money.

bulimia: an eating disorder in which a person has uncontrollable urges to eat excessively and then to rid the body of the food.

bully: a person who hurts or frightens people who are weaker or smaller.

bullying: an attempt by a person to hurt or frighten people who are weaker or smaller.

burn: an injury caused by heat, electricity, chemicals, or radiation.

bypass surgery: surgery to create a detour around a narrowed artery or vein so that blood can reach and leave the heart.

C

caffeinism: a kind of poisoning due to heavy caffeine intake.

calculus: hardened dental plaque.

callus: a thickened layer of skin due to excess rubbing.

calorie: a unit of measure for both the energy supplied by food and the energy used by the body.

cancer: a group of diseases in which cells divide in an uncontrolled manner.

candidiasis (kan·duh·DY·uh·suhs): an STD caused by fungi that produce itching and burning.

capillaries: tiny blood vessels that connect arteries and veins.

carbohydrates: nutrients that provide energy to the body.

carbon monoxide (KAR·buhn muh·NAHK·syd) **(CO):** an odorless, tasteless, colorless, poisonous gas.

carbon monoxide detector: a device that sounds an alarm when there is a dangerous level of CO in the air.

carcinogen (kar·SIN·uh·juhn): a substance that causes cancer.

carcinomas (kar·si·NOH·muhs): cancers of tissues that cover the body surfaces and linings of body organs.

cardiac arrest: the death of the heart muscle.

cardiac output: the amount of blood pumped by the heart each minute.

cardiologist (kar·dee·AH·luh·jist): a physician who specializes in the treatment of disorders of the heart and blood vessels.

cardiopulmonary resuscitation (CPR): a first aid technique that is used to restore heartbeat and breathing.

cardiorespiratory endurance: the ability to do activities that require increased oxygen intake for extended periods of time.

cardiovascular (KAR·dee·oh·VAS·kyoo·ler) **diseases:** diseases of the heart and blood vessels.

cartilage (KAR·tuhl·ij): a soft material that is on the ends of some bones.

catalog store: a store that sells products and services from a book containing pictures, descriptions, and prices.

cataract: a loss of transparency of the lens of the eye.

cavity: a hole in a tooth.

CD-ROM: a computer disc that stores computer programs, text, graphics, music, and animation.

cell: the smallest living part of the body.

Centers for Disease Control and Prevention (CDC): an agency within the United States Public Health Service responsible for tracking diseases, coordinating disease control and prevention efforts, and taking action in response to epidemics and natural disasters.

central nervous system (CNS): the part of the nervous system that consists of the brain and spinal cord.

cerebellum (ser·uh·BEL·uhm): the part of the brain that controls the coordination of muscle activity.

cerebral palsy: a nervous system disorder that interferes with muscle coordination.

cerebrum (suh·REE·bruhm): the part of the brain that controls the ability to memorize, think, and learn.

cesarean section: a surgical procedure in which the baby and the placenta are delivered through an incision in the abdominal wall and uterus.

chancre (SHAN·ker): a hard, round, painless sore.

character: a person's use of self-control to act on responsible values.

chemical addiction: term used for drug dependence.

chemical burn: a burn that occurs when chemicals in a laboratory or in products get on the skin or into the eyes or body.

chemical dependence: term used for drug dependence.

chemotherapy: treatment with anti-cancer drugs.

chewing tobacco: a tobacco product made from chopped tobacco leaves that is placed between the cheek and gums.

child abuse: the harmful treatment of a minor.

child safety restraint: a seat designed for a small child that is to be secured in the back seat of a motor vehicle.

childbirth: the process by which a baby moves from the uterus to the outside world.

chlamydial (kluh·MI·dee·uhl) **infection:** an STD caused by a bacterium that produces inflammation of the reproductive organs.

chlorofluorocarbons (CFCs): a group of gases that are easy to compress and expand.

choking: an emergency in which the airway is blocked.

cholesterol (kuh·LES·tuh·rawl): a fat-like substance made by the body and found in many foods.

chronic bronchitis (brahn·KY·tis): a disease in which too much mucus lines the bronchial tubes.

chronic disease: an illness that develops and lasts over a long period of time.

chronic fatigue syndrome (CFS): a condition in which severe tiredness recurs and makes it difficult for a person to function in normal ways.

chronic health conditions: recurring or persistent conditions.

chronological age: the number of years a person has lived.

cilia (SIH·lee·uh): hair-like structures in the respiratory tract that trap dust and other particles and remove them.

circulatory system: the body system that transports nutrients, oxygen, and cellular waste products throughout the body.

circumcision: the surgical removal of the foreskin.

cirrhosis (suh·ROH·sis): a disease in which the liver tissue is destroyed and replaced with scar tissue.

closed fracture: a fracture in which there is no break in the skin.

closed wound: an injury to the soft tissues under the skin.

cocaine (koh·KAYN): a highly addictive stimulant drug obtained from the leaves of the coca bush.

codeine (KOH·deen): a narcotic painkiller produced from morphine.

codependence: a mental disorder in which a person denies feelings and copes in harmful ways.

cold-temperature related illnesses: physical conditions that result from exposure to low temperatures, either below or above freezing.

color blindness: a condition in which a person sees colors differently than other people.

commercial: an advertisement on television or radio.

commitment: a pledge or promise to do something.

communicable (kuh·MYOO·ni·kuh·buhl) **disease:** an illness caused by a pathogen.

communication: the sharing of feelings, thoughts, and information with another person.

comparison (kuhm·PEHR·i·suhn) **shopping:** evaluating products and services using objective criteria, such as price, convenience, features, quality, and warranty.

compassion: showing concern and a desire to be helpful.

competition: the act of trying to win or gain something from another or others.

complete proteins: proteins from animal sources that contain all of the essential amino acids.

complex carbohydrates: starches.

composting: the breakdown of plant remains and once-living materials into simpler substances.

compulsive: to have an irresistible urge to repeat a behavior.

concealed weapon: a weapon that is hidden from view.

conception: the union of an egg and a sperm.

conditioner: a product that coats the hair shaft making it feel smooth.

conflict: a disagreement between two or more people or between two or more choices.

conflict resolution skills: steps that can be used to resolve a disagreement in a healthful, safe, legal, respectful, and nonviolent way.

congenital (kuhn·JEN·uh·tuhl) **syphilis:** syphilis that is transmitted to a fetus from an infected pregnant female.

conservation: the saving of resources.

consumer (kuhn·SOO·mer): a person who chooses sources of health-related information and buys or uses health products and services.

627

Consumer Product Safety Commission (CPSC): an agency that establishes and enforces product safety standards and receives consumer complaints about the safety of products.

consumerism: the practice of choosing reliable and tested products, services, and information.

Consumers' Research: an organization that tests products and provides ratings for consumers to make comparisons with regard to products' performance and safety.

Consumers' Union: an organization that tests products and publishes a magazine which provides ratings for consumers to make comparisons with regard to products' performance and safety.

controlled drug: a drug whose possession, manufacture, distribution, and sale are controlled by law.

convalescent (kahn·vuh·LE·sent) **home:** a facility where people can recover from illness or surgery; similar to a hospital, but that does not provide intensive care, surgical, and emergency treatment facilities.

convenience: anything that saves time or effort.

cool-down: at least three to five minutes of reduced activity, such as after a workout.

coordination: the ability to use body parts and senses together for movement.

corn: a growth that results from excess rubbing of a shoe against the foot, or from toes being squeezed together.

cornea: the clear tissue over the front of the eye that covers the iris and pupil.

Council of Better Business Bureaus: a nonprofit organization that monitors consumer complaints and advertising and selling practices.

couple family: a family that consists of two adults who do not have children.

coupon (KOO·pahn): a ticket that can be used to reduce the price of something a person plans to buy.

Cowper's glands: glands that secrete a clear, lubricating fluid.

crack: a purified form of cocaine that produces a rapid and intense reaction.

crank: an illegal amphetamine-like stimulant.

credentials: preparations for performing a certain job.

credit card: a card used for payment in which the owner of the card agrees to pay later.

D

daily value: the amount of a nutrient that is needed each day for optimal health.

daily values/calories footnote: the amount of each nutrient needed each day based on a 2,000 and a 2,500 calorie diet.

dandruff: flakes of dead skin cells on the scalp.

DDI: a drug that slows the multiplication of HIV.

debt (DET): the condition of owing.

decibel (dB): a unit used to measure the loudness of sounds.

deductible: a specific amount that must be paid by the individual when insurance payments are needed.

dehydration: a condition in which the body does not have enough water.

dementia: a condition in which thinking and memory are not sharp.

dental hygienist: an allied health professional who provides oral health services, such as cleaning teeth and educating others about proper care of teeth.

dental plaque: an invisible, sticky film of bacteria on teeth, especially near the gum line.

dentist: either a doctor of dental surgery (DDS) or a doctor of medical dentistry (DMD) who specializes in the treatment of teeth.

deodorant: a product that reduces the amount of body odor and might reduce the amount of perspiration.

depression: the feeling of being sad, unhappy, or discouraged.

dermatologist (duhr·muh·TAH·luh·jist): a physician who specializes in the care of the skin.

dermis: the thick layer of living cells below the epidermis.

desensitization (dee·sen·suh·tuh·ZAY·shun): the effect of reacting less and less to the exposure to something.

desirable weight: the weight that is recommended for a person's age, height, sex, and body frame.

developmental tasks: achievements that need to be mastered as a person grows toward maturity.

diabetes (dy·uh·BEE·teez): a disease in which the body produces little or no insulin or cannot use insulin.

diagnosis: the act of finding out what is wrong by having a physical examination, studying symptoms, and having tests.

diastolic (dy·uh·STAH·lik) **blood pressure:** the force of blood against the artery walls between heart beats.

Dietary Guidelines: recommendations for diet choices for healthy Americans who are two years of age or more.

digestion: the process by which food is broken down so that it can be used by the body's cells.

digestive (dy·JES·tiv) **system:** the body system that breaks down food so that nutrients can be used by the body.

dioxins: a group of chemicals used in insecticides.

direct contact: the transfer of pathogens from an infected person to another person.

disability insurance: insurance that replaces lost income should a person have an accident or illness requiring a period of recovery.

discount store: a store that sells products and services lower than the regular price.

discriminate (dis·KRIM·uh·nayt): to treat some people or groups of people differently from others.

disease: an illness.

dislocation: the movement of a bone from its joint.

distress: a harmful response to a stressor.

divorce: the legal end of a marriage.

domestic shelter: a place where family members can stay to be safe.

domestic violence: violence that occurs within a family.

dose: the amount of a drug that is taken at one time.

drownproofing: a floating technique that helps a person float without using much energy.

drug: a substance other than food that changes the way the body or mind works.

drug abuse: the use of an illegal drug or the intentional misuse of a prescription or over-the-counter drug.

drug dependence: the continued use of a drug even though it harms the body, mind, and relationships.

drug-free lifestyle: a lifestyle in which people do not use harmful and illegal drugs.

drug misuse: the incorrect use of a prescription or over-the-counter drug.

drug slipping: placing a drug into someone's food or beverage without that person's knowledge.

drug trafficking: the illegal purchase or sale of drugs.

drug use: a term used to describe drug-taking behavior.

dynamic blood pressure: the measure of the changes in blood pressure during the day.

dysfunctional family: a family in which members behave in ways that are not responsible or loving.

E

earthquake: a violent shaking of Earth's surface caused by the shifting of plates that make up Earth's crust.

eating disorder: a food-related dysfunction in which a person changes eating habits in a way that is harmful to the mind and body.

ecologists: people who study ecology.

ecology: the study of the relationship between living organisms and the environment.

ecosystem: a system made up of living organisms, air, water, soil, and sunlight.

effacement: the thinning and shortening of the cervix.

egg cells: female reproductive cells.

ejaculation: a series of muscular contractions that expel semen from the penis.

elder abuse: the harmful treatment of an aged family member.

electrical burn: a burn that occurs when electricity travels through the body.

electrical storm: a storm in which there are bolts of lightning.

electricity: a current that provides a source of energy.

electrocardiogram (EKG): a measure of the electrical activity of the heart.

ELISA: a blood test used to check for antibodies for HIV.

e-mail (electronic mail): a message delivered quickly from one computer to another.

embryo: the mass of cells during the first eight weeks after conception.

emergency: a serious situation that occurs without warning and calls for quick action.

emergency dispatcher: a person who decides who to contact when there is a call for help.

emergency room: a facility within a hospital where emergency services are provided without an appointment; used at night or on weekends when other care is not available.

emotional abuse: "putting down" another person and making the person feel worthless.

empathy: the ability to share in another person's emotions or feelings.

emphysema (em·fuh·SEE·muh)**:** a disease in which air sacs in the lungs lose most of their ability to function.

empowered: to be inspired because a person feels some sense of control over behavior and decisions.

enabler: a person who knowingly or unknowingly supports the harmful behavior of another person.

endocrine (EN·duh·krin) **system:** the body system that consists of glands that produce hormones.

energy: the ability to do work.

energy conservation: actions to save heat and electricity.

entertainment addiction: a strong desire to be amused or interested in something at the expense of mental-emotional, family-social, and physical health.

environment: everything living and non-living that is around a person.

Environmental Protection Agency (EPA): a regulatory agency responsible for reducing and controlling environmental pollution.

epidermis: the outer layer of dead cells of the skin.

epididymis (e·puh·DI·duh·mus)**:** a comma-shaped structure on the rear upper surface of each testis where sperm are stored.

epiglottis (e·puh·GLAH·tis)**:** a flap that covers the entrance to the trachea.

epilepsy: a disorder in which abnormal electrical activity in the brain causes a temporary loss of control of the mind and body.

esophagus (i·SAH·fuh·guhs)**:** a tube through which food passes to the stomach.

essential amino acids: the nine amino acids the body cannot produce.

essential body fat: the fat that is located around such organs as the heart, lungs, liver, spleen, kidneys, and intestines.

essential hypertension: high blood pressure with no specific cause.

estrogen (ES·truh·juhn)**:** a female sex hormone that controls the development of secondary sex characteristics during puberty.

ethnic restaurant: a restaurant that serves food eaten by people of a specific culture.

eustachian (yoo·STAY·shun) **tube:** a tube that helps keep the air pressure on both sides of the eardrum equal.

eustress (YOO·stres): a healthful response to a stressor.

exhaustion stage: the third stage of the GAS in which wear and tear on the body increases the risk of diseases and accidents.

expenses: the amounts of money needed to buy or do something.

extended care facility: a facility that provides nursing, personal, and residential care; also provides care for people who need assistance in daily living.

extended family: a family that consists of family members from three or more generations who live together.

F

fad: something that is very popular for a short period of time.

Fallopian tube: a four-inch-long tube that extends from the ovary to the uterus.

false image appeal: an advertising appeal that tries to convince a person that (s)he will have a certain image if (s)he buys a specific product or service.

family relationship: the connection a person has with family members.

family-social health: the condition of one's relationships with others.

farsightedness: a visual problem in which close objects appear blurred while distant objects are seen clearly.

fast foods: foods that can be served quickly.

fats: nutrients that are a source of energy and make certain vitamins available for use in the body.

fat-soluble vitamins: vitamins that can be stored in the body.

features: the important or outstanding characteristics of a product or service.

Federal Communications Commission (FCC): an agency charged with regulating interstate and international communications by radio, television, wire, satellite, and cable.

Federal Trade Commission (FTC): an organization that monitors trade practices; the advertising of foods, drugs, and cosmetics, and advertising that appears on television.

feelings: emotions, such as excitement, sadness, happiness, and anger.

female reproductive system: the body system that consists of the female organs involved in producing offspring.

fertilization: the union of an egg and a sperm.

fetal alcohol syndrome (FAS): the presence of severe birth defects in babies born to mothers who drink alcohol during pregnancy.

fetus: the developing of cells from the eighth week of conception until birth.

fever: an increase in the body temperature of 98.6°F.

fiber: the part of grains and plant foods that cannot be digested.

fighting: taking part in a physical struggle.

firearm: a weapon from which shot is ejected when gunpowder explodes.

first aid: the immediate and temporary care given to a person who has been injured or suddenly becomes ill.

first-degree burn: a burn which affects the top layer of skin.

fitness skills: skills that can be used in physical activities, sports, and games.

five stages of dying: stages of dying that include denial, anger, bargaining, depression, and acceptance.

fixed joint: a joint that does not move.

flashback: a sudden illusion that a person has long after having used certain drugs.

flexibility: the ability to bend and move the joints through a full range of motion.

flood: a rising and overflowing of a body of water onto normally dry land.

Food Guide Pyramid: daily guidelines for the number of servings of each major food group.

food label: a nutrition panel of information that is required on all processed foods regulated by the Food and Drug Administration.

Food and Drug Administration (FDA): an agency within the Department of Health and Human Services that monitors the safety and effectiveness of new drugs, medical devices, and the safety of cosmetics and food.

foodborne illness: an illness caused by eating foods that have been contaminated by germs or by toxins produced by germs.

formal intervention: an action by people, such as family members, who want a person to get treatment.

formaldehyde (for·MAL·duh·hyd)**:** a colorless gas with a strong odor.

fossil fuels: coal, oil, and natural gas burned to provide energy.

foster family: a family in which an adult(s) who cares for a child or children who do not live with the birth parents.

fracture: a break or a crack in a bone.

frequency: the number of times a person participates in physical activity each week.

frostbite: the freezing of body parts, often the tissues of the extremities.

fungi (FUHN·jy)**:** single-celled or multicellular plantlike organisms, such as yeast and molds.

G

gallbladder: an organ that stores bile.

gangs: groups of young people who band together and participate in violent or criminal behavior.

gastric ADH: an enzyme the liver needs in order to oxidize or break down alcohol for excretion.

gastroenterologist (gas·tro·en·tuh·RAH·luh·jist)**:** a physician who specializes in disorders of the digestive tract.

general adaptation syndrome (GAS): a series of changes that occur in the body when stress occurs.

generic (jeh·NEHR·ik) **name:** a product or service that meets certain standards, but does not have fancy packaging.

generic-name drug: a drug that contains the same active ingredients as a brand-name drug.

genital herpes: an STD caused by a virus that produces cold sores or fever blisters in the genital area and/or mouth.

genital warts: dry wartlike growths that are caused by a virus.

geriatrician (jer·ee·uh·TRI·shun)**:** a physician who specializes in medical care for the elderly.

gingivitis (jihn·juh·VY·tis)**:** a condition in which the gums are red, swollen, and tender.

gland: a group of cells or an organ that secretes hormones.

glittering generality appeal: an advertising appeal that includes a general statement that is exaggerated to appeal to the emotions.

global warming: an ongoing increase in Earth's temperature.

gonorrhea (gah·nuh·REE·uh)**:** an STD caused by bacteria that produce a discharge from the urethra and/or vagina.

Good Samaritan laws: laws that protect people who give first aid in good faith and without gross negligence or misconduct.

government hospital: a hospital run by the federal government for the benefit of a specific population, such as veterans.

grand mal: a major seizure in which a person might have a convulsion.

greenhouse effect: the trapping of heat from the sun by gases, such as CO_2, in Earth's atmosphere.

grief: the discomfort caused by the death of another person.

grooming: taking care of the body so that a person appears at his or her best.

gynecologist (gy·nuh·KAH·luh·jist)**:** a physician who specializes in treatment of the disorders of the female reproductive tract.

H

hallucinogens (huh·LOO·suhn·uh·juhnz)**:** a group of drugs that interfere with the senses, causing people to see and hear things that are not real.

harmful relationship: a relationship that harms self-respect and includes harmful behavior.

hashish: a drug that comes from the marijuana plant.

headache: a pain in the head.

health: the quality of life that includes physical, mental-emotional, and family-social health.

health awareness: the knowledge a person gains about his or her health behavior.

health behavior contract: a written plan to develop the habit of following a specific life skill.

Health Behavior Inventory: a personal assessment tool that contains a list of life skills to which a person responds, "YES, I practice this life skill," or "NO, I do not practice this life skill."

health care facility: a place where people receive health care.

health care practitioner: a professional whose practice is restricted to a specific area of the body.

health care provider: a professional who helps people obtain optimal health.

health care system: a system that includes health care providers, health care facilities, and payment for health care.

health center: a facility that provides routine health care to a special population, such as low income families.

health department clinic: a facility in most state and local health departments that keeps records and performs services, such as immunizations and testing for sexually transmitted diseases.

health history: a record of a person's health habits, past health conditions, past medical care, allergies, and family's health.

health insurance (in·SHUR·ens) **policy:** a plan that helps pay the cost of health care.

health knowledge: the information and understanding a person has about health.

health literate person: a person who is skilled in effective communication; self-directed learning; critical thinking; and responsible citizenship.

health maintenance (MAYN·te·nuhns) **organization (HMO):** a business that organizes health care services for its members.

healthful behaviors: actions that promote health; prevent illness, injury, and premature death; and improve the quality of the environment.

healthful body composition: a high ratio of lean tissue to fat tissue.

healthful entertainment: entertainment that promotes physical, mental, or social health.

healthful family: a family in which members behave in ways that are loving and responsible.

healthful family relationship: one in which family members relate well and make necessary adjustments to family changes.

healthful friendship: a balanced relationship that promotes mutual respect and healthful behavior.

healthful relationship: a relationship that promotes mutual respect and responsible behavior.

health-related fitness: the ability of the heart, lungs, muscles, and joints to perform well.

heart: a four-chambered muscle that pumps blood throughout the body.

heart attack: the death of part of the heart muscle caused by a lack of blood flow to the heart.

heat cramps: painful muscle spasms that occur most often in the legs and arms due to excessive fluid loss through sweating.

heat detector: a device that sounds an alarm when the room temperature rises above a certain level.

heat exhaustion: extreme tiredness due to the inability of the body temperature to be regulated.

heat-related illnesses: physical conditions that can result when a person is exposed to higher than normal temperatures.

heat stroke: a sudden attack of illness from exposure to high temperatures.

633

heredity: the sum of the traits that have been transmitted from parents.

heroin: an illegal narcotic drug derived from morphine.

hidden anger: anger that is not expressed or that is expressed in a harmful way.

high density lipoproteins (HDLs): substances that carry cholesterol to the liver for breakdown and excretion.

hinge joint: a joint that allows bones to move back and forth.

homicide (HAHM·uh·syd): the accidental or purposeful killing of another person.

honest talk: the straightforward sharing of a person's thoughts and feelings about a situation, a person, or a person's behavior.

hormone: a chemical messenger that is released into the bloodstream.

hospital: a health care facility where people can receive medical care, diagnosis, and treatment on an inpatient or outpatient basis.

hospitalization insurance: insurance that pays the cost of a hospital stay.

huffing: inhaling fumes from substances to get a high.

human immunodeficiency (IM·yoo·noh·di·FI·shuhn·see) **virus (HIV):** a pathogen that destroys infection-fighting T cells in the body.

humor appeal: an advertising appeal that contains a catchy slogan, jingle, or cartoon that grabs attention.

hunger: the physiological need for food.

hurricane: a tropical storm with heavy rains and winds in excess of 74 miles per hour.

hyperopia (hy·puh·ROH·pee·uh): a visual problem in which close objects appear blurred while distant objects are seen clearly.

hypertension: a condition in which the pressure exerted by the blood on the artery walls when the heart beats is above normal for a long period of time; also called high blood pressure.

hypnotic drugs: drugs that promote drowsiness and sleep.

hypoglycemia (hy·poh·gly·SEE·mee·uh): a condition in which the pancreas produces too much insulin and the blood sugar level becomes low.

hypothermia (hy·poh·THUHR·mee·uh): a reduction of the body temperature so that it is lower than normal.

I

ice: a smokeable form of pure meth.

identity: a sense of who one is.

illegal drug use: the wrong use, possession, manufacture, or sale of controlled drugs, and the use, possession, manufacture, or sale of illegal drugs.

I-message: a statement that contains a specific behavior or event; the effect that the behavior or event has on the individual; and the feeling that results.

immune system: the body system that contains cells and organs that fight disease.

immunity (i·MYOO·nuh·tee): a resistance to disease.

immunotherapy: a process in which the immune system is stimulated to fight cancer cells.

implied consent: unspoken understanding that first aid may be given if no one who can give actual consent is consious or present.

inactive decision-making style: a decision-making style in which a person fails to make choices, and this failure determines what will happen.

income: money received from different sources.

incest: sexual abuse between family members.

incision: a cut caused by a sharp-edged object, such as a knife, razor, scissors or broken glass.

incomplete proteins: proteins from plant sources that do not contain all of the essential amino acids.

indirect contact: contact with an object that has been used by an infected person.

infection: a condition in which pathogens enter the body and multiply.

ingredients listing: the list of ingredients in a food.

ingrown toenail: a toenail that grows into the skin.

inhalants: chemicals that are breathed in and produce immediate effects.

injecting drug users: people who inject illegal drugs into their blood vessels with syringes and needles.

injury: harm or damage done to a person.

inner ear: the part of the ear that sends messages to the brain and helps a person keep his or her balance.

inpatient: a person who stays at the hospital while receiving health care.

inpatient care: treatment that is given to a person during a stay at a facility, such as a hospital.

insomnia: a condition in which a person has difficulty sleeping.

insulin: a hormone that regulates the blood sugar level.

integumentary (in·TEH·gyuh·ment·tuh·ree) **system:** the body system composed of parts that cover and protect the body.

interest: money that is paid for the use of a larger sum of money.

intergroup conflict: a conflict that occurs between two or more groups of people.

Internet: a worldwide collection of networks that connect millions of people worldwide.

interpersonal conflict: a conflict that involves two or more people.

intrapersonal conflict: a conflict that occurs within a person.

involuntary muscles: muscles that function without a person's control.

ionizing radiation: radiation that has enough energy to separate electrons from their atoms, forming atoms or ions.

iris: the colored part of the eye that adjusts to the size of the pupil to regulate the amount of light that enters the eye.

irradiation: the use of radiation to kill microorganisms and insects, prevent spoiling, and delay ripening in foods.

isokinetic exercise: an exercise in which a weight is moved through an entire range of motion.

isometric exercise: an exercise in which muscles are tightened for five to ten seconds without movement of body parts.

isotonic exercise: an exercise in which there is a muscle contraction that causes movement.

joint: the point at which two bones meet.

joint-custody family: two parents living apart sharing custody of their children.

junk foods: foods that are high in fat, sugar, or salt.

juvenile offender: a legal minor who commits a criminal act.

Kaposi's (KA·poh·seez) **sarcoma (KS):** a type of cancer in people who have AIDS.

kidney: an organ through which blood circulates as wastes are filtered.

knocked-out tooth: a tooth that has been knocked out of its socket.

labor: a series of three stages that result in the birth of the baby.

laceration: a cut that causes a jagged or irregular tearing of the skin.

land conservation: actions to save land.

landfill: a place where wastes are dumped and buried.

large intestine (colon): a tube extending below the small intestine where undigested food is prepared for elimination from the body.

laser disc: a disc that presents computer programs, text, images, music and animation onto a television or computer monitor.

law: a rule of conduct or action that represents the beliefs of a majority of people in a community, state, or nation.

lead: a toxic metal that may be present in air or water.

learning disability: a disorder that causes a person to have difficulty learning.

learning style: the way a person acquires basic skills.

lens: the part of the eye that focuses light rays entering the pupil on the retina.

leukemia (loo·KEE·mee·uh): a cancer of the blood-forming parts of the body.

lice: insects that pierce the skin and secrete a substance that causes itching and swelling.

license: a document granted by a government agency to a person for the right to practice or to use a certain title.

life skills: healthful actions that are learned and practiced for a lifetime.

lifetime sports and physical activities: sports and physical activities in which a person can participate as a person grows older.

ligaments: the fibers that connect bones together.

lightning: the flashing of light caused by electricity in the air.

lipoproteins: substances that transport cholesterol in the bloodstream.

list of nutrients: the Percent Daily Value for the nutrients that must be considered when planning a healthful diet.

liver: a gland that produces and releases bile to help break down fats; maintains blood sugar levels; and filters poisonous wastes.

local health department: the official agency that has responsibility for providing health services and programs for people living within a community.

lockjaw: a bacteria that grows in the body and produces a strong poison that affects the nervous system and muscles.

look-alike drug: a tablet or capsule manufactured to resemble amphetamines and mimic their effects.

loving person: someone who is respectful, responsible, understanding, and self-disciplined.

low density lipoproteins (LDLs): substances that carry cholesterol to body cells.

LSD: a hallucinogen that is often sold illegally in powder, tablet, or capsule form.

Lyme disease: a bacterial disease transmitted through a tick.

lymphomas (lim·FOH·muhs): cancers that develop and metastasize in the lymph system.

M

major medical insurance: insurance that pays for extra expenses not covered by other insurance policies.

male reproductive system: the body system that consists of the male organs involved in producing offspring.

malignant melanoma (muh·LIG·nuhnt mel·uh·NOH·muh): a form of skin cancer that is often fatal.

malnutrition: a condition in which the body does not get the nutrients required for good health.

malocclusion (ma·luh·KLEW·zhun): the abnormal fitting together of teeth when the jaws are closed.

managed care: an organized system of health care services designed to control health care costs.

marijuana: a drug containing THC that impairs short-term memory and changes mood.

mature: to become fully grown or developed.

maximum heart rate: a heart rate of 220 beats per minute minus age.

media: the various forms of mass communication.

media literacy: the ability to recognize and evaluate the messages in media.

mediation: a process in which a third person helps people in conflict reach a solution.

mediator: a person who helps people in conflict reach a solution.

Medic Alert tag: a medical identification tag that provides information about the person wearing it.

Medicaid (MED·i·kayd): a health insurance plan for the needy that is managed and paid for by the state and federal government.

medical doctor: a physician who is trained in a medical school and who has a doctor of medicine degree (MD).

medical insurance: insurance that pays physicians' fees, laboratory fees from outside the hospital, and fees for prescription drugs.

Medicare (MED·i·kehr): a government health insurance plan for people 65 years of age and older and people who receive Social Security disability benefits for more than two years.

medicine: a drug that is used to treat, prevent, or diagnose illness.

Medline: a bibliographic medical data base created by the National Institutes of Health.

medulla (muh·DUH·luh): the part of the brain that controls involuntary actions, such as heart rate and breathing.

melanin (MEL·uh·nin): a pigment that gives the skin its color and provides protection from the ultraviolet rays of the sun.

menarche (MEN·are·kee): the first menstrual cycle.

menstrual cycle: the monthly series of changes that take place in the female reproductive system.

menstruation: the part of the menstrual cycle in which an unfertilized egg and the inner lining of the uterus leave the body.

mental alertness: the ability to think clearly, to reason, and to solve problems.

mental-emotional health: the condition of the mind and the ways that a person expresses feelings.

mental health clinic: a facility that provides services for people having difficulty coping; might be open daily for 24 hours to help with crises.

mental rehearsal: a technique that involves imagining a stressful conversation or situation, pretending to say and do specific things, and imagining how the other person will respond.

mentor: a responsible, trusted person who guides and helps a younger person.

mercury: a metal contained in some latex paints that might cause poisoning.

mescaline (MES·kuh·leen): a hallucinogen made from the peyote cactus plant.

metabolism (muh·TA·buh·li·zuhm): the rate at which food is converted to energy in the cells.

metastasis (muh·TAS·tuh·sis): the spreading of cancer cells to other body parts from an original source.

methamphetamines (meth·am·FE·tuh·meenz): stimulant drugs within the amphetamine family.

middle ear: the part of the ear in which sound waves push against the eardrum causing it to vibrate.

migraine headache: severe head pain that is caused by dilation of blood vessels in the brain.

minerals: nutrients that regulate many chemical reactions in the body.

miscarriage: a natural ending of a pregnancy before a baby is developed enough to survive on its own.

mixed message: a message that conveys two different meanings.

Model for Using Resistance Skills*™ *The: a list of suggested ways to resist negative peer pressure.

modem: a device that allows a computer to talk to another computer over the telephone lines.

monovision: wearing one contact lens to see close objects and the other to see at a distance.

morphine: a narcotic that is used to control pain.

motor vehicle emissions: products of the combustion of motor fuels, such as gasoline.

mucous membranes: the tissues that line the body openings and secret mucus.

mucus: a thick secretion that coats the mucous membranes.

multiple addiction: a condition in which a person has more than one addiction.

multiple sclerosis (MS): a disease in which the protective covering of nerve fibers in the brain and spinal cord is destroyed.

murder: killing someone on purpose.

muscular endurance: the ability to use muscles for an extended period of time.

muscular strength: the ability to lift, pull, push, kick, and throw with force.

muscular (MUHS·kyuh·ler) **system:** the body system that consists of muscles that provide motion and maintain posture.

mutagen: an environmental agent that causes changes in the genetic material of living cells.

myopia (my·OH·pee·uh): a visual problem in which distant objects appear blurred while close objects are seen clearly.

N

narcotics: a group of drugs that slow down the central nervous system, cause drowsiness, and can be used as painkillers.

National Health Information Center (NHIC): a health information referral agency that sponsors a toll-free hotline which refers consumers to organizations that can provide health-related information.

National Institute for Occupational Safety and Health (NIOSH): is an agency that makes recommendations for workplace safety.

National Institutes on Drug Abuse (NIDA): an agency that focuses on improving the understanding, treatment, and prevention of drug abuse and addiction through research, training, and community programs.

National Institutes of Health (NIH): an agency within the Public Health Service that supports and conducts research into the causes and prevention of diseases and provides information to the public.

National Safety Council: an organization that focuses on the prevention of accidental deaths, injuries, and preventable illnesses through training programs and publications.

National School Health Education Coalition (NaSHEC): an organization for health educators that distributes health information through publications and other resources.

natural disaster: an event caused by nature that results in damage or loss.

nearsightedness: a visual problem in which distant objects appear blurred while close objects are seen clearly.

neglect: failure to provide proper care and guidance.

nervous system: the body system that carries messages to and from the brain and spinal cord and all other parts of the body.

neurologist (nu·RAH·luh·jist): a physician who specializes in the diagnosis and treatment of diseases of the brain, spinal cord, and nerves.

neurons (NOO·rahnz): nerve cells.

nicotine: a colorless, odorless drug in tobacco that stimulates the nervous system and is highly addictive.

noise: sound that produces discomfort or annoyance.

noise pollution: loud or constant noise that causes hearing loss, stress, fatigue, irritability, and tension.

noncommunicable disease: an illness that is caused by something other than a pathogen.

nongonococcal (nahn·gahn·uh·KAH·kuhl) **urethritis (NGU):** an STD that produces an infection and inflammation of the urethra.

nonrenewable resources: resources that cannot be replaced once they are used.

nonverbal behavior: the use of actions rather than words to express thoughts and feelings.

norepinephrine (nor·eh·puh·NEH·frun): a substance that helps transmit brain messages along certain nerves.

nosebleed: a loss of blood from the mucous membranes that line the nose.

nurse practitioner: a specially trained registered nurse who can function as a primary care provider in some states.

nurturing environment: surroundings that help a person grow, develop, and succeed.

nutrient (NOO·tree·ent): a chemical substance in foods that builds, repairs, and maintains body tissues; regulates body processes; and provides energy (measured in calories).

Nutrition Facts: the title of the food label that is required on all processed foods regulated by the Food and Drug Administration.

obesity: excessive body fat.

obstetrician (ahb·stuh·TRI·shun): a physician who specializes in the care of a mother-to-be and her developing baby.

Occupational Safety and Health Administration (OSHA): a regulatory agency responsible for the workplace environment.

occupational therapist: an allied health professional who helps people with disabilities learn to adapt to their disabilities.

online: the interactive use of computers using telecommunications technology.

open fracture: a fracture in which there is a break in the skin.

open wound: an injury in which the skin's surface is broken.

ophthalmologist (ahf·thuhl·MAHL·uh·jist): a physician who specializes in the medical and surgical treatment of the eyes.

opportunistic infection: an infection that develops in a person with a weak immune system.

optic nerve: the nerve that carries the electrical messages from the retina to the brain.

optometrist (ahp·TAHM·uh·trist): a doctor of optometry (OD) who specializes in examining the eyes and prescribing lenses.

oral hairy leukoplakia (loo·koh·PLAK·ee·uh): an infection in which fuzzy white patches are found on the tongue.

organ: a body part consisting of several kinds of tissues that do a particular job.

orthodontist: a dentist who treats malocclusion.

orthopedist (or·thuh·PEE·dist): a physician who specializes in the surgical care of muscle, bone, and joint injuries and disorders.

osteoarthritis (ah·stee·oh·ahr·THRY·tuhs): a condition in which the movable parts of a joint break down.

osteopath (AH·stee·oh·path): a physician trained in a college of osteopathic medicine who has a doctor of osteopathy degree (DO).

osteoporosis (ah·stee·oh·puh·ROH·sis): a bone disease in which bone tissue becomes thin.

outer ear: the part of the ear that collects sound waves.

outpatient: a person who comes to the hospital or other health care facility for treatment, but does not stay overnight.

outpatient care: treatment that does not require an overnight stay at a facility.

ova: female reproductive cells.

ovaries (OH·vuh·reez): two female reproductive glands that produce egg cells and estrogen.

overload: an additional activity that increases the body's capacity to do work.

over-the-counter drug (OTC): a drug that can be purchased without a prescription.

ovulation (ahv·yuh·LAY·shun): the release of a mature egg from an ovary and is part of the menstrual cycle.

oxidation (AHK·suh·DAY·shuhn): the process by which alcohol is changed to carbon dioxide and water.

ozone: a form of oxygen created by the energy of sunlight acting upon oxygen.

ozone layer: a layer in the upper atmosphere where ozone traps dangerous ultraviolet radiation from the sun and prevents it from reaching Earth's surface.

pancreas (PAN·kree·uhs): a gland that produces digestive enzymes and chemicals that control blood sugar levels.

pancreatitis (pan·kree·uh·TY·tis): the inflammation of the pancreas.

parathyroid (pehr·uh·THY·royd) **glands:** four glands that control the amount of calcium and phosphorus in the body.

parent abuse: the harmful treatment of a parent.

parent support group: a group formed by parents to help one another cope with problems.

particulates: tiny particles in the air.

passive immunity: immunity that results from introducing antibodies into the bloodstream.

pathogen: a disease-causing organism.

PCBs: chemicals containing chlorine.

PCP: also known as angel dust, a hallucinogen that can act as a stimulant or a depressant.

pedestrian: a person who is walking.

pediatrician (pee·dee·uh·TRI·shuhn): a physician who specializes in the care of children and adolescents.

peer: a person who is similar in age or status.

peer pressure: influence that people of similar age or status place on others to encourage them to make certain decisions or to behave in certain ways.

pelvic inflammatory disease (PID): an infection of the internal female reproductive organs.

penis: the male sex organ for reproduction and urination.

people pleaser: a person who is more concerned about having the approval of others than doing what (s)he believes to be best.

Percent Daily Value: the portion of the daily value of a nutrient provided by one serving of the food.

perfectionism (per·FEK·shuh·ni·zum): an addiction in which a person is obsessed with doing things without fault.

periodontal disease: a disease of the gums and other tissues that support the teeth.

periosteum (per·ee·AHS·tee·um): a thin sheet of outer tissue that covers bone.

peripheral (puh·RIF·uh·rul) **nervous system (PNS):** the part of the CNS that consists of all of the nerves that branch out from the CNS to the muscles, skin, internal organs, and glands.

personal health management: self-care that promotes optimal well-being.

personal health record: a record of a person's health, health care, and health care providers.

personality: a person's unique blend of physical, mental, social, and emotional traits.

pesticides: chemicals that are used to kill unwanted insects, weeds, or fungi.

petit mal: a small seizure in which a person loses consciousness for a few seconds.

phagocytes: white blood cells that surround and kill pathogens by ingesting them.

pharmacist: an allied health professional who dispenses medications prescribed by physicians.

physical abuse: harmful treatment that results in physical injury to the victim.

physical activities: activities that require the use of muscles and energy.

physical dependence: a condition in which a person develops tolerance and a drug becomes necessary, or the person has withdrawal symptoms.

physical examination: a series of tests that measure health status.

physical fitness: the condition of the body that results from regular physical activity.

physical fitness plan: a written schedule of physical activities to do to develop health-related fitness and skill-related fitness.

physical health: the condition of the body.

physical profiling: a method of testing a person's physical limits to determine what types of physical activities are best.

physical therapist: an allied health professional who works with people who have physical disabilities and are in need of rehabilitation.

physician (fuh·ZI·shun): a professional who is licensed to practice medicine and, with special training, surgery in all branches of medicine.

pinkeye: an inflammation of the membranes covering the white of the eye and eyelid.

pituitary (pi·TOO·i·tehr·ree) **gland:** a gland that produces hormones that control other glands.

placenta: an organ that attaches the egg to the inner wall of the uterus.

plaque: hardened fatty deposits in blood vessels.

plasma: the liquid component of blood.

plastic surgeon (SUHR·juhn): a physician who specializes in surgery to correct, repair, or improve body features.

platelets: the smallest parts of blood that help blood clot.

pleasant sounds: sounds that promote health.

pneumocystis (noo·muh·SIS·tus) **carinii pneumonia (PCP):** a form of pneumonia often found in people who have AIDS.

podiatrist (puh·DY·uh·trist): a doctor of podiatric medicine (DPM) who specializes in problems of the feet.

poison: a substance that causes injury, illness, or death if it enters the body.

poisoning: a harmful chemical reaction that can occur when a drug or other substance enters the body.

pollutant: something that causes pollution.

pollutant standard index (PSI): a measure of air quality based on the sum of the levels of five different pollutants.

pollution: any change in the air, water, soil, noise level, or temperature that has a negative effect on life and health.

postpartum period: the six- to eight-week period after the birth of a baby.

post traumatic stress disorder (PTSD): a condition in which a person relives a stressful experience again and again.

power: the ability to combine strength and speed.

power eating: eating the appropriate number of servings of food needed for optimal health.

precycling: the process of reducing waste by: buying recycled products; buying products in packages or containers that can be recycled; buying products with less packaging; repairing products rather than buying new ones.

preferred provider: a health care provider who appears on the approved list for payments from the health insurance company.

pregnancy: the time period from conception to birth.

premature birth: the birth of a baby before it is fully developed.

premature delivery: the birth of a baby before the 37th week of the pregnancy.

premature heart attack: a heart attack that occurs before age 55 in males and before age 65 in females.

premenstrual syndrome (PMS): a group of changes that can affect a female before her menstrual period.

premium: the required amount of money that will guarantee that an insurance company will help pay for health services.

prenatal care: the care given to both the mother-to-be and her unborn baby.

prescription (pri·SKRIP·shuhn): a written order from a certain licensed health professional.

prescription drug: a medicine that can be obtained only with a written order from a licensed health professional.

price: the cost of a product or service.

primary care provider: a physician or other health care provider who provides general care.

private hospital: a hospital owned by private individuals; operates as a profit-making business.

proactive decision-making style: a decision-making style in which a person examines the decision to be made, identifies and evaluates action to take, selects an action, and takes responsibility for the consequences of this action.

probation: a sentence in which an offender remains in the community under the supervision of a probation officer for a specific period of time.

problem drinker: a person who causes problems for himself or herself or others when drinking.

problem drinking: a pattern of drinking that produces difficulties in a person's life.

products: material goods, such as food, medicine, and clothing, that are made for consumers to purchase.

progress appeal: an advertising appeal that emphasizes that a product is "new and improved."

progression: the gradual increase in intensity and duration of physical activity.

prolactin: a hormone that causes the mammary glands in the mother's breasts to produce milk.

prostate gland: a gland that makes a fluid that helps keep sperm alive.

protective factors: ways that a person might behave and characteristics of the environment in which a person lives that promote health, safety, and well-being.

protein: a nutrient needed to build, repair, and maintain body tissues.

protozoa (proh·tuh·ZOH·uh): tiny, single-celled parasite.

psychiatrist (sy·KY·uh·trist): a physician who specializes in the diagnosis and treatment of mental and emotional problems.

psychological dependence: a strong desire to continue using a drug for emotional reasons.

puberty: the stage of growth and development when secondary sex characteristics appear.

pubic lice: an infestation with pubic, or crab, lice.

puncture: a wound produced when a pointed instrument pierces the skin.

pupil: the black opening in the center of the iris that changes size to regulate the amount of light that enters the eye.

Q

quackery: consumer fraud, or deception that involves the practice of promoting or selling useless products or services.

quality: the degree of excellence of a product or service.

R

radiation therapy: treatment of cancer with high-energy rays to kill or damage cancer cells.

radon: an odorless, colorless radioactive gas that is given off by rocks and soil.

radwaste: radioactive waste material.

rain forest: a group of trees and plants covering a warm, wet area.

rape: the threatened or actual use of physical force to get someone to have sex without giving consent.

reaction time: the period of time it takes to move after a person hears, sees, feels, or touches a stimulus.

reactive decision-making style: a decision-making style in which a person allows others to make decisions.

realistic standard: is a requirement a person sets for himself or herself that can reasonably be achieved.

receptor site: the part of a cell where the chemical substance in a drug fits.

recreational activities: activities that involve play, amusement, and relaxation.

recycling: the process of reforming or breaking down waste products so that they can be used again.

red blood cells: cells that carry oxygen.

reflex action: an involuntary action in which a message is sent to the spinal cord where it is interpreted and responded to immediately.

registered dietitian: an allied health professional who counsels people about healthful dietary principles and designs special diets.

registered nurse: a nurse who is certified for general practice or for any one or more of several nurse specialties.

regulatory agencies: government agencies that enforce laws to protect the general public.

rehabilitation: the process of helping people change negative behavior to positive behavior.

rejection: the feeling of being unwanted.

relapse: the return to addictive behavior after a period of having stopped it.

relationship: the connection a person has with others.

remarriage: a marriage in which a previously married person has married again.

renewable resources: resources that can be replaced.

reproductive system: the body system that consists of the organs involved in producing offspring.

rescue breathing: a way of breathing air into an unconscious victim who is not breathing, but has a pulse.

resilient: to be able to prevent or "bounce back" from misfortune, change, or pressure.

resistance skills: skills that are used when a person wants to say NO to an action or to leave a situation.

resistance stage: the second stage of the GAS in which the body attempts to return to normal.

respiratory system: the body system that provides body cells with oxygen and removes the carbon dioxide that cells produce as waste.

respiratory therapist: an allied health professional who tests for and treats breathing disorders according to a physician's orders.

responsibility: the quality of being reliable and dependable.

Responsible Decision-Making Model*™*, The: a series of steps to follow to assure that decisions lead to actions that promote health; protect safety; follow laws; show respect for self and others; follow guidelines set by responsible adults such as parents or a guardian; and demonstrate good character.

responsible drug use: the correct use of legal drugs to promote health and well-being.

retainer: a plastic device with wires that keep the teeth from moving back to their original places.

retina: the inner lining of the eyeball where light rays are absorbed and changed to electrical messages.

reward appeal: an advertising appeal that offers a special prize, gift, or coupon when a specific product or service is purchased.

Rh factor: the presence (Rh positive) or absence (Rh negative) of a special substance in the blood.

RICE treatment: a technique for treating musculoskeletal injuries.

rickettsia (ri·KET·see·uh): pathogens that grow inside living cells and resemble bacteria.

risk behaviors: voluntary actions that threaten health; increase the likelihood of illness and premature death; and harm the quality of the environment.

risk factors: ways that a person might behave and characteristics of the environment in which a person lives that threaten health, safety, and well-being.

role model: a person who is an example or shows others how to behave.

S

safe and drug-free school zone: a defined area around a school for the purpose of sheltering young people from weapons and the sale of drugs.

safety belt: a seat belt and shoulder strap.

salivary (SA·luh·vehr·ee) **glands:** glands that produce saliva.

salmonella (sal·muh·NE·luh): bacteria that contaminates foods.

sarcomas (sar·KOH·muhs): cancers that form in middle tissues such as bones and muscles.

saturated fats: fats from dairy products, solid vegetable fats, and animal products.

savings: money set aside for future use.

scientific evidence appeal: an advertising appeal that includes the results of surveys and laboratory tests.

scoliosis (skoh·lee·OH·sis): a deformity of the spine in which the spine develops an S-shaped curve.

scrotum: a sac-like pouch that holds each testis and helps regulate temperature for sperm production.

sebaceous (si·BAY·shuhs) **glands:** glands that secrete an oil to keep skin soft.

secondary hypertension: high blood pressure caused by specific factors.

second-degree burn: a burn that involves the top layers of the skin.

secondhand smoke: exhaled smoke and sidestream smoke.

sedative-hypnotic drugs: a group of drugs that depress the activities of the central nervous system.

sedatives: drugs that have a calming effect on behavior.

seizure: the period in which a person loses control over mind and body.

self-control: the degree to which a person regulates his or her own behavior.

self-discipline: the effort or energy with which a person follows through on intentions or promises.

self-esteem: what a person thinks or believes about himself or herself.

selfish: to care about oneself without thinking about others.

self-protection strategies: strategies that can be practiced to protect oneself and decrease the risk of becoming a victim.

self-respect: a high regard for oneself because one behaves in responsible ways.

self-responsibility for health: the priority a person assigns to being healthy.

self-statements: words a person says to remind himself or herself to stay in control.

semen: the fluid that consists of a combination of sperm and fluids from the seminal vesicles, prostate gland, and Cowper's glands.

seminal vesicles: two small glands that secrete a fluid that nourishes and helps the sperm to move.

seminiferous (se·muh·NI·fuh·ruhs) **tubules:** a network of coiled tubes in which sperm are produced.

separation: an agreement between a couple to live apart, but remain married.

service learning: an educational experience that combines learning with community service without pay.

services: work that is provided by people.

Serving Size: the amount of a food that is considered a serving.

Servings Per Container: the number of servings that are in the container or package.

sewage: waste liquids or matter carried off by sewers.

sex appeal: an advertising appeal that tries to convince a person that others will find him or her irresistible if a specific product or service is used.

sex role: the way a person acts and the feelings and attitudes (s)he has about being a male or a female.

sexual abuse: sexual contact that is forced on a person.

sexual harassment: unwanted sexual behavior that ranges from making unwanted sexual comments to forcing another person into unwanted sex acts.

sexuality: the feelings and attitudes a person has about his or her body, sex role, and relationships.

sexually transmitted disease (STD): a disease caused by pathogens that are transmitted from an infected person to an uninfected person during intimate sexual contact.

shadowing: spending time with a mentor as (s)he performs work activities.

shock: a dangerous reduction in blood flow to the body tissues.

shopping addiction: the uncontrollable urge to shop and buy.

shyness: withdrawing from contact with other people or activities.

sick building syndrome (SBS): an illness that results from indoor air pollution.

sickle-cell anemia: an inherited blood disease in which the red blood cells have less oxygen.

side effect: an unwanted body change that is not related to the main purpose of a drug.

sidestream smoke: the smoke that enters the air from a burning cigarette or cigar.

simple carbohydrates: sugars that enter the bloodstream rapidly and provide quick energy.

single-custody family: a family that consists of two parents living apart and a child or children living with only one parent.

single-parent family: a family that consists of one parent and a child or children.

skeletal system: the body system that serves as a support framework, protects vital organs, works with muscles to produce movement, and produces blood cells.

skill-related fitness: the ability to perform well in sports and physical activities.

sleep: a restful state in which there is little or no conscious thought.

small intestine: a coiled tube in which the greatest amount of digestion and absorption take place.

smog: a combination of smoke and fog.

smoke detector: a device that sounds an alarm when smoke is detected.

sniffing: inhaling fumes from substances to get a high.

snuff: a tobacco product made from powdered tobacco leaves and stems that is placed between the cheek and gums.

social age: a measure of a person's involvement in leisure activities.

social-emotional environment: the quality of the contacts one has with the people with whom one interacts.

social skills: skills a person can use to relate well with others.

Society of Public Health Education (SOPHE): an organization for public health educators that focuses on promoting health and preventing disease.

solid waste: discarded solid material such as paper, metals, and yard waste.

solubility: the ability of a substance to be dissolved.

sound waves: vibrations or movements of air.

specialist: a physician who has additional training in a particular aspect of health care.

specificity: choosing a physical activity for its desired benefit.

speech pathologist (pa·THAH·luh·jist)**:** an allied health care professional who helps people overcome speech disorders.

speed: the ability to move quickly.

sperm: the male reproductive cells.

spinal cord: a thick band of nerve cells that extends through the backbone.

spirochete (SPY·roh·keet)**:** a spiral-shaped bacterium.

splint: material or a device used to protect and immobilize a body part.

sports participant: a person who plays sports.

sports spectator: a person who watches and supports sports without actively participating in them.

spouse abuse: the harmful treatment of a husband or wife.

sprain: an injury to the ligaments, tendons, and soft tissue around a joint caused by undue stretching.

state health department: the official agency that has responsibility for the health services and programs for people living within the state.

stepfamily: a family that is formed as a result of the remarriage of one of the parents.

sterile: unable to produce children.

stimulants: a group of drugs that increase the activities of the central nervous system.

stomach: an organ that releases acids and juices that mix with the food and produces a thick paste called chyme (KYM).

strain: an overstretching of muscles and/or tendons.

stress: the response of the body to the demands of daily living.

stress management skills: techniques to cope with the body changes produced by stress.

stressor: a source or cause of stress.

stroke: a condition caused by a blocked or broken blood vessel in the brain.

stroke volume: the amount of blood the heart pumps with each beat.

student assistance program: a school-based approach to the prevention and treatment of alcohol and other drugs.

subcutaneous (suhb·kyoo·TAY·nee·uhs) **layer:** a layer of fatty tissue located below the dermis.

sudden illness: an illness that occurs without warning signals of what is actually happening.

suffocation (su·fuh·KAY·shun)**:** a condition in which a person lacks oxygen due to an obstruction to the passage of air into the lungs.

suicide: the intentional taking of one's own life.

suicide prevention skills: steps to take when a person shows signs of suicide.

support network: a group of people who help and encourage a person.

suppository (suh·PAH·zuh·toh·ree)**:** a wax-coated form of a drug that is inserted into the anus or vagina.

surgical insurance: insurance that pays surgeons' fees.

symptom: a change in a body function or behavior from the usual pattern.

syphilis (SI·fuh·lis)**:** an STD caused by spirochetes that produce a chancre, skin rash, and damage to body organs.

systemic lupus erythematosus (er·uh·THEE·muh·TOH·suhs) **(SLE):** a chronic disease that causes inflammation of the connective tissue.

systolic (si·STAH·lik) **blood pressure:** the force of blood against the artery walls when the heart is beating.

T

T cells: white blood cells that regulate the action of the immune system.

tamper-resistant package: a package with an unbroken seal that assures the buyer that the package has not been previously opened.

tar: a thick, sticky fluid that is produced when tobacco burns.

target heart rate: a heart rate of 75 percent of maximum heart rate.

teaching hospital: a hospital that is associated with a medical school and/or school of nursing; provides training in addition to the regular services of most hospitals.

tendons: tough tissue fibers that connect muscles to bones.

tension headache: pain that results from muscle contractions in the neck or head.

teratogen: an environmental agent that crosses the placenta of a pregnant female and causes miscarriage or birth defects in offspring.

terminal illness: an illness that is incurable and will cause death.

testes (TES·teez): two male reproductive glands that produce sperm cells and testosterone.

testimonial appeal: an advertising appeal that focuses on a person who gives a statement about the benefits of a specific product or service.

testosterone (te·STAHS·tuh·rohn): a male sex hormone that controls the development of the secondary sex characteristics during puberty.

tetanus: a bacteria that grows in the body and produces a strong poison that affects the nervous system and muscles.

thermal inversion: a condition that occurs when a layer of warm air forms above a cooler layer.

thermal pollution: pollution of water with heat.

third-degree burn: a burn that involves all layers of the skin and some underlying tissues.

thrush: a fungal infection of the mucous membranes of the tongue and mouth.

thyroid gland: a gland that produces thyroxin.

thyroxin (thy·RAHK·sin): a hormone that controls metabolism.

time management plan: a plan that shows how a person will set aside time for activities done regularly and leisure activities.

tissue: a group of cells that are similar in form or function.

tobacco cessation programs: programs to help people stop smoking cigarettes and cigars or using smokeless tobacco.

tobacco use: the use of any nicotine-containing tobacco products, such as cigarettes, cigars, and smokeless tobacco.

tolerance: a condition in which the body becomes used to a drug and larger amounts are needed to produce the same effect.

tornado: a violent, rapidly spinning windstorm that has a funnel-shaped cloud.

tornado warning: a caution that a tornado has been sighted.

tornado watch: a caution issued by the National Weather Service that the weather conditions are such that a tornado is possible.

toxemia: a condition in which high blood pressure, sudden weight gain, blurred vision, headaches, and swelling of the hands and feet occur.

toxic shock syndrome (TSS): an illness caused by the presence of harmful bacteria in the body.

toxic waste: waste that is poisonous.

trachea (TRAY·kee·uh): the windpipe through which air travels to the lungs.

traditional family: a family that consists of a husband and wife and their children.

training principles: guidelines to follow to derive the maximum benefits from physical activity and to prevent injury.

tranquilizers: sedatives that are prescribed by a physician to treat anxiety.

transfusion: the transfer of blood from one person to another.

trichomoniasis (trik·oh·moh·NY·uh·sis): an STD caused by protozoa that infect the vagina, urethra, or prostate.

trihalomethanes (try·ha·luh·ME·thaynz): harmful chemicals that are produced when chlorine attacks pollutants in the water.

tumor: a growth of cells that form a lump.

U

umbilical cord: a ropelike structure through which the mother and the developing baby exchange oxygen, nutrients, and waste.

unintentional injury: an injury caused by an accident.

United States Department of Agriculture (USDA): an agency that enforces standards to ensure that food is processed safely, and that oversees the distribution of food information to the public.

United States Office of Consumer Affairs: an organization that coordinates federal consumer complaints, coordinates research, and provides information to the public on consumer issues.

United States Postal Service (USPS): an organization that offers postal services throughout the country and protects the public when products and services are sold through the mail.

United States Public Health Service: an agency within the Department of Health and Human Services that consists of many smaller agencies which promote the protection and advancement of physical and mental health.

universal distress signal: a warning that a person has difficulty breathing and is shown by clutching at the throat with one or both hands.

universal precautions: steps taken to prevent the spread of disease by treating all human blood and body fluids as if they contain HIV, HBV, and other pathogens.

unsaturated fats: fats from fish and plant products.

ureter (YU·ruh·ter): a narrow tube that connects the kidney to the bladder.

urethra (yu·REE·thruh): the tube leading from the bladder and through which urine passes out of the body.

urgent care center or trauma center: a facility separate from a hospital that offers immediate care; more expensive than a private physician and less expensive than an emergency room.

urinary system: the body system that removes liquid wastes from the body.

urine: a pale yellow liquid composed of water, salts, and other waste substances.

urologist (yur·AH·luh·jist): a physician who specializes in the treatment of urinary disorders and the male reproductive system.

uterus: a muscular organ that supports the fertilized egg during pregnancy.

V

vaccine (vak·SEEN): dead or weakened pathogens that are introduced into the body to give a person more immunity.

vagina: a muscular tube that connects the uterus to the outside of the body.

validation: a statement that is true.

vas deferens: two long, thin tubes that function as a passageway for sperm and as a place for sperm storage.

veins (VAYNZ): blood vessels that return blood to the heart.

ventricle: one of the lower two chambers of the heart.

victim assessment: a check of the injured or medically ill person to determine if: the victim has an open airway; the victim is breathing; the victim's heart is beating; the victim is severely bleeding; the victim has other injuries.

victim of violence: a person who is harmed or killed by violence.

victim recovery: a person's return to physical and emotional health after being harmed by violence.

violence: the use of physical force to injure, damage, or destroy oneself, others, or property.

violent behavior: behavior that threatens or uses force to injure, damage, or destroy a person or property.

viruses (VY·rus·es): the smallest pathogens.

visual environment: everything a person sees regularly.

visual pollution: sights that are unattractive.

visual validation: something placed in the environment that reminds a person of his or her successes.

vitamins: nutrients that help chemical reactions take place in the body.

vitamins and minerals required on a food label: vitamins A and C and the minerals calcium and iron.

voluntary hospital: a hospital owned by a community and not operated for profit.

voluntary muscles: muscles that a person can control.

volunteer: a person who provides a service without pay.

W

walk-in surgery center: a facility where surgery is performed on an outpatient basis.

warm-up: three to five minutes of easy activity to prepare the muscles for more work.

warranty: a written assurance that a product or service will be replaced or repaired if it is not satisfactory.

water: a nutrient that makes up a part of blood; helps the process of digestion; helps remove body wastes; regulates body temperature; and cushions the spinal cord and joints.

water conservation: actions to save water.

water pollution: the contamination of water with sewage, waste, gases, or chemicals that harm health.

water runoff: water that runs off the land into a body of water, and contains solids and dissolved substances.

water-soluble vitamins: vitamins that cannot be stored by the body in significant amounts.

weapon: an instrument or device used for violence.

weather: the condition of the atmosphere at a particular time or place.

weight management: a diet and exercise plan that helps a person achieve and maintain his or her desirable weight and a healthful percentage of body fat.

wellness: another term for health.

Wellness Scale, The: a scale that shows the ranges of health from optimal health to premature death.

Western blot: a blood test used to check for the presence and size of antibodies for HIV.

white blood cells: cells that attack, surround, and destroy pathogens that enter the body and prevent them from causing infection.

wind-chill factor: a measure of the air temperature which takes into account the chilling effect of the wind.

withdrawal symptoms: unpleasant reactions that occur when the drug is no longer taken.

World Health Organization (WHO): an agency of the United Nations that focuses on improving the quality of health by coordinating health services throughout the world.

World Wide Web (WWW): a computer system that allows a person to view information as text and/or graphics.

wound: an injury to the body's soft tissues.

Y

you-message: a statement that blames or shames another person.

youth gang: a group of young people who band together and participate in violent and unlawful behavior.

Z

zygote: the single cell that is formed from the union of the sperm and egg.